Dictionary of Medical Acronyms & Abbreviations

2nd edition

Compiled and edited by
Stanley Jablonski

HANLEY & BELFUS, INC./Philadelphia
MOSBY–YEAR BOOK, INC./St. Louis • Baltimore • Boston
Chicago • London • Philadelphia • Sydney • Toronto

Publisher: HANLEY & BELFUS, INC.
                  210 South 13th Street
                  Philadelphia, PA 19107
                  (215) 546-7293

North American and worldwide sales and distribution:

                  MOSBY-YEAR BOOK, INC.
                  11830 Westline Industrial Drive
                  St. Louis, MO 63146

In Canada: THE C.V. MOSBY COMPANY
                  5240 Finch Avenue East
                  Unit 1
                  Scarborough, Ontario M1S 4P2

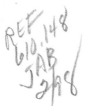

**Dictionary of Medical Acronyms
& Abbreviations**   ISBN 1-56053-052-9

Last digit is the print number: 9   8   7   6   5   4   3   2   1

Preface to the First Edition

Acronyms and abbreviations are used extensively in medicine, science and technology for good reason—they are more essential in such fields. It would be difficult to imagine how one could write down chemical and mathematical formulas and equations without using abbreviations or symbols. In medicine, they are used as a convenient shorthand in writing medical records, instructions, and prescriptions, and as space-saving devices in printed literature. It is easier and more economical to write down the acronyms HETE and RAAS than their full names 12-L-hydroxy-5,8,10,14-eicosatetraenoic acid and renin-angiotensin-aldosterone system, respectively.

The main reason for abbreviations is said to be economy. Some actually save space in print, such as acronyms for the names of institutions and organizational units, as well as being convenient to use. Many are used for other reasons, as for instance, when trying to be delicate, we may euphemistically refer to bowel movement as BM, an unprincipled individual as SOB, and body odor as BO. Also, it is sometimes difficult to fathom the reasoning of bureaucratic acronym makers, who have created some tongue-twisting monstrosities, such as ADCOMSUBORDCOMPHIBSPAC (for Administrative Command, Amphibious Forces, Pacific Fleet, Subordinate Command).

Abbreviations and acronyms used in medicine can be grouped into two broad categories. The first consists of official abbreviations and symbols used in chemistry, mathematics, and other sciences, and those designating weights and measures, whose exact form, capitalization, and punctuation have been determined by official governing bodies. In this category, they mean only one thing (e.g., kg is the symbol for kilogram and Hz for hertz), and their form, capitalization, and punctuation have been established by the International System of Units (Système International d'Unités). Abbreviations in the second group, on the other hand, may appear in a variety of forms, the same abbreviation having a different number of letters, sometimes capitalized, at other times not, with or without punctuation. Moreover, they may also have numerous meanings. The abbreviation AP may mean alkaline phosphatase, acid phosphatase, action potential, angina pectoris, and many other things.

Editors of individual scientific publications make an effort to standardize the form of abbreviations and symbols in their journals and books, but they generally vary from one publication to another.

This dictionary lists acronyms and abbreviations occurring with a reasonable frequency in the medical literature that were identified by a systematic scanning of collections of books and periodicals at the National Library of Medicine. Except as they take the form of Greek letters, pure geometric symbols are not included. Although we have attempted to be as inclusive as possible, a book such as this one can never be complete, in spite of the most diligent effort, and it is expected that some abbreviations and acronyms may have escaped detection and others have been introduced since completion of the manuscript.

ACKNOWLEDGMENTS

I wish to express my appreciation to the following members of the staff of the National Library of Medicine for their assistance in the preparation of this Dictionary: Mary Hantzes, Robert Mehnert, Edith Calhoun, Regina Broadhurst, Daniel Carangi, and especially, Dr. Maria Farkas.

Stanley Jablonski
Bethesda, Maryland

Preface to the Second Edition

It is a reality of medicine and science that the number of acronyms and abbreviations is increasing dramatically. Despite the efforts of teachers and editors to contain them, clinicians and researchers constantly introduce new ones, as perusal of any current journal demonstrates. This growth attests to the fact that acronyms and abbreviations are necessary and useful in medical writing and speaking, conserving space and preventing needless repetition.

This edition, like its predecessor, is a selective collection of the most frequently used acronyms and abbreviations. Over 2,000 entries have been added. We trust you will find it to be a handy reference to be kept within easy reach.

Stanley Jablonski

Symbols

°	degree	$>$	greater than
′	foot	$<$	less than
″	inch	$\sqrt{\ }$	root; square root
/	per	χ^2	chi square (test)
%	per cent	σ	1/1000 of a second standard deviation
:	ratio		
∞	infinity	Σ	sum of
+	positive	π	3.1416—ratio of circumference of a circle to its diameter
−	negative		
±	positive or negative		
#	number; fracture	τ	life (time)
÷	divided by	$\tau\frac{1}{2}$	half-life (time)
×	multiplied by; magnification	λ	wavelength
		$\bar{a}$	before
=	equals	$\bar{c}$	with
≠	does not equal	$\sqrt{\bar{c}}$	check with
∼	approximate	$\bar{p}$	after
↓	decreased	$\bar{s}$	without
↑	increased	24°	24 hours
∅	normal	Δt	time interval
∨	systolic blood pressure	2d	second
∧	diastolic blood pressure	2°	secondary

Greek Alphabet

Letter	Lower Case	Capital
alpha	α	A
beta	β	B
chi	χ	X
delta	δ	Δ
epsilon	ϵ	E
eta	η	H
gamma	γ	Γ
iota	ι	I
kappa	κ	K
lambda	λ	Λ
mu	μ	M
nu	ν	N
omega	ω	Ω
omicron	o	O
phi	ϕ	Φ
pi	π	Π
psi	ψ	Ψ
rho	ρ	P
sigma	σ	Σ
tau	τ	T
theta	θ	Θ
upsilon	υ	Υ
xi	ξ	Ξ
zeta	ζ	Z

The placement of Greek letters throughout this dictionary is as though they were spelled out (for example, for π look under pi).

A abnormal; abortion; absolute temperature; absorbance; acceptor; accommodation; acetone; acetum; acid; acidophil; acidophilic; acromion; actin; *Actinomyces*; activity [radiation]; adenine; adenoma; adenosine; admittance; adrenalin; adult; age; akinetic; alanine; albino [guinea pig]; albumin; allergologist; allergy; alpha [cell]; alveolar gas; ampere; amphetamine; ampicillin; anaphylaxis; androsterone; anesthetic; angstrom, Ångström unit; anode; *Anopheles*; antagonism; anterior; antrectomy; aqueous; area; argon; artery [Lat. *arteria*]; atomic weight; atrium; atropine; auricle; auscultation; axial; axilla, axillary; before [Lat. *ante*] blood group A; ear [Lat. *auris*]; mass number; subspinale; total acidity; water [Lat. *aqua*]; year [Lat. *annum*]

A [band] the dark-staining zone of a striated muscle

Å Ångström unit

Ã cumulated activity; antinuclear antibody

A₁ aortic first sound

A₂ aortic second sound

A₂₋ₒₛ aortic second sound, opening snap

A₂ P₂ aortic second sound; pulmonary second sound

AI, AII, AIII angiotensin I, II, III

a absorptivity; acceleration; accommodation; ampere; anode; ante [before]; anterior; arterial blood; artery [Lat. *arteria*]; atto-; thermodynamic activity; total acidity; water [Lat. *aqua*]

ā before [Lat. *ante*]

A see *alpha*

α see *alpha*

AA acetic acid; achievement age; active alcoholic; active assistive [range of motion]; active avoidance; acupuncture analgesia; adenine arabinoside; adenylic acid; adjuvant arthritis; adrenal androgen; agranulocytic angina; Alcoholics Anonymous; allergic alveolitis; alopecia areata; alveolo-arterial; amino acid; amyloid A; anticipatory avoidance; antigen aerosol; aortic arch; aplastic anemia; arachidonic acid; arteries; ascending aorta; atlanto-axial; atomic absorption; Australia antigen; autoanalyzer; automobile accident; axonal arborization; so much of each [Gr. *ana*]

aa arteries [Lat. *arteriae*]; so much of each [Gr. *ana*]

A&A aid and attendance; awake and aware

aA abampere

AAA abdominal aortic aneurysm/aneurysmectomy; acne-associated arthritis; acquired aplastic anemia; acute anxiety attack; American Academy of Allergy; American Association of Anatomists; androgenic anabolic agent; aneurysm of ascending aorta; Area Agency on Aging; aromatic amino acid

AAAD aromatic amino acid decarboxylase

AAAE amino acid activating enzyme

AAAHE American Association for the Advancement of Health Education

AAAI American Academy of Allergy and Immunology

AAALAC American Association for Accreditation of Laboratory Animal Care

AAAS American Association for the Advancement of Science

AAB American Association of Bioanalysts; aminoazobenzene

AABB American Association of Blood Banks

AABCC alertness (consciousness), airway, breathing, circulation, cervical spine

AABS automobile accident, broadside

AAC antibiotic-associated pseudomembranous colitis; antimicrobial agent-induced colitis; augmentative and alternative communication

AACA acylaminocephalosporanic acid

AACC American Association for Clinical Chemistry

AACCN American Association of Critical Care Nurses

AACG acute angle closure glaucoma

AACHP American Association for Comprehensive Health Planning

AACIA American Association for Clinical Immunology and Allergy

AACN American Association of Colleges of Nursing

AACP American Academy of Cerebral Palsy; American Association of Colleges of Pharmacy

AACPDM American Academy for Cerebral Palsy and Developmental Medicine

AACSH adrenal androgen corticotropic stimulating hormone

AACT American Association for Clinical Chemistry

AAD acute agitated delirium; alloxazine adenine dinucleotide; alpha-1-antitrypsin deficiency; American Academy of Dermatology; antibiotic-associated diarrhea; aromatic acid decarboxylase

AADC amino acid decarboxylase

AADE American Association of Dental Editors; American Association of Dental Examiners

AADGP American Academy of Dental Group Practice

(A-a)D$_{N_2}$ alveolo–arterial nitrogen tension difference

AAD$_{O_2}$, (a-A) D$_{O_2}$ arterio-alveolar oxygen tension difference

AADP American Academy of Denture Prosthetics; amyloid A-degrading protease

AADPA American Academy of Dental Practice Administration

AADR American Academy of Dental Radiology

AADS American Academy of Dental Schools

AAE active assistive exercise; acute allergic encephalitis; American Associ-

ation of Endodontists; annuloaortic ectasia

AAEE American Association of Electromyography and Electrodiagnosis

AAEM American Academy of Environmental Medicine

AA ex active assistive exercise

AAF acetylaminofluorene; ascorbic acid factor

AAFP American Academy of Family Physicians

AAG allergic angiitis and granulomatosis; alpha-1-acid glycoprotein; alveolar arterial gradient; autoantigen

AAGP American Academy of General Practice; American Association for Geriatric Psychiatry

AAHD American Association of Hospital Dentists

AAHE Association for the Advancement of Health Education

AAHPER American Association for Health, Physical Education, and Recreation

AAHS American Association for Hand Surgery

AAI acute alveolar injury; Adolescent Alienation Index; American Association of Immunologists; atrial inhibited [pacemaker]

AAIB alpha-1-aminoisobutyrate

AAID American Academy of Implant Dentures

AAIN American Association of Industrial Nurses

AAK allo-activated killer

AAL anterior axillary line

AALAS American Association of Laboratory Animal Science

AALL American Association for Labor Legislation

AAM acute aseptic meningitis; American Academy of Microbiology; amino acid mixture

AAMA American Academy of Medical Administrators; American Association of Medical Assistants

AAMC American Association of Medical Clinics; Association of American Medical Colleges

AAMD American Association of Mental Deficiency

AAME acetylarginine methyl ester

AAMFT American Association for Marriage and Family Therapy

AAMI Association for the Advancement of Medical Instrumentation

AAMIH American Association for Maternal and Infant Health

AAMMC American Association of Medical Milk Commissioners

AAMP American Academy of Maxillofacial Prosthetics; American Academy of Medical Prevention

AAMR American Academy of Mental Retardation

AAMRL American Association of Medical Record Librarians

AAMRS automated ambulatory medical record system

AAMS acute aseptic meningitis syndrome

AAMSI American Association for Medical Systems and Informatics

AAMT American Association for Medical Transcription

AAN AIDS-associated nephropathy; alpha-amino nitrogen; American Academy of Neurology; American Academy of Nursing; American Academy of Nutrition; American Association of Neuropathologists; amino acid nitrogen; analgesic-associated nephropathy; attending's admission notes

AANA American Association of Nurse Anesthetists

AANM American Association of Nurse-Midwives

AANPI American Association of Nurses Practicing Independently

AAO American Academy of Ophthalmology; American Academy of Optometry; American Academy of Osteopathy; American Academy of Otolaryngology; American Association of Ophthalmologists; American Association of Ortho-

dontists; amino acid oxidase; awake, alert, and oriented

A-a O_2 alveolo-arterial oxygen tension

AAOC antacid of choice

AAofA Ambulance Association of America

AAOM American Academy of Oral Medicine

AAOO American Academy of Ophthalmology and Otolaryngology

AAOP American Academy of Oral Pathology

AAOS American Academy of Orthopedic Surgeons

AAP air at atmospheric pressure; American Academy of Pediatrics; American Academy of Pedodontics; American Academy of Periodontology; American Academy of Psychoanalysts; American Academy of Psychotherapists; American Association of Pathologists; Association for the Advancement of Psychoanalysis; Association for the Advancement of Psychotherapy; Association of American Physicians

AAPA American Academy of Physician Assistants; American Association of Pathologist Assistants

AAPB American Association of Pathologists and Bacteriologists

AAPC antibiotic-associated pseudomembranous colitis

AaP$_{CO_2}$, (A-a) P$_{CO_2}$ alveolo-arterial carbon dioxide tension difference

AAPF anti-arteriosclerosis polysaccharide factor

AAPHD American Association of Public Health Dentists

AAPHP American Association of Public Health Physicians

AAPMC antibiotic-associated pseudomembranous colitis

AAPM&R American Academy of Physical Medicine and Rehabilitation

AaP$_{O_2}$, (A-a) P$_{O_2}$ alveolo-arterial oxygen tension difference

AAPS American Association of Plastic Surgeons; Arizona Articulation Proficiency Scale; Association of American Physicians and Surgeons

AAR active avoidance reaction; acute articular rheumatism; antigen-antiglobulin reaction

aar against all risks

AARE automobile accident, rear end

AAROM active assertive range of motion

AART American Association for Rehabilitation Therapy; American Association for Respiratory Therapy

AAS acid aspiration syndrome; alcoholic abstinence syndrome; American Academy of Sanitarians; American Analgesia Society; aneurysm of atrial septum; anthrax antiserum; aortic arch syndrome; atomic absorption spectrophotometry

AASD American Academy of Stress Disorders

aa seq amino acid sequence

AASH adrenal androgen stimulating hormone

AASP acute atrophic spinal paralysis; American Association of Senior Physicians; ascending aorta synchronized pulsation

AASS American Association for Social Security

AAT Aachen Aphasia Test; academic aptitude test; alanine aminotransferase; alkylating agent therapy; alpha-1-antitrypsin; atrial triggered [pacemaker]; auditory apperception test; automatic atrial tachycardia

A1AT alpha-1-antitrypsin

AATS American Association for Thoracic Surgery

AAU acute anterior uveitis

AAV adeno-associated virus

AAVMC Association of American Veterinary Medical Colleges

AAVP American Association of Veterinary Parasitologists

AAW anterior aortic wall

AB abdominal; abnormal; abortion; Ace bandage; active bilaterally; aid to the blind; alcian blue; antibiotic; antibody; antigen binding; asbestos body; asth-

matic bronchitis; axiobuccal; Bachelor of Arts [Lat. *Artium Baccalaureus*]; blood group AB

A/B acid-base ratio

A&B apnea and bradycardia

A>B air greater than bone [conduction]

Ab abortion; antibody

aB azure B

ab abortion; antibody; from [Lat.]

3AB 3-aminobenzamide

ABA abscissic acid; allergic bronchopulmonary aspergillosis; American Board of Anesthesiologists; antibacterial activity

ABB Albright-Butler-Bloomberg [syndrome]; American Board of Bioanalysis

ABBQ Acquired Immunodeficiency Syndrome Beliefs and Behavior Questionnaire

abbr abbreviation, abbreviated

ABC absolute basophil count; absolute bone conduction; acid balance control; aconite-belladonna-chloroform; airway, breathing, and circulation; alternative birth center; alum, blood, and charcoal [purification and deodorizing method]; alum, blood, and clay [sludge deodorizing method]; American Blood Commission; aneurysmal bone cyst; antigen-binding capacity; apnea, bradycardia, cyanosis; aspiration biopsy cytology; assessment of basic competency; atomic, biological, and chemical [warfare]; axiobuccocervical

A&BC air and bone conduction

ABCC Atomic Bomb Casualty Commission

ABCDE botulism toxin pentavalent

ABCIL antibody-mediated cell-dependent immunolympholysis

ABCN American Board of Clinical Neuropsychology

ABD; abdomen; aged, blind, and disabled; aggressive behavioral disturbance; average body dose

Abd abdomen, abdominal; abduction, abductor

abd abdomen, abdominal; abduct, abductor

abdom abdomen, abdominal

ABDPH American Board of Dental Public Health

ABE acute bacterial endocarditis; American Board of Endodontics; botulism equine trivalent antitoxin

ABEPP American Board of Examiners in Professional Psychology

aber aberrant

ABF aortobifemoral

ABG arterial blood gas; axiobucco-gingival

ABI ankle/brachial index; atherothrombotic brain infarct

ABIC Adaptive Behavior Inventory for Children

ABIM American Board of Internal Medicine

ABIMCE American Board of Internal Medicine certifying examination

ABK aphakic bullous keratopathy

ABL abetalipoproteinemia; African Burkitt's lymphoma; Albright-Butler-Lightwood [syndrome]; angioblastic lymphadenopathy; antigen-binding lymphocyte; Army Biological Laboratory; automated biological laboratory; axiobuccolingual

ABLB alternate binaural loudness balance

ABM adjusted body mass; alveolar basement membrane; autologous bone marrow

ABMI autologous bone marrow transplantation

ABMS American Board of Medical Specialties

ABMT autologous bone marrow transplantation

AbN antibody nitrogen

Abn, abn abnormal; abnormality(ies)

ABNMP alpha-benzyl-N-methyl phenethylamine

abnor abnormal

ABO abortion; absent bed occupancy; American Board of Orthodontists; blood

group system consisting of groups A, AB, B, and O

ABOHN American Board for Occupational Health Nurses

ABOMS American Board of Oral and Maxillofacial Surgery

ABOP American Board of Oral Pathology

Abor, abor abortion

ABP ambulatory blood pressure; American Board of Pedodontics; American Board of Periodontology; American Board of Prosthodontists; antigen-binding protein; androgen-binding protein; arterial blood pressure; avidin-biotin peroxidase

ABPA allergic bronchopulmonary aspergillosis

ABPC antibody-producing cell

ABPE acute bovine pulmonary edema

ABR abortus Bang ring [test]; absolute bed rest; auditory brainstem response

ABr agglutination test for brucellosis

Abr, Abras abrasion

ABS abdominal surgery; acute brain syndrome; Adaptive Behavior Scale; admitting blood sugar; adult bovine serum; aging brain syndrome; alkylbenzene sulfonate; aloin, belladonna, strychnine; American Board of Surgery; amniotic band sequence; amniotic band syndrome; anti-B serum; Antley-Bixler syndrome; arterial blood sample; at bed side

Abs absorption

abs absent; absolute

absc abscess; abscissa

abs conf absolute configuration

ABSe ascending bladder septum

abs feb while fever is absent [Lat. *absente febre*]

absorp absorption

AbSR abnormal skin reflex

abst, abstr abstract

abt about

ABU asymptomatic bacteriuria

ABV actinomycin D-bleomycin-vincristine; arthropod-borne virus

ABVD Adriamycin, bleomycin, vinblastine, and dacarbazine

ABW average body weight

ABY acid bismuth yeast [medium]

AC abdominal circumference; abdominal compression; absorption coefficient; abuse case; acetate; acetylcholine; acidified complement; *Acinetobacter calcoaceticus;* acromioclavicular; activated charcoal; acupuncture clinic; acute; acute cholecystitis; adenocarcinoma; adenylate cyclase; adherent cell; adrenal cortex; adrenocorticoid; air chamber; air conditioning; air conduction; alcoholic cirrhosis; alternating current; alveolar crest; ambulatory care; anesthesia circuit; angiocellular; anodal closure; antecubital; anterior chamber; anterior column; anterior commissure; antibiotic concentrate; anticoagulant; anticomplement; antiphlogistic corticoid; aortic closure; aortocoronary; arm circumference; ascending colon; atriocarotid; axiocervical; before meals [Lat. *ante cibum*]

A-C adult-versus-child; aortocoronary bypass

A/C albumin/coagulin [ratio]; anterior chamber of eye

Ac accelerator [globulin]; acetate; acetyl; actinium; arabinosyl cytosine

aC abcoulomb; arabinsyl cytosine

ac acceleration; acid; acute; alternating current; antecubital; anterior chamber; axiocervical; before meals [Lat. *ante cibum*]

5-AC azacitidine

ACA abnormal coronary artery; acrodermatitis chronica atrophicans; acute cerebellar ataxia; adenocarcinoma; adult child of an alcoholic; American Chiropractic Association; American College of Allergists; American College of Anesthesiologists; American College of Angiology; American College of Apothecaries; American Council on Alcoholism; aminocephalosporanic acid; ammonia, copper, and acetate; amyotrophic choreo-acanthocytosis; anterior cerebral

artery; anterior communicating aneurysm [or artery]; anticardiolipin antibody; anticentromere antibody; anticollagen antibody; anticomplement activity; anticytoplasmic antibody; Automatic Clinical Analyzer

AC/A accommodative convergence/accommodation [ratio]

ACAC activated charcoal artificial cell

ACACN American Council of Applied Clinical Nutrition

ACAD asymptomatic coronary artery disease

Acad academy

A-CAH autoimmune chronic active hepatitis

ACAO acyl coenzyme A oxidase

ACAT automated computerized axial tomography

ACB antibody-coated bacteria; aortocoronary bypass; arterialized capillary blood; asymptomatic carotid bruit

AC/BC air conduction/bone conduction [time ratio]

ACBE air contrast barium enema

ACBG aortocoronary bypass graft

ACC accommodation; acetyl coenzyme A carboxylase; acinic cell carcinoma; acute care center; adenoid cystic carcinoma; administrative control center; adrenocortical carcinoma; alveolar cell carcinoma; ambulatory care center; anodal closure contraction; antitoxin-containing cell; aplasia cutis congenita; articular chondrocalcinosis

Acc adenoid cystic carcinoma; acceleration

acc acceleration, accelerator; accident; accommodation

ACCESS Ambulatory Care Clinic Effectiveness Systems Study

ACCH Association for the Care of Children's Health

AcCh acetylcholine

AcChR acetylcholine receptor

AcCHS acetylcholinesterase

accid accident, accidental

acc insuff accommodation insufficiency

ACCL, Accl anodal closure clonus

ACCME Accreditation Council for Continuing Medical Education

AcCoA acetyl coenzyme A

accom accommodation

ACCP American College of Chest Physicians; American College of Clinical Pharmacology

accum accumulation

accur accurately [lat. *accuratissime*]

ACD absolute cardiac dullness; absolute claudication distance; acid-citrate-dextrose [solution]; actinomycin D; adult celiac disease; advanced care directive; allergic contact dermatitis; American College of Dentists; angiokeratoma corporis diffusum; anterior chest diameter; anticoagulant citrate dextrose; area of cardiac dullness

AC-DC, ac/dc alternating current or direct current

ACE acetonitrile; acute cerebral encephalopathy; acute coronary event; adrenocortical extract; alcohol, chloroform, and ether; angiotensin-converting enzyme

ace acentric; acetone

ACED anhydrotic congenital ectodermal dysplasia

ACEDS angiotensin-converting enzyme dysfunction syndrome

ACEH acid cholesterol ester hydrolase

ACEI angiotensin-converting enzyme inhibitor

ACEP American College of Emergency Physicians

AcEst acetyl esterase

ACET, acet acetone; vinegar [*Lat.* acetum]

acetab acetabular, acetabulum

acetyl-CoA acetyl coenzyme A

ACF accessory clinical findings; acute care facility; anterior cervical fusion; area correction factor

ACFO American College of Foot Orthopedists

ACFS American College of Foot Surgeons

ACG accelerator globulin; American

College of Gastroenterology; angiocardiography, angiocardiogram; aortocoronary graft; apexcardiogram

AC-G, AcG accelerator globulin

ACGIH American Conference of Governmental Industrial Hygienists

ACGME Accreditation Council for Graduate Medical Education

ACGP American College of General Practitioners

ACGPOMS American College of General Practitioners in Osteopathic Medicine and Surgery

ACGT antibody-coated grid technique

ACH acetylcholine; achalasia; active chronic hepatitis; adrenocortical hormone; amyotrophic cerebellar hypoplasia; arm girth, chest depth, and hip width [nutritional index]

ACh acetylcholine

ACHA American College of Hospital Administrators

AChA anterior choroidal artery

AChE acetylcholinesterase

ACHOO autosomal dominant compelling helio-ophthalmic outburst [syndrome]

AChR acetylcholine receptor

AChRAb acetylcholine receptor antibody

AChRP acetylcholine receptor protein

AC&HS before meals and at bedtime [Lat. *ante cibum* & *hora somni*]

ACI acoustic comfort index; acute coronary infarction; acute coronary insufficiency; adenylate cyclase inhibitor; adrenocortical insufficiency; anticlonus index

ACID Arithmetic, Coding, Information, and Digit Span; automatic implantable cardioverter defibrillator

ACIF anticomplement immunofluorescence

ACIP acute canine idiopathic polyneuropathy; Advisory Committee on Immunization Practices [CDC]

ACIR Automotive Crash Injury Research

AcK francium [actinium K]

ACL Achievement Check List; acromegaloid features, cutis verticis gyrata, corneal leukoma [syndrome]; anterior cruciate ligament

ACl aspiryl chloride

ACLA American Clinical Laboratory Association

ACLC Assessment of Children's Language Comprehension

ACLD Association for Children with Learning Disabilities

ACLI American Council on Life Insurance

ACLM American College of Legal Medicine

ACLPS Academy of Clinical Laboratory Physicians and Scientists

ACLS advanced cardiac life support; Assessment of Children's Language Comprehension

AcLV avian acute leukemia virus

ACM acute cerebrospinal meningitis; Adriamycin, cyclophosphamide, methotrexate; albumin-calcium-magnesium; alveolar capillary membrane; anticardiac myosin; Arnold-Chiari malformation

ACMA American Occupational Medical Association

ACME Advisory Council on Medical Education; Automated Classification of Medical Entities

ACMF arachnoid cyst of the middle fossa

ACML atypical chronic myeloid leukemia

ACMP alveolar-capillary membrane permeability

ACMR Advisory Committee on Medical Research

ACMS American Chinese Medical Society

ACMT artificial circus movement tachycardia

ACMV assist-controlled mechanical ventilation

ACN acute conditioned neurosis; American College of Neuropsychiatrists; American College of Nutrition

ACNM American College of Nuclear Medicine; American College of Nurse-Midwives

ACNP American College of Nuclear Physicians

ACO acute coronary occlusion; alert, cooperative, and oriented; anodal closure odor

ACoA anterior communicating artery

ACOG American College of Obstetricians and Gynecologists

ACOHA American College of Osteopathic Hospital Administrators

ACO-HNS American Council of Otolaryngology-Head and Neck Surgery

ACOI American College of Osteopathic Internists

ACOM American College of Occupational Medicine

ACOMS American College of Oral and Maxillofacial Surgeons

ACOOG American College of Osteopathic Obstetricians and Gynecologists

ACOP American College of Osteopathic Pediatricians

ACORDE A Corsortium on Restorative Dentistry Education

ACOS American College of Osteopathic Surgeons

Acous acoustics, acoustic

ACP accessory conduction pathway; acid phosphatase; acyl carrier protein; American College of Pathologists; American College of Pharmacists; American College of Physicians; American College of Prosthodontists; American College of Psychiatrists; Animal Care Panel; anodal closure picture; aspirin-caffeine-phenacetin; Association for Child Psychiatrists; Association of Clinical Pathologists; Association of Correctional Psychologists

ACPA American Cleft Palate Association

ACPC aminocyclopentane carboxylic [acid]

AC-PH, ac phos acid phosphatase

ACPM American College of Preventive Medicine

ACPP adrenocortical polypeptide

ACPS acrocephalopolysyndactyly

ACR abnormally contracting region; absolute catabolic rate; acriflavine; adenomatosis of colon and rectum; American College of Radiology; anticonstipation regimen; axillary count rate

Acr acrylic

ACRF ambulatory care research facility

ACRM American Congress of Rehabilitation Medicine

ACS acrocallosal syndrome; acrocephalosyndactyly; acute chest syndrome; acute confusional state; Alcon Closure System; American Cancer Society; American Chemical Society; American College of Surgeons; anodal closure sound; antireticular cytotoxic serum; aperture current setting; Association of Clinical Scientists

ACSA adenylate cyclase-stimulating activity

ACS AO ascending aorta

ACSM American College of Sports Medicine

ACSP adenylate cyclase-stimulating protein

ACSV aortocoronary saphenous vein

ACSVBG aortocoronary saphenous vein bypass graft

ACT achievement through counseling and treatment; actinomycin; activated clotting time; advanced coronary treatment; anterocolic transposition; antichymotrypsin; anticoagulant therapy; anxiety control training; atropine coma therapy

act actinomycin; activity, active

ACTA automatic computerized transverse axial [scanning]

Act-C actinomycin C

Act-D actinomycin D

ACTe anodal closure tetanus

ACTG AIDS Clinical Treatment Group

ACTH adrenocorticotropic hormone

ACTH-LI adrenocorticotropin-like immunoreactivity

ACTH-RF adrenocorticotropic hormone releasing factor

activ active, activity

ACTN adrenocorticotropin

ACTP adrenocorticotropic polypeptide

ACTS acute cervical traumatic sprain or syndrome; Auditory Comprehension Test for Sentences

ACU acquired cold urticaria; acute care unit; agar colony-forming unit; ambulatory care unit

ACV acute cardiovascular [disease]; acyclovir; atrial/carotid/ventricular

ACVB aortocoronary venous bypass

ACVD acute cardiovascular disease, atherosclerotic cardiovascular disease

AD accident dispensary; acetate dialysis; active disease; acute dermatomyositis; addict, addiction; adenoid degeneration [agent]; adjuvant disease; admitting diagnosis; adrenostenedione; adult disease; advanced directive; aerosol deposition; affective disorder; after discharge; alcohol dehydrogenase; Aleutian disease; alveolar diffusion; alveolar duct; Alzheimer's dementia; Alzheimer's disease; analgesic dose; anodal duration; anterior division; antigenic determinant; appropriate disability; arthritic dose; Associate Degree; atopic dermatitis; attentional disturbance; autonomic dysreflexia; autosomal dominant; average deviation; axiodistal; axis deviation; right ear [Lat. *auris dextra*]

A/D analog-to-digital [converter]

A&D admission and discharge; ascending and descending

Ad adenovirus; adrenal; anisotropic disk

ad add [Lat. *adde*] let there be added [up to a specified amount] [Lat. *addetur*]; axiodistal; right ear [Lat. *auris dextra*]

ADA adenosine deaminase; American Dental Association; American Dermatological Association; American Diabetes Association; American Dietetic Association; anterior descending artery; antideoxyribonucleic acid antibody; approved dietary allowance

ADAA American Dental Assistants Association

ADAM amniotic deformity, adhesion, mutilation [syndrome]

ADAMHA Alcohol, Drug Abuse, and Mental Health Administration

ADAP American Dental Assistant's Program; Assistant Director of Army Psychiatry

ADAS-COG cognitive portion of the Alzheimer's Disease Assessment Scale

ADase adenosine deaminase

ADAU adolescent drug abuse unit

ADB accidental death benefit

ADC affective disorders clinic; Aid to Dependent Children; AIDS-dementia complex; albumin, dextrose, and catalase [medium]; ambulance design criteria; analog-to-digital converter; anodal duration contraction; average daily census; axiodistocervical

AdC adenylate cyclase; adrenal cortex

ADCC acute disorder of cerebral circulation; antibody-dependent cell-mediated cytotoxicity

ADCP adenosine deaminase complexing protein

ADCS Argonz del Castillo syndrome

ADD adduction; adenosine deaminase; attentional deficit disorder; average daily dose

add addition; adductor, adduction; let there be added [Lat. *addatur*]

add c trit add with trituration [Lat. *adde cum tritu*]

ad def an to the point of fainting [Lat. *ad defectionem animi*]

ad deliq to fainting [Lat. *ad deliquium*]

addend to be added [Lat. *addendus*]

ADDH attention deficit disorder with hyperactivity

ADD/HA attention deficit disorder/ hyperactivity

addict addiction, addictive

addn addition

add poll adductor pollicis

ADDS American Digestive Disease Society

ADDU alcohol and drug dependence unit

ADE acute disseminated encephalitis; antibody-dependent enhancement; apparent digestible energy

Ade adenine

AdeCbl adenosyl cobalamine

ADEE age-dependent epileptic encephalopathy

ad effect until effective [Lat. *ad effectum*]

ADEM acute disseminated encephalomyelitis

adeq adequate

ad feb fever being present [Lat. *adstante febre*]

ADFN albinism–deafness syndrome

ADG atrial diastolic gallop; axiodistogingival

ad gr acid to an agreeable acidity [Lat. *ad gratum aciditatem*]

ad gr gust to an agreeable taste [Lat. *ad gratum gustum*]

ADH Academy of Dentistry for the Handicapped; adhesion; alcohol dehydrogenase; antidiuretic hormone; arginine dihydrolase

adh adhesion, adhesive; antidiuretic hormone

ADHA American Dental Hygienists Association

ADHD attention deficit–hyperactivity disorder

adhib to be administered [Lat. *adhibendus*]

ADI Academy of Dentistry International; acceptable daily intake; allowable daily intake; artificial diverticulum of the ileum; atlas–dens interval; axiodistoincisal

ad int meanwhile [Lat. *ad interim*]

adj adjacent; adjoining; adjuvant

ADK adenosine kinase

ADKC atopic dermatitis with keratoconjunctivitis

ADL activities of daily living; Amsterdam Depression List

ADLC antibody-dependent lymphocyte-mediated cytotoxicity

ad lib as desired [Lat. *ad libitum*]

ADM administrative medicine; Adriamycin

AdM adrenal medulla

adm administration; admission; apply [Lat. *admove*]

Adm Dr admitting doctor

Admin administration

admov let there be applied [Lat. *admove, admoveatur*]

Adm Ph admitting physician

ADMR average daily metabolic rate

ADMX adrenal medullectomy

ADN antideoxyribonuclease; aortic depressor nerve

ad naus to the point of producing nausea [Lat. *ad nauseam*]

ADN-B antideoxyribonuclease B

ad neut to neutralization [Lat. *ad neutralizandum*]

ADO adolescent medicine; axiodisto-occlusal

Ado adenosine

ADOD arthrodentosteodysplasia

AdoDABA adenosyldiaminobutyric acid

AdoHcy *S*-adenosylhomocysteine

AdoMet *S*-adenosylmethionine

Adox oxidized adenosine

ADP adenopathy; adenosine diphosphate; administrative psychiatry; approved drug product; area diastolic pressure; automatic data processing

AdP adductor pollicis

ad part dolent to the painful parts [Lat. *ad partes dolentes*]

ADPase adenosine diphosphatase

ADPKD autosomal dominant polycystic kidney disease

ADPL average daily patient load

ad pond om to the weight of the whole [Lat. *ad pondus omnium*]

ADPR adenosine diphosphate ribose

ADQ abductor digite quinte

ADR adrenodoxin reductase; Adriamycin; adverse drug reaction; airway dilation reflex; arrested development of righting response; ataxia-deafness-retardation [syndrome]

Adr adrenalin; Adriamycin

adr adrenal, adrenalectomy

ad rat as reasonable [Lat. *ad rationem*]

ADRBR adrenergic beta-receptor

ADS acute death syndrome; acute diarrheal syndrome; Alcohol Dependence Scale; alternative delivery system; anatomical dead space; anonymous donor's sperm; antibody deficiency syndrome; antidiuretic substance; Army Dental Service

ad sat to saturation [Lat. *ad saturandum*]

adst feb while fever is present [Lat. *adstante febre*]

ADT Accepted Dental Therapeutics; adenosine triphosphate; admission, discharge, transfer; agar-gel diffusion test; alternate day therapy; any, what you desire, thing (a placebo); Alzheimer's-type dementia; Auditory Discrimination Test

ADTA American Dental Trade Association

ADTe anodal duration tetanus

ad us according to custom [Lat. *ad usum*]

ad us ext for external application [Lat. *ad usum externum*]

ADV adenovirus; adventitia; Aleutian disease virus

Adv adenovirus

adv advanced; against [Lat. *adversum*]

ad 2 vic at two times, for two doses [Lat. *ad duas vices*]

ADVIRC autosomal dominant vitreoretinochoroidopathy

ADW assault with deadly weapon

A5D5W alcohol 5%, dextrose 5%, in water

ADX adrenalectomized

AE above-elbow [amputation]; acrodermatitis enteropathica; activation energy; adult erythrocyte; after-effect; agarose electrophoresis; air embolism; air entry; alcoholic embryopathy; anoxic encephalopathy; autiepileptic; antitoxic unit [Ger. *Antitoxineinheit*]; apoenzyme; aryepiglottic; atherosclerotic encephalopathy; avian encephalomyelitis

A + E accident and emergency [department]; analysis and evaluation

AEA alcohol, ether, and acetone [solution]; apocrine membrane antigen

AEB acute erythroblastopenia; avian erythroblastosis

AEC ankyloblepharon, ectodermal defects, and cleft lip [syndrome]; at earliest convenience; Atomic Energy Commission

AECD allergic eczematous contact dermatitis

AED antiepileptic drug; antihidrotic ectodermal dysplasia

AEDP automated external defibrillator pacemaker

AEE atomic energy establishment

AEF allogenic effect factor; amyloid enhancing factor

AEG air encephalography, air encephalogram; atrial electrogram

aeg patient [Lat. *aeger, aegra*]

AEGIS Aid for the Elderly in Government Institutions

AEI arbitrary evolution index; atrial emptying index

AEM analytical electron microscopy; ambulatory electrocardiographic monitoring; avian encephalomyelitis

AEMIS Aerospace and Environmental Medicine Information System

AEN aseptic epiphyseal necrosis

AEP acute edematous pancreatitis; artificial endocrine pancreas; auditory evoked potential; average evoked potential

AEq age equivalent

aeq equal [Lat. *aequales*]

AER abduction/external rotation; acoustic evoked response; acute exertional rhabdomyolysis; agranular endoplasmic reticulum; albumin excretion rate; aldosterone excretion rate; apical ectodermal ridge; auditory evoked response; average electroencephalic response; average evoked response

AERE Atomic Energy Research Establishment

Aero Aerobacter

AERP antegrade effective refractory period; atrial effective refractory period

AERPAP antegrade effective refractory period accessory pathway

AES acetone-extracted serum; American Electroencephalographic Society; American Encephalographic Society; American Endocrine Society; American Endodontic Society; American Epidemiological Society; American Equilibration Society; anterior esophageal sensor; antiembolic stockings; antral ethmoidal sphenoidectomy; aortic ejection sound; Auger's electron spectroscopy; autoerythrocyte sensitization

AEST aeromedical evacuation support team

AET absorption-equivalent thickness; S-(2-aminoethyl) isothiuronium

aet age [Lat. *aetas*]

aetat aged [Lat. *aetatis*]

aetiol etiology [Brit. *aetiology*]

AEV avian erythroblastosis virus

AF abnormal frequency; acid-fast; adult female; afebrile; aflatoxin; albumin-free; albumose-free; aldehyde fuchsin; amaurosis fugax; aminophylline; amniotic fluid; angiogenesis factor; anteflexion; anterior fontanelle; antibody-forming; anti-fog; aortic flow; Arthritis Foundation; artificial feeding; ascitic fluid; atrial fibrillation; atrial flutter; atrial fusion; attenuation factor; attributable fraction; audio frequency

aF abfarad

af audio frequency

AFA acromegaloid facial syndrome; advanced first aid; alcohol-formaldehyde-acetic [fixative]

AFAFP amniotic fluid alpha-fetoprotein

AFAR American Foundation for Aging Research

AFB acid-fast bacillus; aflatoxin B; air fluidized bed; aortofemoral bypass

AFBG aortofemoral bypass graft

AFC antibody-forming cell

AFCI acute focal cerebral ischemia

AFCR American Federation for Clinical Research

AFD accelerated freeze drying

AFDC Aid to Families with Dependent Children

AFDH American Fund for Dental Health

AFDW ash-free dry weight

AFE amniotic fluid embolism

afeb afebrile

AFF atrial fibrillation; atrial filling fraction; atrial flutter

aff afferent

AFG aflatoxin G; amniotic fluid glucose

AFH angiofollicular hyperplasia; anterior facial height

AFI amaurotic familial idiocy

AFib atrial fibrillation

AFIP Armed Forces Institute of Pathology

AFIS amniotic fluid infection syndrome

AFL antifibrinolysin; artificial limb; atrial flutter

AFLNH angiofollicular lymph node hyperplasia

AFLP acute fatty liver of pregnancy

AFM aflatoxin M

AFN afunctional neutrophil

AFNC Air Force Nurse Corps

AFND acute febrile neutrophilic dermatosis

AFO ankle-foot orthrosis

AFP alpha-fetoprotein; anterior faucial pillar; atypical facial pain

AfP affiliate physician

aFP alpha-fetoprotein

AfPh affiliate physician

AFPP acute fibropurulent pneumonia

AFQ aflatoxin Q

AFR aqueous flare response; ascorbic free radical

AFRAX autism–fragile X [syndrome]

AFRD acute febrile respiratory disease

AFRI acute febrile respiratory illness

AFS acquired or adult Fanconi syndrome; American Fertility Society; antifibroblast serum

AFSAM Air Force School of Aviation Medicine

AFSP acute fibrinoserous pneumonia

AFT aflatoxin; agglutination-flocculation test

AFTA American Family Therapy Association

AFTN autonomously functioning thyroid nodule

AFV amniotic fluid volume

AG agarose; analytical grade; antigen; antiglobulin; antigravity; atrial gallop; attached gingiva; axiogingival; azurophilic granule

AG, A/G albumin-globulin [ratio]

Ag antigen; silver [Lat. *argentum*]

ag antigen

AGA accelerated growth area; allergic granulomatosis and angiitis; American Gastroenterological Association; American Genetic Association; American Geriatrics Association; American Goiter Association; anti-IgG autoantibody; antiglomerular antibody; appropriate for gestational age

Ag-Ab antigen-antibody complex

AGAG acidic glycosaminoglycans

AGBAD Alexander Graham Bell Association for the Deaf

AGC absolute granulocyte count; automatic gain control

AGCT antiglobulin consumption test; Army General Classification Test

AGD agar gel diffusion; agarose diffusion

AGDD agar gel double diffusion

AGE acrylamide gel; acute gastroenteritis; agarose gel electrophoresis; angle of greatest extension

AGED automated general experimental device

AGEPC acetyl glyceryl ether phosphorylcholine

AGF adrenal growth factor; angle of greatest flexion

ag feb when the fever is coming on [Lat. *aggrediente febre*]

AGG agammaglobulinemia

agg agglutination; aggravation; aggregation

aggl, agglut agglutination
aggrav aggravated, aggravation
aggred feb while the fever is coming on [Lat. *aggrediente febre*]
aggreg aggregated, aggregation
AGGS anti-gas gangrene serum
agit agitated, agitation; shake [Lat. *agita*]
agit ante sum shake before taking [Lat. *agita ante sumendum*]
agit vas the vial being shaken [Lat. *agitato vase*]
AGL acute granulocytic leukemia; agglutination; aminoglutethimide
AGMK African green monkey kidney [cell]
AGMkK African green monkey kidney [cell]
AGN acute glomerulonephritis; agnosia
VIII_{AGN} factor VIII antigen
agn agnosia
AgNOR silver-staining nucleolar organizer region
AGOS American Gynecological and Obstetrical Society
AGP acid glycoprotein; agar gel precipitation
AGPA American Group Practice Association; American Group Psychotherapy Association
AGPI agar gel precipitin inhibition
AGPT agar-gel precipitation test
AGR aniridia, genitourinary abnormalities, and mental retardation; anticipatory goal response
agri agriculture
AGS adrenogenital syndrome; American Geriatrics Society; audiogenic seizures
AGT abnormal glucose tolerance; activity group therapy; acute generalized tuberculosis; antiglobulin test
agt agent
AGTH adrenoglomerulotropic hormone
AGTr adrenoglomerulotropin
AGTT abnormal glucose tolerance test
AGV aniline gentian violet
AH abdominal hysterectomy; absorptive hypercalciuria; accidental hypothermia; acetohexamide; acid hydrolysis; acute

hepatitis; adrenal hypoplasia; after hyperpolarization; agnathia-holoprosencephaly; alcoholic hepatitis; amenorrhea and hirsutism; aminohippurate; anterior hypothalamus; antihyaluronidase; arcuate hypothalamus; Army Hospital; arterial hypertension; artificial heart; ascites hepatoma; astigmatic hypermetropia; ataxic hemiparesis; autonomic hyperreflexia; axillary hair
A/H amenorrhea-hyperprolactinemia
A+H accident & health [policy]
A•h ampere hour
aH abhenry
ah hyperopic astigmatism
AHA acetohydroxamic acid; acquired hemolytic anemia; acute hemolytic anemia; American Heart Association; American Hospital Association; anterior hypothalamic area; anti-heart antibody; antihistone antibody; area health authority; arthritis-hives-angioedema [syndrome]; aspartyl-hydroxamic acid; Associate, Institute of Hospital Administrators; autoimmune hemolytic anemia
AHB alpha-hydroxybutyric acid
AHC academic health care; acute hemorrhagic conjunctivitis; acute hemorrhagic cystitis; antihemophilic factor C
AHCA American Health Care Association
AHCPR Agency for Health Care Policy and Research
AHCy adenosyl homocysteine
AHD acquired hepatocerebral degeneration; acute heart disease; antihyaluronidase; antihypertensive drug; arteriohepatic dysplasia; arteriosclerotic heart disease; atherosclerotic heart disease; autoimmune hemolytic disease
AHDMS automated hospital data management system
AHDP azacycloheptane diphosphonate
AHE acute hemorrhagic encephalomyelitis
AHEA area health education activity
AHEC area health education center
AHES artificial heart energy system

AHF acute heart failure; American Health Foundation; American Hepatic Foundation; American Hospital Formulary; antihemolytic factor; antihemophilic factor; Argentinian hemorrhagic fever; Associated Health Foundation
AHFS American Hospital Formulary Service
AHG aggregated human globulin; antihemophilic globulin; antihuman globulin
AHGG antihuman gammaglobulin; aggregated human gammaglobulin
AHGS acute herpetic gingival stomatitis
AHH alpha-hydrazine analog of histidine; anosmia and hypogonadotropic hypogonadism [syndrome]; arylhydrocarbon hydroxylase; Association for Holistic Health
AHI active hostility index; Animal Health Institute; apnea-plus-hypopnea index
AHIP assisted health insurance plan
AHIS automated hospital information system
AHJ artificial hip joint
AHL apparent half-life
AHLE acute hemorrhagic leukoencephalitis
AHLG antihuman lymphocyte globulin
AHLS antihuman lymphocyte serum
AHM allied health manpower; ambulatory Holter monitor
AHMA American Holistic Medicine Association; antiheart muscle autoantibody
AHMC Association of Hospital Management Committees
AHN Army Head Nurse; assistant head nurse
AHO Albright's hereditary osteodystrophy
AHP acute hemorrhagic pancreatitis; after hyperpolarization; air at high pressure; Assistant House Physician
AHPA American Health Planning Association
AHPO anterior hypothalamic preoptic [area]

AHR antihyaluronidase reaction; Association for Health Records
AHRA American Hospital Radiology Administration
AHRF acute hypoxemic respiratory failure; American Hearing Research Foundation
AHS Academy of Health Sciences; African horse sickness; alveolar hypoventilation syndrome; American Hearing Society; American Hospital Society; assistant house surgeon
AHSDF area health service development fund
AHSN Assembly of Hospital Schools of Nursing
AHSR Association for Health Services Research
AHT aggregation half time; antihyaluronidase titer; augmented histamine test; autogenous hamster tumor
AHTG antihuman thymocyte globulin
AHTP antihuman thymocyte plasma
AHTS antihuman thymus serum
AHU acute hemolytic uremic [syndrome]; arginine, hypoxanthine, and uracil
AHuG aggregated human IgG
AHV avian herpes virus
AI accidental injury; accidentally incurred; adiposity index; aggregation index; allergy and immunology; anaphylatoxin inactivator; angiogenesis inhibitor; angiotensin I; anxiety index; aortic incompetence; aortic insufficiency; apical impulse; articulation index; artificial insemination; artificial intelligence; atherogenic index; atrial insufficiency; autoimmune, autoimmunity; axio-incisal
A&I allergy and immunology
aI active ingredient
AIA allylisopropylacetamide; amylase inhibitor activity; anti-immunoglobulin antibody; anti-insulin antibody; aspirin-induced asthma; automated image analysis
AIB aminoisobutyrate; avian infectious bronchitis

AIBA aminoisobutyric acid

AIBS American Institute of Biological Sciences

AIC aminoimidazole carboxamide; Association des Infirmières Canadiennes

A-IC average integrated concentration

AICA anterior inferior cerebellar artery; anterior inferior communicating artery

AI-CAH autoimmune-type chronic active hepatitis

AICAR aminoimidazole carboxamide ribonucleotide

AICD automatic implantable cardioverter defibrillator

AICE angiotensin I converting enzyme

AICF autoimmune complement fixation

AID acquired immunodeficiency disease; acute infectious disease; acute ionization detector; Agency for International Development; argon ionization detector; artificial insemination donor; autoimmune deficiency; autoimmune disease; automatic implantable defibrillator; average interocular difference

AIDP acute inflammatory demyelinating polyradiculopathy

AIDS acquired immune deficiency syndrome

AIDSDRUGS clinical trials of acquired immunodeficiency drugs [MEDLARS data base]

AIDS-KS acquired immune deficiency syndrome with Kaposi's sarcoma

AIDSLINE on-line information on acquired immunodeficiency syndrome [MEDLARS data base]

AIDSTRIALS clinical trials of acquired immunodeficiency syndrome drugs [MEDLARS data base]

AIE acute inclusion-body encephalitis; acute infectious encephalitis; acute infective endocarditis

AIEP amount of insulin extractable from pancreas

AIF anemia-inducing factor; anti-inflammatory; anti-invasion factor

AIFD acute intrapartum fetal distress

AIG anti-immunoglobulin

AIH American Institute of Homeopathy; artificial insemination, homologous; artificial insemination by husband

AIHA American Industrial Hygiene Association; autoimmune hemolytic anemia

AIHC American Industrial Health Conference

AIHD acquired immune hemolytic disease

AII acute intestinal infection

AIIS anterior inferior iliac spine

AIIT amiodarone-iodine-induced thyrotoxicosis

AIL acute infectious lymphocytosis; angiocentric immunoproliferative lesion; angioimmunoblastic lymphadenopathy

AILD alveolar interstitial lung disease; angioimmunoblastic lymphadenopathy

AIM Abridged Index Medicus; acute transverse myelopathy; artificial intelligence in medicine

AIMD abnormal involuntary movement disorder

AIMS abnormal involuntary movement scale

AIN acute interstitial nephritis; American Institute of Nutrition; anterior interosseons nerve

AINA automated immunonephelometric assay

AINS anti-inflammatory nonsteroidal

A Insuf aortic insufficiency

AION anterior ischemic optic neuropathy

AIP acute idiopathic pericarditis; acute infectious polyneuritis; acute intermittent porphyria; aldosterone-induced protein; automated immunoprecipitation; average intravascular pressure; integral anatuberculin, Petragnani

AIPE acute interstitial pulmonary emphysema

AIPFP acute idiopathic peripheral facial nerve palsy

AIPS American Institute of Pathologic Science

AIR amino-imidazole ribonucleotide; average impairment rating

AIRA anti-insulin receptor antibody

AIRF alterations in respiratory function

AIRS Amphetamine Interview Rating Scale

AIS Abbreviated Injury Scale; amniotic infection syndrome; androgen insensitivity syndrome; anterior interosseous nerve syndrome; anti-insulin serum

AISA acquired idiopathic sideroblastic anemia

AIS/MR Alternative Intermediate Services for the Mentally Retarded

AIT acute intensive treatment

AITP autoimmune idiopathic thrombocytopenic purpura

AITT arginine insulin tolerance test; augmented insulin tolerance test

AIU absolute iodine uptake; antigen-inducing unit

AIUM American Institute of Ultrasound in Medicine

AIVR accelerated idioventricular rhythm

AIVV anterior informal vertebral vein

AJ, A/J ankle jerk

AJCCS American Joint Committee on Cancer Staging

AJS acute joint syndrome

AK above knee; acetate kinase; adenosine kinase; adenylate kinase; artificial kidney

A/K, ak above knee

A→K ankle to knee

AKA above-knee amputation; alcoholic ketoacidosis; also known as; antikeratin antibody

AK amp above-knee amputation

AKE acrokeratoelastoidosis

A/kg amperes per kilogram

AKP alkaline phosphatase

AKS alcoholic Korsakoff syndrome; auditory and kinesthetic sensation

AL absolute latency; acinar lumen; acute leukemia; adaptation level; albumin; alcoholism; alignment; amyloidosis; antihuman lymphocytic [globulin]; avian

leukosis; axial length; axillary loop; axiolingual; left ear [Lat. *auris laeva*]

Al allantoic; allergic, allergy; aluminum

al left ear [Lat. *auris laeva*]

ALA American Laryngological Association; American Lung Association; aminolevulinic acid; axiolabial

ALa axiolabial

Ala alanine

AL-Ab antilymphocyte antibody

ALAD abnormal left axis deviation

ALAD, ALA-D aminolevulinic acid dehydrase

ALAG, ALaG axiolabiogingival

ALAL, ALaL axiolabiolingual

AlaP, ala-P alafosfalin

ALARA as low as reasonably achievable [radiation exposure]

ALARM adjustable leg and ankle repositioning mechanism

ALAS aminolevulinic acid synthetase

ALAT alanine aminotransferase

ALB albumin; avian lymphoblastosis

alb albumin; white [Lat. *albus*]

ALBC albumin clearance

ALB/GLOB albumin/globulin [ratio]

ALC absolute lymphocyte count; acute lethal catatonia; Alternative Lifestyle Checklist; approximate lethal concentration; avian leukosis complex; axiolinguocervical

alc alcohol, alcoholism, alcoholic

ALCA anomalous left coronary artery

ALCAPA anomalous origin of left coronary artery from pulmonary artery

ALCEQ Adolescent Life Change Event Questionnaire

alcoh alcohol, alcoholic, alcoholism

AlcR, alcR alcohol rub

AlCr aluminum crown

ALD adrenoleukodystrophy; alcoholic liver disease; aldolase; anterior latissimus dorsi; Appraisal of Language Disturbance

Ald aldolase

ALDH aldehyde dehydrogenase

Aldo, ALDOST aldosterone

ALE allowable limits of error

ALEC artificial lung-expanding compound

ALEP atypical lymphoepithelioid cell proliferation

ALF acute liver failure; American Liver Foundation

ALFT abnormal liver function test

ALG antilymphocytic globulin; axiolinguogingival

alg allergy

ALGOL algorithmic oriented language

ALH angiolymphoid hyperplasia; anterior lobe hormone; anterior lobe of hypophysis

ALHE angiolymphoid hyperplasia with eosinophilia

ALI annual limit of intake

ALIP abnormal localized immature myeloid precursor

ALK, alk alkaline; alkylating

ALK-P alkaline phosphatase

ALL acute lymphoblastic leukemia; acute lymphocytic leukemia

all allergy, allergic

ALLA acute lymphocytic leukemia antigen

ALLO atypical *Legionella*-like organism

ALM aerial lentiginous melanoma; alveolar living material

ALME acetyl-lysine methyl ester

ALMI anterior lateral myocardial infarct

ALMV anterior leaflet of the mitral valve

ALN allylnitrile; anterior lymph node

ALO average lymphocyte output; axiolinguo-occlusal

ALOS average length of stay

ALOSH Appalachian Laboratory for Occupational Safety and Health

ALOX aluminum oxide

ALP acute leukemia protocol; acute lupus pericarditis; alkaline phosphatase; alveolar proteinosis; anterior lobe of pituitary; antilymphocytic plasma; argon laser photocoagulation

AlPase alkaline phosphatase

α Greek letter alpha; angular acceleration; first [carbon atom next to the carbon

atom bearing the active group in organic compounds]; optical rotation; probability of type I error; solubility coefficient

alpha₂-AP alpha 2-antiplasmin

alpha-GLUC alpha-glucosidase

alpha₂M alpha₂-macroglobulin

ALPS angiolymphoproliferative syndrome; Aphasia Language Performance Scale

ALRI anterolateral rotatory instability

ALROS American Laryngological, Rhinological, and Otological Society

ALS acute lateral sclerosis; advanced life support; afferent loop syndrome; amyotrophic lateral sclerosis; angiotensin-like substance; anterolateral sclerosis; anticipated life span; antilymphocyte serum

ALSD Alzheimer's-like senile dementia

ALS-PD amyotrophic lateral sclerosis-parkinsonism-dementia [complex]

ALT alanine aminotransferase; argon laser trabeculoplasty; avian laryngotracheitis

Alt, alt aluminum tartrate; alternate; altitude

AlT aluminum tartrate

ALTB acute laryngotracheobronchitis

alt dieb every other day [Lat. *alternis diebus*]

ALTE apparent life-threatening event

ALTEE acetyl-*L*-tyrosine ethyl ester

alt h, alt hor every other hour [Lat. *alternis horis*]

alt noct every other night [Lat. *alternis nocta*]

ALTS acute lumbar traumatic sprain [or syndrome]

ALU arithmetic and logic unit

ALV Abelson leukemia virus; adeno-like virus; alveolar, alveolus; ascending lumbar vein; avian leukosis virus

Alv alveolus, alveolar

ALVAD abdominal left ventricular assist device

alv adst when the bowels are constipated [Lat. *alvo adstricta*]

alv deject discharge from the bowels [Lat. *alvi dejectiones*]

ALV M alveolar mucosa
ALVT aortic and left ventricular tunnel
alv vent alveolar ventilation
ALVX alveolectomy
ALW arch-loop whorl
ALWMI anterolateral wall myocardial infarct
AM actomyosin; acute myelofibrosis; adult male; adult monocyte; aerospace medicine; akinetic mutism; alveolar macrophage; alveolar mucosa; amacrine cell; ambulatory; amethopterin; ametropia; ammeter; amperemeter; ampicillin; amplitude modulation; amyl; anovular menstruation; arithmetic mean; arousal mechanism; articular manipulation; aviation medicine; axiomesial; before noon [Lat. *ante meridiem*]; Master of Arts [Lat. *artium magister*]; meter angle; myopic astigmatism
Am americium; amnion; amyl
A/m amperes per meter
A-m² ampere-square meter
am ametropia; amyl; amplitude; before noon [Lat. *ante meridiem*]; meter angle; myopic astigmatism
AMA against medical advice; American Medical Association; antimitochondrial antibody; antimyosin antibody; antithyroid microsomal antibody; Australian Medical Association
AMA-DE American Medical Association Drug Evaluation
AMAL Aero-Medical Acceleration Laboratory
AMAP as much as possible
A-MAT amorphous material
AMB avian myeloblastosis; amphotericin B; anomalous muscle bundle
Amb ambulance; ambulatory, ambulation
amb ambient; ambiguous; ambulance; ambulatory
ambig ambiguous
AMBL acute megakaryoblastic leukemia
ambul ambulatory
AMC acetylmethyl carbinol; Animal

Medical Center; antibody-mediated cytotoxicity; antimalaria campaign; arm muscle circumference; Army Medical Corps; arthrogryposis multiplex congenita; automated mixture control; axiomesiocervical
AMCHA aminomethylcyclohexane-carboxylic acid
AMCN anteromedial caudate nucleus
AMD acid maltase deficiency; acromandibular dysplasia; actinomycin D; adrenomyelodystrophy; age-related macular degeneration; Aleutian mink disease; alpha-methyldopa; Association for Macular Diseases; axiomesiodistal
AMDGF alveolar macrophage-derived growth factor
AMDS Association of Military Dental Surgeons
AME amphotericin methyl ester; aseptic meningoencephalitis
AMEA American Medical Electroencephalographic Association
AMEAE acute monophasic experimental autoimmune encephalomyelitis
AMEDS Army Medical Service
AMEGL, AMegL acute megakaryoblastic leukemia
AMet adenosyl-*L*-methionine
AMF antimuscle factor
AMFAR American Foundation for AIDS Research
AMG amyloglucosidase; antimacrophage globulin; axiomesiogingival
A₂MG alpha-2-macroglobulin
AMH anti-müllerian hormone; automated medical history
Amh mixed astigmatism with myopia predominating
AMHA Association of Mental Health Administrators
AMHT automated multiphasic health testing
AMI acquired monosaccharide intolerance; acute myocardial infarction; amitriptyline; anterior myocardial infarction; Association of Medical Illustrators;

Athletic Motivation Inventory; axiomesioincisal

AMIA American Medical Informatics Association

AMKL acute megakaryoblastic leukemia

AML acute monocytic leukemia; acute mucosal lesion; acute myeloblastic leukemia; acute myelocytic leukemia; anatomic medullary locking; anterior mitral leaflet; automated multitest laboratory

AMLB alternate monoaural loudness balance

AMLC adherent macrophage-like cell; autologous mixed lymphocyte culture

AMLR autologous mixed lymphocyte reaction

AMLS antimouse lymphocyte serum

AMLSGA acute myeloblastic leukemia surface glycoprotein antigen

AMM agnogenic myeloid metaplasia; ammonia; antibody to murine cardiac myosin; World Medical Association [Fr. *Association Médicale Mondiale*]

amm, ammonia

AMML acute myelomonocytic leukemia

AMMoL acute myelomonoblastic leukemia

ammon ammonia

AMN adrenomyeloneuropathy; alloxazine mononucleotide; aminonucleoside; anterior median nucleus

AMNS aminonucleoside

AMO assistant medical officer; axiomesio-occlusal

A-mode amplitude modulation

AMOL acute monoblastic leukemia

amo, amor amorphous

AMP accelerated mental processes; acid mucopolysaccharide; adenosine monophosphate; amphetamine; ampicillin; ampule; amputation; average mean pressure

amp ampere; amplification; ampule; amputation, amputee

AMPA American Medical Publishers Association

AMPAC American Medical Political Action Committee

AMP-c cyclic adenosine monophosphate

AMPH, amphet amphetamine

amp-hr ampere-hour

ampl large [Lat. *amplus*]

A-M pr Austin-Moore prosthesis

AMPS abnormal mucopolysacchariduria; acid mucopolysaccharide

AMPT alpha-methylparatyrosine

ampul ampule

AMR acoustic muscle reflex; activity metabolic rate; alternate motion rate; alternating motion reflex

AMRA American Medical Record Association

AMRI anteromedial rotatory instability

AMRL Aerospace Medical Research Laboratories

AMRNL Army Medical Research and Nutrition Laboratory

AMRS automated medical record system

AMS acute mountain sickness; aggravated in military service; altered mental status; American Microscopical Society; amount of substance; amylase; antimacrophage serum; Army Medical Service; aseptic meningitis syndrome; Association of Military Surgeons; auditory memory span; automated multiphasic screening

ams amount of a substance

AMSA acridinylamine methanesulfon-m-anisidide; American Medical Society on Alcoholism; American Medical Students Association; amsacrine

AMSC Army Medical Specialist Corps

AMSRDC Army Medical Service Research and Development Command

AMT acute miliary tuberculosis; alpha-methyltyrosine; American Medical Technologists; amethopterin; amitriptyline; amphetamine; anxiety management training

amt amount

AMU Army Medical Unit

amu atomic mass unit

AmuLV Abelson murine leukemia virus; amphotrophic murine leukemia virus

AMV assisted mechanical ventilation; avian myeloblastosis virus

AMVI acute mesenteric vascular insufficiency

aMVL anterior mitral valve leaflet

AMWA American Medical Women's Association; American Medical Writers' Association

AMX amoxicillin

AMY, amy amylase

AN acanthosis nigricans; acne neonatorum; acoustic neuroma; adult, normal; ala nasi; amyl nitrate; aneurysm; anisometropia; anode; anorexia nervosa; antenatal; anterior; antineuraminidase; aseptic necrosis; atmosphere normal; atrionodal; autonomic neuropathy; avascular necrosis

A/N as needed

An actinon; anisometropia; anode, anodal; atmosphere normal

A$_n$ atmosphere normal

ANA acetylneuraminic acid; American Narcolepsy Association; American Neurological Association; American Nurses Association; anesthesia [*anaesthesia*]; antibody to nuclear antigens; antinuclear antibody; aspartyl naphthylamide

ANAD anorexia nervosa with associated disorders

ANAE alpha-naphthyl acetate esterase

anal analgesia, analgesic; analysis, analytic

ANAG acute narrow angle glaucoma

ANAL, anal analgesia, analgesic; analysis, analytic

ANAP agglutination negative, absorption positive [reaction]

ANAS anastomosis; auditory nerve activating substance

anast anastomosis

Anat, anat anatomy, anatomist

ANB avascular necrosis of bone

ANC absolute neutrophil count; acid neutralization capacity; antigen-neutralizing capacity; Army Nurse Corps

ANCA antineutrophil cytoplasm antibody

ANCC, AnCC anodal closure contraction

ANCOVA analysis of covariance

AND algoneurodystrophy; anterior nasal discharge

ANDA Abbreviated New Drug Application

ANDRO, andro androsterone

ANDTE, AnDTe anodal duration tetanus

anes, anesth anesthesia, anesthetic

ANESR apparent norepinephrine secretion rate

AnEx, an ex anodal excitation

ANF alpha-naphthoflavone; American Nurses' Foundation; antineuritic factor; antinuclear factor; atrial natriuretic factor

ANG angiogram, angiography; angiotension

ang angiogram; angiography, angle, angular

Ang GR angiotensin generation rate

ang pect angina pectoris

anh anhydrous

ANI acute nerve irritation

ANIA automated nephelometric immunoassay

ANIS Anorexia Nervosa Inventory for Self-rating

aniso anisocytosis

ANIT alpha-naphthyl-isothiocyanate

ank ankle

ANL acute nonlymphoblastic leukemia

ANLI antibody-negative with latent infection

ANLL acute nonlymphocytic leukemia

Ann annual

ann fib annulus fibrosus

ANOC, AnOC anodal opening contraction

ANOCL anodal opening clonus

ANOV, ANOVA analysis of variance

ANP acute necrotizing pancreatitis

A-norprogesterone; atrial natriuretic peptide

A-NPP absorbed normal pooled plasma

ANRC American National Red Cross

ANRL antihypertensive neutral renomedullary lipid

ANS acanthion; American Nutrition Society; 8-anilino-1-naphthalene-sulfonic acid; anterior nasal spine; antineutrophilic serum; antirat neutrophil serum; Army Nursing Service; arterionephrosclerosis; Associate in Nursing Science; autonomic nervous system

ANSCII American National Standard Code for Information Interchange

ANSI American National Standards Institute

ANT acoustic noise test; aminonitrothiazole; anterior

ant anterior; antimycin

AntA antimycin A

antag antagonist

anti-HB$_c$ antibody to hepatitis B core antigen

anti-HB$_e$ antibody to hepatitis B early antigen

anti-HB$_s$ antibody to hepatitis B surface antigen

anti-PNM Ab anti-peripheral nerve myelin antibody

ant jentac before breakfast [Lat. *ante jentaculum*]

ANTR apparent net transfer rate

ANTU alpha-naphthylthiourea

ANuA antinuclear antibody

ANUG acute necrotizing ulcerative gingivitis

ANV avian nephritis virus

anx anxiety

AO abdominal aorta; achievement orientation; acid output; acridine orange; ankle orthosis; anodal opening; anterior oblique; aorta; aortic opening; atomic orbital; atrioventricular valve opening; average optical [density]; axio-occlusal

Ao aorta

A&O, A/O alert and oriented

AOA Administration on Aging; American Optometric Association; American Orthopedic Association; American Orthopsychiatric Association; American Osteopathic Association

AOAA amino-oxyacetic acid

AOAC Association of Official Agricultural Chemists

AOAP as often as possible

AOAS American Osteopathic Academy of Sclerotherapy

AOB accessory olfactory bulb; alcohol on breath

AOBS acute organic brain syndrome

AOC abridged ocular chart; amyloxycarbonyl; anodal opening contraction; area of concern

AOCA American Osteopathic College of Anesthesiologists

AOCD American Osteopathic College of Dermatology

AOCl anodal opening clonus

AOCPA American Osteopathic College of Pathologists

AOCPR American Osteopathic College of Proctology

AOCR American Osteopathic College of Radiology; American Osteopathic College of Rheumatology

AOD Academy of Operative Dentistry; Academy of Oral Dynamics; adult onset diabetes; arterial oxygen desaturation; arteriosclerotic occlusive disease; auriculo-osteodysplasia

AODM adult onset diabetes mellitus

AODME Academy of Osteopathic Directors of Medical Education

AODP alcohol and other drug problems

AOHA American Osteopathic Hospital Association

AOIVM angiographically occult intracranial vascular malformation

AOL acro-osteolysis

AOM acute otitis media; alternatives of management; azoxymethane

AOMA American Occupational Medical Association

AOMP, AoMP aortic mean pressure

AOO anodal opening odor; atrial asynchronous (competitive, fixed-rate) [pacemaker]

AOP anodal opening picture; aortic pressure

AOPA American Orthotics and Prosthetics Association

AOPW, AoPW aortic posterior wall

AOR Alvarado Orthopedic Research [instruments]; auditory oculogyric reflex

AOS American Ophthalmological Society; American Otological Society; anodal opening sound; anterior [o]esophageal sensor

AOSSM American Orthopedic Society for Sports Medicine

AOT accessory optic tract; anodal opening tetanus; Association of Occupational Therapists

AOTA American Occupational Therapy Association

AOTe anodal opening tetanus

AOU apparent oxygen utilization

AOV, AoV aortic valve

AP accessory pathway; acid phosphatase; acinar parenchyma; action potential; active pepsin; acute pancreatitis; acute phase; acute pneumonia; acute proliferative; adenomatous polyposis; adolescent psychiatry; alkaline phosphatase; alum precipitated; aminopeptidase; amyloid P-component; angina pectoris; antepartal [Lat. *ante partum*]; anterior pituitary; anteroposterior; antidromic potential; antipyrine; antral peristalsis; aortic pressure; aortopulmonary; apical pulse; apothecary; appendectomy; appendicitis; appendix; apurinic acid; area postrema; arithmetic progression; arterial pressure; artificial pneumothorax; aspiration pneumonia; assessment and plans; association period; atherosclerotic plaque; atrial pacing; atrioventricular pathway; axiopulpal; before dinner [Lat. *ante prandium*]; before parturition [Lat. *ante partum*]

A-P anteroposterior

A/P ascites/plasma [ratio]

A&P anterior and posterior; assessment and plans; auscultation and percussion

Ap apex

ap attachment point; before dinner [Lat. *ante prandium*]

APA action potential amplitude; aldosterone-producing adenoma; American Pancreatic Association; American Pharmaceutic Association; American Physiotherapy Association; American Podiatric Association; American Psychiatric Association; American Psychoanalytic Association; American Psychological Association; American Psychopathological Association; American Psychotherapy Association; aminopenicillanic acid; antipernicious anemia [factor]

APAAP alkaline phosphatase-antialkaline phosphatase [labeling]

APAB antiphospholipid antibody

APACHE Acute Physiology and Chronic Health Evaluation [severity-of-illness index]

APAF antipernicious anemia factor

APAP acetaminophen

APB abductor pollicis brevis; atrial premature beat

APC acetylsalicylic acid, phenacetin, and caffeine; adenoidal-pharyngeal-conjunctival [agent]; adenomatous polyposis coli; all-purpose capsule; antigen-presenting cell; antiphlogistic corticoid; aperture current; apneustic center; aspirin-phenacetin-caffeine; atrial premature contraction

APCC aspirin-phenacetin-caffeine-codeine

APCD acquired prothrombin complex deficiency [syndrome]; adult polycystic kidney disease

APCF acute pharyngoconjunctival fever

APCG apex cardiogram

APCKD adult-type polycystic kidney disease

APD action potential duration; acute polycystic disease; anteroposterior diameter; antipsychotic drug; atrial premature depolarization; autoimmune progesterone dermatitis; automated peritoneal dialysis

A-PD anteroposterior diameter

APDER anterior-posterior dual energy radiography

APDI Adult Personal Data Inventory

APE acetone powder extract; acute polioencephalitis; acute psychotic episode; airway pressure excursion; aminophylline, phenobarbital, and ephedrine; anterior pituitary extract; asthma of physical effort; avian pneumoencephalitis

APECED autoimmune polyendocrinopathy-candidosis-ectodermal dystrophy

APF acidulated phosphofluoride; American Psychological Foundation; anabolism-promoting factor; animal protein factor; antiperinuclear factor

APG acid-precipated globulin; animal pituitary gonadotropin

APGAR American Pediatric Gross Assessment Record

APGL alkaline phosphatase activity of granular leukocytes

APH alcohol-positive history; alternative pathway hemolysis; aminoglycoside phosphotransferase; antepartum hemorrhage; anterior pituitary hormone; Association of Private Hospitals

Aph aphasia

APHA American Protestant Hospital Association; American Public Health Association

APhA American Pharmaceutical Association

APHP anti-Pseudomonas human plasma

API alkaline protease inhibitor; Analytical Profile Index; arterial pressure index; atmospheric pressure ionization; Autonomy Preference Index

APIC Association for Practitioners in Infection Control

APIE assessment, plan, implementation, and evaluation

APIM Association Professionnelle Internationale des Médecins

APIP additional personal injury protection

APIVR artificial pacemaker-induced ventricular rhythm

APKD adult-onset polycystic kidney disease

APL abductor pollicis longus; accelerated painless labor; acute premyelocytic leukemia; animal placenta lactogen; anterior pituitary-like

APLA antiphospholipid antibody

APM Academy of Parapsychology and Medicine; Academy of Physical Medicine; Academy of Psychosomatic Medicine; acid precipitable material; alternating pressure mattress; anteroposterior movement; aspartame; Association of Professors of Medicine

APMR Association for Physical and Mental Retardation

APN acute pyelonephritis; average peak noise

APO abductor pollicis obliguus; acquired pendular oscillation; aphoxide; apolipoprotein; apomorphine; apoprotein

Apo, apo apolipoprotein

apoC apolipoprotein C

APORF acute postoperative renal failure

apoE apolipoprotein E

apoth apothecary

APP acute phase protein; alum-precipitated pyridine; aminopyrazolopyrimidine; amyloid peptide precursor; antiplatelet plasma; aqueous procaine penicillin; automated physiologic profile; avian pancreatic polypeptide

App, app appendix

APPA American Psychopathological Association

appar apparatus

APPG aqueous procaine penicillin G

appl appliance; application, applied

approx approximate

appt appointment

Appx appendix

appy appendectomy

APR abdominoperineal resection; absolute proximal reabsorption; acute phase reactant; amebic prevalence rate; anatomic porous replacement; anterior pituitary reaction

aprax apraxia

APRL American Prosthetic Research Laboratory

AProL acute promyelocytic leukemia

APRP acidic proline-rich protein; acute phase reactant protein

APRT adenine phosphoribosyl transferase

APS adenosine phosphosulfate; American Pediatric Society; American Physiological Society; American Proctologic Society; American Prosthodontic Society; American Psychological Society; American Psychosomatic Society; attending physician's statement; autoimmune polyglandular syndrome; automated patient system

APSAC anisoylated plasminogen streptokinase activator complex

APSD aorticopulmonary septal defect

APSGN acute poststreptococcal glomerulonephritis

APSQ Abbreviated Parent Symptom Questionnaire

APSS Association for the Psychophysiological Study of Sleep

APT alum-precipitated toxoid; aminophenylthioether

APTA American Physical Therapy Association

APTD Aid to Permanently and Totally Disabled

APTT, aPTT activated partial thromboplastin time

APUD amine precursor uptake and decarboxylation

APV abnormal posterior vector

APVC anomalous pulmonary venous connection

APW alkaline peptone water

AQ achievement quotient; any quantity; aphasia quotient

aq aqueous; water [Lat. *aqua*]

aq ad add water [Lat. *aquam ad*]

aq bull boiling water [Lat. *aqua bulliens*]

aq cal hot water [Lat. *aqua calida*]

aq dest distilled water [Lat. *aqua destillata*]

aq ferv hot water [Lat. *aqua fervens*]

aq frig cold water [Lat. *aqua frigata*]

aq pur pure water [Lat. *aqua pura*]

AQS additional qualifying symptoms

aq tep tepid water [Lat. *aqua tepida*]

aqu aqueous

AR achievement ratio; actinic reticuloid [syndrome]; active resistance; adherence ratio; admitting room; airway resistance; alarm reaction; alcohol related; alkali reserve; allergic rhinitis; alloy restoration; amplitude ratio; analytical reagent; androgen receptor; anterior root; aortic regurgitation; apical–radial; Argyll Robertson [pupil]; aromatase; arsphenamine; articulare; artificial respiration; assisted respiration; at risk; atrial rate; atrophic rhinitis; autoradiography; autosomal recessive

Ar argon; articulare

ar aromatic

A/R apical/radial

A&R advised and released

ARA Academy of Rehabilitative Audiometry; acetylene reduction activity; American Rheumatism Association; antireticulin antibody; aortic root angiogram; arabinose; Associate of the Royal Academy

ara arabinose

ara-A adenine arabinoside

ara-C cytosine arabinoside

ARAMIS American Rheumatism Association Medical Information System

ARAS ascending reticular activating system

ara-U arabinosyluracil

ARB adrenergic receptor binder

arb arbitrary unit

ARBD alcohol-related birth defects

ARC accelerating rate calorimetry; acquired immunodeficiency syndrome-related complex; active renin concentration; AIDS-related complex; American Red Cross; anomalous retinal correspondence; antigen reactive cell; arcuate; Arthritis Rehabilitation Center; Association for Retarded Children

ARCA acquired red cell aplasia

ARCI Addiction Research Center Inventory

ARCS Associate of the Royal College of Science

ARD absolute reaction of degeneration; acute radiation disease; acute respiratory disease; adult respiratory distress; allergic respiratory disease; anorectal dressing; arthritis and rheumatic diseases; atopic respiratory disease

ARDS adult respiratory distress syndrome

ARE active-resistive exercises; AIDS-related encephalitis

AREDYLD acrorenal field defect, ectodermal dysplasia, lipoatrophic diabetes [syndrome]

ARES antireticulo-endothelial serum

ARF acute renal failure; acute respiratory failure; acute rheumatic fever; Addiction Research Foundation; area resource file

ARFC active rosette-forming T-cell; autologous rosette-forming cell

ARG, Arg arginine

arg arginine; silver [Lat. *argentum*]

ARI acute respiratory illness; airway reactivity index; anxiety reaction, intense

ARIA automated radioimmunoassay

Ar Kr argon-krypton [laser]

ARL average remaining lifetime

ARLD alcohol related liver disease

ARM adrenergic receptor material; aerosol rebreathing method; anorectal manometry; anxiety reaction, mild; Armenian [hamster]; artificial rupture of membranes; atomic resolution microscopy

ARMS Adverse Reaction Monitoring System

ARN acute renal necrosis; acute retinal necrosis; arcuate nucleus; Association of Rehabilitation Nurses

ARNMD Association for Research in Nervous and Mental Diseases

ARNP Advanced Registered Nurse Practitioner

ARO Associate for Research in Ophthalmology

AROA autosomal recessive ocular albinism

AROM active range of motion; artificial rupture of membranes

arom aromatic

ARP absolute refractory period; American Registry of Pathologists; assay reference plasma; assimilation regulatory protein; at risk period; automaticity recovery phase

ARPES angular resolved photoelectron spectroscopy

ARPKD autosomal recessive polycystic kidney disease

ARPT American Registry of Physical Therapists

ARR aortic root replacement

arr arrest, arrested

ARRC Associate of the Royal Red Cross

ARRS American Roentgen Ray Society

ARRT American Registry of Radiologic Technologists

ARS acquiescence response scale; adult Reye's syndrome; alizarin red S; American Radium Society; American Rhinologic Society; antirabies serum; arsphenamine; arylsulfatase; autonomously replicating sequence

Ars arsphenamine

ARSA American Reye's Syndrome Association

ARSACS autosomal recessive spastic ataxia of Charlevoix-Saguenay

ARSC Associate of the Royal Society of Chemistry

ARSM acute respiratory system malfunction

ARSPH Associate of the Royal Society for the Promotion of Health

ART absolute retention time; Accredited

Record Technician; acoustic reflex test; algebraic reconstruction technique; artery; assisted reproductive technique; automated reagin test; automaticity recovery time

art artery, arterial; articulation; artificial

arth arthritis

artic articulation, articulated

artif artificial

ARV AIDS-associated retrovirus; anterior right ventricle; avian reovirus

AS acetylstrophanthidin; acidified serum; acoustic stimulation; active sarcoidosis; active sleep; Adams-Stokes [disease]; Alport syndrome; alveolar sac; amyloid substance; anal sphincter; androsterone sulfate; Angelman syndrome; ankylosing spondylitis; anovulatory syndrome; antiserum; antisocial; antistreptolysin; antral spasm; anxiety state; aortic sound; aortic stenosis; aqueous solution; aqueous suspension; arteriosclerosis; artificial sweetener; aseptic meningitis; astigmatism; asymmetric; atrial septum; atrial stenosis; atropine sulfate; audiogenic seizure; Auto-Suture; left ear [Lat. *auris sinistra*]

As arsenic; astigmatism; asymptomatic

A(s) asplenia syndrome

A•s ampere second

A x s ampere per second

aS absiemens

as left ear [Lat. *auris sinistra*]

ASA acetylsalicylic acid; active systemic anaphylaxis; Adams-Stokes attack; American Society of Anesthesiologists; American Standards Association; American Surgical Association; antibody to surface antigen; argininosuccinic acid; arylsulfatase-A; aspirin-sensitive asthma

ASAAD American Society for the Advancement of Anesthesia in Dentistry

ASAC acidified serum-acidified complement

ASAH antibiotic sterilized aortic valve homograft

ASAHP American Society of Allied Health Professions

ASAIO American Society for Artificial Internal Organs

ASAP American Society for Adolescent Psychology; as soon as possible

ASAS argininosuccinate synthetase

ASAT aspartate aminotransferase

ASB American Society of Bacteriologists; anencephaly spina bifida [syndrome]; anesthesia standby; Anxiety Scale for the Blind; asymptomatic bacteriuria

ASBV avocado sunblotch viroid

ASC acetylsulfanilyl chloride; altered state of consciousness; ambulatory surgical center; American Society of Cytology; antigen-sensitive cell; ascorbate, ascorbic acid; asthma symptom checklist

asc ascending; anterior subcapsular

ASCAD atherosclerotic coronary artery disease

ASCAo ascending aorta

ASCH American Society of Clinical Hypnosis

ASCI American Society for Clinical Investigation

ASCII American Standard Code for Information Interchange

ASCLT American Society of Clinical Laboratory Technicians

ASCMS American Society of Contemporary Medicine and Surgery

ASCO American Society of Clinical Oncology; American Society of Contemporary Ophthalmology

ASCP American Society of Clinical Pathologists; American Society of Consulting Pharmacists

ASCR American Society of Chiropodical Roentgenology

ascr ascribed to [Lat. *ascriptum*]

ASCT autologous stem cell transplantation

ASCVD arteriosclerotic cardiovascular disease; atherosclerotic cardiovascular disease

ASD aldosterone secretion defect; Alzheimer senile dementia; antisiphon device; arthritis syphilitica deformans; arthroscopic subacromial decompression; atrial septal defect

ASDC American Society of Dentistry for Children; Association of Sleep Disorders Centers

ASDH acute subdural hematoma

ASE acute stress erosion; axilla, shoulder, and elbow

ASF African swine fever; aniline-sulfur-formaldehyde [resin]

ASFR age-specific fertility rate

ASG American Society for Genetics; Army Surgeon General; advanced cell group

ASGBI Association of Surgeons of Great Britain and Ireland

ASGE American Society for Gastrointestinal Endoscopy

AS/GP antiserum, guinea pig

ASH aldosterone-stimulating hormone; American Society of Hematology; alkylosing spinal hyperostosis; antistreptococcal hyaluronidase; asymmetric septal hypertrophy

AsH astigmatism, hypermetropic

A&Sh arm and shoulder

ASHA American School Health Association; American Social Health Association; American Speech and Hearing Association

ASHBM Associate Scottish Hospital Bureau of Management

ASHCVD atherosclerotic hypertensive cardiovascular disease

ASHD arteriosclerotic heart disease; atrioseptal heart disease

ASHET American Society for Health Manpower Education and Training

ASHG American Society for Human Genetics

ASHI Association for the Study of Human Infertility

ASHN acute sclerosing hyaline necrosis

AS/Ho antiserum, horse

ASHP American Society of Hospital Pharmacists; American Society for Hospital Planning

ASHPA American Society for Hospital Personnel Administration

ASHT American Society of Hand Therapists

ASI addiction severity index; anxiety status inventory; arthroscopic screw installation

ASII American Science Information Institute

ASIM American Society of Internal Medicine

ASIS anterior superior iliac spine

ASK antistreptokinase

ASL antistreptolysin; argininosuccinate lyase

ASLIB Association of Special Libraries and Information Bureau

ASLM American Society of Law and Medicine

ASLO antistreptolysin O

ASLT antistreptolysin test

ASM airway smooth muscle; American Society for Microbiology; anterior scalenus muscle

AsM astigmatism, myopic

ASMA antismooth muscle antibody

ASMC arterial smooth muscle cell

ASMD atonic sclerotic muscle dystrophy

ASME Association for the Study of Medical Education

ASMI anteroseptal myocardial infarct

As/Mk antiserum, monkey

ASMPA Armed Services Medical Procurement Agency

ASMR age-standardized mortality ratio

ASMT American Society for Medical Technology

ASN alkali-soluble nitrogen; American Society of Nephrology; American Society of Neurochemistry; arteriosclerotic nephritis; asparagine; Associate in Nursing

Asn asparagine

ASO allele-specific oligonucleoside; antistreptolysin O; arteriosclerosis obliterans

ASOS American Society of Oral Surgeons

ASOT antistreptolysin-O test

ASP abnormal spinal posture; acute symmetric polyarthritis; African swine pox; aged substrate plasma; alkali-stable pepsin; American Society of Parasitology; ankylosing spondylitis; anorectal malformation, sacral bony abnormality, presacral mass [association]; antisocial personality; aortic systolic pressure; area systolic pressure; asparaginase; aspartic acid

Asp aspartic acid; asparaginase

asp aspartate, aspartic acid; aspiration

ASPA American Society of Physician Analysts; American Society of Podiatric Assistants

ASPAT antistreptococcal polysaccharide test

ASPDM American Society of Psychosomatic Dentistry and Medicine

ASPG antispleen globulin

ASPM American Society of Paramedics

ASPO American Society for Psychoprophylaxis in Obstetrics

ASPP Association for Sane Psychiatric Practices

ASPRS American Society of Plastic and Reconstructive Surgeons

ASPS advanced sleep phase syndrome

ASPVD atherosclerotic peripheral vascular disease

ASQ Abbreviated Symptom Questionnaire; Anxiety Scale Questionnaire

ASR aldosterone secretion rate; antistreptolysin reaction

AS/Rab antiserum, rabbit

ASRT American Society of Radiologic Technologists

ASS acute serum sickness; acute spinal stenosis; anterior superior spine

ASSA, ASSAS aminopterin-like syndrome sine aminopterin

ASSC acute splenic sequestration crisis

ASSH American Society for Surgery of the Hand

ASSI Accurate Surgical and Scientific Instruments

ASSIM assiimilate, assimilation

ASSO American Society for the Study of Orthodontics

Assoc association, associate

ASSR adult situation stress reaction

AST allergy serum transfer; angiotensin sensitivity test; anterior spinothalamic tract; antistreptolysin test; aspartate aminotransferase (SGOT); Association of Medical Technologists; astigmatism; atrial overdrive stimulation rate; audiometry sweep test

Ast astigmatism

ASTA anti-alpha-staphylolysin

ASTH, Asth asthenopia

ASTHO Association of State and Territorial Health Officers

ASTI antispasticity index

ASTM American Society for Testing and Materials

ASTMH American Society of Tropical Medicine and Hygiene

ASTO antistreptolysin O

as tol as tolerated

ASTZ antistreptozyme

ASV anodic stripping voltammetry; antisiphon valve; antisnake venom; avian sarcoma virus

ASVO American Society of Veterinary Ophthalmology

ASVPP American Society of Veterinary Physiologists and Pharmacologists

ASW artificial sweetener

Asx amino acid that gives aspartic acid after hydrolysis; asymptomatic

asym asymmetry, asymmetric

AT achievement test; Achilles tendon; Achard-Thiers [syndrome]; adaptive thermogenesis; adenine-thyronine; adipose tissue; adjunctive therapy; air temperature; allergy treatment; aminotransferase; amitriptyline; anaerobic threshold; anaphylotoxin; anterior tibia; antithrombin; antitrypsin; antral transplantation; applanation tonometry; ataxia–telangiectasia; atmosphere; atraumatic; atresia, tricuspid; atrial tachycardia; atropine; attenuate, attenuation; axonal terminal; old tuberculin [Gr. *alt Tuberkulin*]

A-T ataxia telangiectasia

AT₁₀ dihydrotachysterol

AT I angiotensin I

AT II angiotensin II

AT III angiotensin III; antithrombin III

At acidity, total; astatine; atrium, atrial

at tight; atom, atomic

ATA alimentary toxic aleukia; American Thyroid Association; aminotriazole; antithymic activity; antithyroglobulin antibody; anti-Toxoplasma antibody; atmosphere absolute; aurintricarboxylic acid

ATB at the time of the bomb [A-bomb in Japan]; atrial tachycardia with block

ATC activated thymus cell; around the clock

ATCC American Type Culture Collection

ATCS anterior tibial compartment syndrome

ATD Alzheimer-type dementia; androstatrienedione; anthropomorphic test dummy; antithyroid drug; aqueous tear deficiency; asphyxiating thoracic dystrophy

ATDC Association of Thalidomide Damaged Children

ATE acute toxic encephalopathy; adipose tissue extract; autologous tumor extract

ATEE N-acetyl-1-tyrosyl-ethyl ester

ATEM analytic transmission electron microscopy

Aten atenolol

ATF ascites tumor fluid

At fib atrial fibrillation

ATG adenine-thymidine-guanine anti-human thymocyte globulin; antithrombocyte globulin; antithymocyte globulin; antithyroglobulin

ATGAM antithymocyte gamma-globulin

AT/GC adenine-thymine/guanine-cytosine [ratio]

ATH acetyl-tyrosine hydrazide

ATh Associate in Therapy

Athsc atherosclerosis

ATI abdominal trauma index

ATL Achilles tendon lengthening; adult T-cell leukemia; anterior tricuspid leaflet; antitension line; atypical lymphocyte

ATLA adult T-cell leukemia virus-associated antigen

ATLL adult T-cell leukemia/lymphoma

ATLS acute tumor lysis syndrome; Advanced Trauma Life Support Program

ATLV adult T-cell leukemia virus

ATM abnormal tubular myelin; acute transverse myelopathy; atmosphere

atm standard atmosphere

ATMA antithyroid plasma membrane antibody

atmos atmospheric

ATN acute tubular necrosis; augmented transition network

ATNC atraumatic normocephalic

at no atomic number

ATNR asymmetric tonic neck reflex

ATP adenosine triphosphate; ambient temperature and pressure; autoimmune thrombocytopenic purpura

A-TP adsorbed test plasma

AT-P antitrypsin-Pittsburgh

AtP attending physician

AT-PAS aldehyde-thionine-periodic acid Schiff [test]

ATPase adenosine triphosphatase

ATPD dried at ambient temperature and pressure

ATP-2Na adenosine triphosphate disodium

ATPS ambient temperature and pressure, saturated

ATR Achilles tendon reflex

atr atrophy

Atr fib atrial fibrillation

ATS Achard-Thiers syndrome; acid test solution; alpha-D-tocopherol acid succinate; American Thoracic Society; American Trudeau Society; American Trauma Society; antirat thymocyte serum;

antitetanus serum; antithymocyte serum; anxiety tension state; arteriosclerosis

ATSDR Agency for Toxic Substances and Disease Registry

ATT arginine tolerance test; aspirin tolerance time

att attending

ATV Abelson virus transformed; avian tumor virus

at vol atomic volume

at wt atomic weight

ATx adult thymectomy

atyp atypical

ATZ atypical transformation zone

AU according to custom [Lat. *ad usum*]; allergenic unit; Ångström unit; antitoxin unit; arbitrary unit; Australia antigen; azauridine; both ears together [Lat. *aures unitas*]; each ear [Lat. *auris uterque*]

Au Australia [antigen]; gold [Lat. *aurum*]

AUA American Urological Association

Au Ag Australia antigen

AUB abnormal uterine bleeding

AUC area under the curve

AUD arthritis of unknown diagnosis

aud auditory

aud-vis audiovisual

AUG acute ulcerative gingivitis; adenosine-uracil-guanine

Aug increase [Lat. *augere*]

AUGH acute upper gastrointestinal hemorrhage

AuHAA Australia hepatitis-associated antigen

AUI Alcohol Use Inventory

AUL acute undifferentiated leukemia

AUO amyloid of unknown origin

AuP Australian antigen protein

AUPHA Association of University Programs in Health Administration

aur, auric auricle, auricular

AUS acute urethral syndrome

AuS Australia serum hepatitis

aus, ausc auscultation

AuSH Australia serum hepatitis

Auto-PEEP self-controlled positive end-expiratory pressure

aux auxiliary

AV Adriamycin and vincristine; air velocity; allergic vasculitis; anteroventral; anteversion; anticipatory vomiting; antivirin; aortic valve; arteriovenous; artificial ventilation; assisted ventilation; atrioventricular; audiovisual; augmented vector; average; aviation medicine; avoirdupois

A-V arteriovenous; atrioventricular

A/V ampere/volt; arteriovenous

Av average; avoirdupois

aV abvolt

av air velocity; average; avulsion

AVA activity vector analysis; antiviral antibody; aortic valve atresia; arteriovenous anastomosis

AV/AF anteverted, anteflexed

AVB atrioventricular block

AVC aberrant ventricular conduction; Academy of Veterinary Cardiology; associative visual cortex; Association of Vitamin Chemists; associative visual cortex; atrioventricular canal; automatic volume control

AVCS atrioventricular conduction system

AVD aortic valvular disease; apparent volume of distribution; atrioventricular dissociation; Army Veterinary Department

AVDO$_2$ arteriovenous oxygen saturation difference

AVDP average diastolic pressure

avdp avoirdupois

AVE aortic valve echocardiogram

ave, aver average

AVF antiviral factor; arteriovenous fistula

aV$_F$ unipolar limb lead on the left leg in electrocardiography

avg average

AVH acute viral hepatitis

AVHS acquired valvular heart disease

AVI air velocity index; Association of Veterinary Inspectors

AVJ atrioventricular junction

AVJR atrioventricular junction rhythm

AVJRe atrioventricular junctional reentrant

aV$_L$ unipolar limb lead on the left arm in electrocardiography

AVLINE Audiovisuals On-Line [data base]

AVM arteriovenous malformation; atrioventricular malformation; aviation medicine

AVMA American Veterinary Medical Association

AVN acute vasomotor nephropathy; atrioventricular nodal [conduction]; atrioventricular node

AVND atrioventricular node dysfunction

AVNFH avascular necrosis of the femoral head

AVNFRP atrioventricular node functional refractory period

AVNR atrioventricular nodal reentry

AVO atrioventricular opening

AVP abnormal vasopressin; actinomycin-vincristine-Platinol; ambulatory venous pressure; antiviral protein; aqueous vasopressin; arginine vasopressin; arteriovenous passage time

AVR accelerated ventricular rhythm; antiviral regulator; aortic valve replacement

aV$_R$ unipolar limb lead on the right arm in electrocardiography

AVRI acute viral respiratory infection

AVRP atrioventricular refractory period

AVRT atrioventricular reentrant tachycardia; atrioventricular reciprocating tachycardia

AVS aortic valve stenosis; arteriovenous shunt; auditory vocal sequencing

AVSD atrioventricular septal defect

AVSV aortic valve stroke volume

AVT Allen vision test; arginine vasotocin; Aviation Medicine Technician

Av3V anteroventral third ventricle

AVZ avascular zone

AW able to work; above waist; abrupt withdrawal; alcohol withdrawal; alveolar wall; anterior wall; atomic warfare; atomic weight

A&W alive and well

aw airway; water activity

AWBM alveolar wall basement membrane

AWG American Wire Gauge

AWI anterior wall infarction

AWMI anterior wall myocardial infarction

AWP airway pressure; average of the wholesale prices

AWRS anti-whole rabbit serum

AWRU active wrist rotation unit

AWS alcohol withdrawal syndrome

AWTA aniridia-Wilms' tumor association

awu atomic weight unit

ax axillary; axis, axial

AXF advanced x-ray facility

AXG adult xanthogranuloma

AXL axillary lymphoscintigraphy

AXT alternating exotropia

A^y yellow [mouse]

AYA acute yellow atrophy

AYF antiyeast factor

AYP autolyzed yeast protein

AYV aster yellow virus

AZ Aschheim-Zondek [test]

Az nitrogen [Fr. *azote*]

AZA azathioprine

AzC azacytosine

AzG; azg azaguanine

AZO [indicates presence of the group] –N:N–

AZQ diaziquone

AZR alizarin

AZT Aschheim-Zondek test; azidothymidine; 3'-azido-3'-deoxythymidine; zidovudine (azidothymidine)

AZT-TP 3'azido-3'-deoxythymidine triphosphate

AZU azauracil

AzUr 6-azauridine

B

B bacillus; bands; barometric; base; basophil, basophilic; bath [Lat. *balneum*]; Baumé scale; behavior; bel; Benoist scale; benzoate; beta; biscuspid; black; blood, bloody; blue; body; boils at; Bolton point; bone marrow-derived [cell or lymphocyte]; boron; bound; bovine; break; bregma; bronchial, bronchus; brother; *Brucella*; bruit; buccal; Bucky [film in cassette in Potter-Bucky diaphragm]; bursa cells; bypass; magnetic induction; supramentale [point]

b barn; base; boils at; born; brain; supramentale [point]; twice [Lat. *bis*]

B_0 constant magnetic field in nuclear magnetic resonance

B_1 radiofrequency magnetic field in nuclear magnetic resonance; thiamine

B_2 riboflavin

B_6 pyridoxine

B_7 biotin

B_8 adenosine phosphate

B_{12} cyanocobalamin

β see beta

BA Bachelor of Arts; backache; bacterial agglutination; basilar artery; basion; benzyladenine; best amplitude; betamethasone acetate; bilateral asymmetrical; bile acid; biliary atresia; biological activity; blocking antibody; blood agar; blood alcohol; bone age; boric acid; bovine albumin; brachial artery; breathing apparatus; bronchial asthma; buccoaxial; buffered acetone; sand bath [Lat. *balneum arenae*]

Ba barium; barium enema; basion

ba basion

BAA benzoylarginine amide; branched amino acid

BAB blood agar base

Bab Babinski's reflex; baboon

BabK baboon kidney

BAC bacterial adherent colony; bacterial antigen complex; blood alcohol concentration; British Association of Chemists; bronchoalveolar cells; buccoaxiocervical

Bac, bac *Bacillus*, bacillary

Bact, bact *Bacterium;* bacterium, bacteria

BAD biological aerosol detection; British Association of Dermatologists

BAE bovine aortic endothelium; bronchial artery embolization

BaE barium enema

BAEC bovine arotic endothelial cells

BAEE benzoylarginine ethyl ester

BaEn barium enema

BAEP brainstem auditory evoked potential

BAER brainstem auditory evoked response

BAG buccoaxiogingival

BAGG buffered azide glucose glycerol

BAHS butoctamide hydrogen succinate

BAI basilar artery insufficiency; beta-aminoisobutyrate

BAIB beta-aminoisobutyric [acid]

BAIF bile acid independent flow

BAIT bacterial automated identification technique

BAL blood alcohol level; British anti-lewisite; bronchoalveolar lavage

bal balance; balsam; bath [Lat. *balneum*]

bal aren sand bath [Lat. *balneum arenae*]

BALB binaural alternate loudness balance

BALF bronchoalveolar lavage fluid

bals balsam

BALT bronchus-associated lymphoid tissue

bal vap steam bath [Lat. *balneum vaporis*]

BAM basilar artery migraine; brachial artery mean [pressure]

BaM barium meal

Bam benzamide

BAME benzoylarginine methyl ester

BAN British Approved Name; British Association of Neurologists

BANS back, arms, neck, and scalp

BAO basal acid output; brachial artery output

BAO-MAO basal acid output to maximal acid output [ratio]

BAP bacterial alkaline phosphatase; Behavior Activity Profile; beta-amyloid peptide; blood-agar plate; bovine albumin in phosphate buffer; brachial artery pressure

BAPhysMed British Association of Physical Medicine

BAPI barley alkaline protease inhibitor

BAPN beta-aminoproprionitrile fumarate

BAPS biomechanical ankle platform system; bovine albumin phosphate saline; British Association of Paediatric Surgeons; British Association of Plastic Surgeons

BAPT British Association of Physical Training

BAPV bovine alimentary papilloma virus

BAQ brain-age quotient

BAR bariatrics; barometer, barometric; beta-adrenergic receptor

bar barometric

Barb, barb barbiturate, barbituric

BARN bilateral acute retinal necrosis

BART blood-activated recalcification time

BAS balloon atrial septostomy; benzyl anti-serotinin; beta-adrenergic stimulation; boric acid solution

BaS barium swallow

bas basilar; basophil, basophilic

BASA Boston Assessment of Severe Aphasia

BASE B27–arthritis–sacroiliitis–extra-articular features [syndrome]

BASH body acceleration synchronous with heart rate

BASIC Beginner's All-Purpose Symbolic Introduction Code

baso basophil

BAT basic aid training; best available technology; brown adipose tissue

BAUS British Association of Urological Surgeons

BAV bicuspid aortic valve

BAVCP bilateral abductor vocal cord paralysis

BAVFO bradycardia after arteriovenous fistula occlusion

BAW bronchoalveolar washing

BB bad breath; bed bath; beta blockade, beta blocker; BioBreeding [rat]; blanket bath; blood bank; blood buffer; blow bottle; blue bloaters [emphysema]; both bones; breakthrough bleeding; breast biopsy; brush border; buffer base; bundle branch; isoenzyme of creatine kinase containing two B subunits

bb Bolton point; both bones

BBA born before arrival

BBB blood-brain barrier; blood buffer base; bundle-branch block

BBBB bilateral bundle-branch block

BBC bromobenzycyanide

BBD benign breast disease

BBE *Bacteroides* bile esculin [agar]

BBEP brush border endopeptidase

BBF bronchial blood flow

BBI Bowman-Birk soybean inhibitor

BBM brush border membrane

BBMV brush border membrane vesicle

BBN broad band noise

BBRS Burks' Behavior Rating Scale

BBS Barolet-Biedl syndrome; bashful bladder syndrome; benign breast syndrome; bilateral breath sounds; bombesin; brown bowel syndrome

BBT basal body temperature

BB/W BioBreeding/Worcester [rat]

BC Bachelor of Surgery [Lat. *Baccalaureus Chirurgiae*]; back care; bactericidal concentration; basal cell; basket cell; battle casualty; bicarbonate; biliary colic; bipolar cell; birth control; blastic crisis; blood count; blood culture; Blue Cross [plan]; board certified; bone conduction; brachiocephalic; bronchial carcinoma; buccal cartilage; buccocervical; buffy coat

B&C biopsy and curettage

b/c benefit/cost [ratio]

BCA balloon catheter angioplasty; blood color analyzer; Blue Cross Association; branchial cleft anomaly; breast cancer antigen

BCAA branched chain-enriched amino acid

BCAT brachiocephalic arterial trunk

BCB blood–cerebrospinal fluid barrier; brilliant cresyl blue

BCBR bilateral carotid body resection

BC/BS Blue Cross/Blue Shield [plan]

BCC basal-cell carcinoma; biliary cholesterol concentration; birth control clinic

bcc body-centered-cubic

BCCG British Cooperative Clinical Group

BCCP biotin carboxyl carrier protein

BCD binary-coded decimal; bleomycin, cyclophosphamide, dactinomycin

BCDDP Breast Cancer Detection Demonstration Project

BCDF B-cell differentiation factor

BCDL Brachmann-Cornelia de Lange [syndrome]

BCE basal cell epithelioma; benign childhood epilepsy; bubble chamber equipment

BCF basophil chemotactic factor; bioconcentration factor; breast cyst fluid

BCFP breast cyst fluid protein

BCG bacille Calmette-Guérin [vaccine]; ballistocardiography, ballistocardiogram; bicolor guaiac test; bromcresol green

BCGF B-cell growth factor

BCH basal cell hyperplasia

BCh Bachelor of Surgery [Lat. *Baccalaureus Chirurgiae*]

BChD Bachelor of Dental Surgery

BChir Bachelor of Surgery [Lat. *Baccalaureus Chirurgiae*]

Bchl, bChl bacterial chlorophyll

BCHS Bureau of Community Health Services

BCKA branched-chain keto acid

BCKD branched-chain alpha-keto acid dehydrogenase

BCL basic cycle length

BCLL B-cell chronic lymphocytic leukemia

BCLP bilateral cleft of lip and palate

BCLS basic cardiac life support

BCM birth control medication; blood-clotting mechanism effects; body cell mass

BCME bis-chloromethyl ether

BCN basal cell nevus; bilateral cortical necrosis

BCNS basal cell nevus syndrome

BCNU 1,3-bis-(2-chloroethyl)-1-nitrosourea

BCO biliary cholesterol output

BCP basic calcium phosphate; birth control pill; Blue Cross Plan; bromcresol purple

BCPD bromcresol purple deoxylate

BCPV bovine cutaneous papilloma virus

BCR B-cell reactivity; birth control regimen; bromocriptine

BCRx birth control drug

BCS battered child syndrome; blood cell separator; British Cardiac Society; Budd-Chiari syndrome

BCSI breast cancer screening indicator

BCT brachiocephalic trunk; branched-chain amino acid transferase

BCTF Breast Cancer Task Force

BCtg bovine chymotrypsinogen

BCtr bovine chymotrypsin

BCW biological and chemical warfare

BCYE buffered charcoal-yeast extract [agar]

BD barbital-dependent; barbiturate dependence; base deficit; base of prism down; basophilic degeneration; Batten's disease; behavioral disorder; Behçet's disease; belladonna; bicarbonate dialysis; bile duct; binocular deprivation; birth date; black death; block design [test]; blood donor; blue diaper [syndrome]; borderline dull; bound; brain damage; brain dead, brain death; Briquet disorder; bronchodilation, bronchodilator; buccodistal; Byler's disease

B-D Becton-Dickinson

Bd board; buoyant density

bd band; bundle; twice a day [Lat. *bis die*]

BDA balloon dilation angioplasty; British Dental Association

BDAC Bureau of Drug Abuse Control

BDAE Boston Diagnostic Aphasia Examination

BDC Bazex-Dupré-Christol [syndrome]; burn-dressing change

BDE bile duct examination

BDentSci Bachelor of Dental Science

BDG buccal developmental groove; buffered desoxycholate glucose

BDI Beck Depression Inventory

BDL below detectable limits; bile duct ligation

BDLS Brachmann-de Lange syndrome

BDM Becker's muscular dystrophy

BDP benzodiazepine; bilateral diaphragmatic paralysis; bronchopulmonary dysplasia

BDR background diabetic retinopathy

BDS Bachelor of Dental Surgery; biological detection system; Blessed Dementia Scale

bds to be taken twice a day [Lat. *bid in die summendus*]

BDSc Bachelor of Dental Science

BDUR bromodeoxyuridine

BDW buffered distilled water

BE bacillary emulsion; bacterial endocarditis; barium enema; Barrett's esophagus; base excess; below-elbow; bile-esculin [test]; bovine enteritis; brain edema; bread equivalent; breast examination; bronchoesophagology

B/E below-elbow

B&E brisk and equal

Be beryllium

Bé Baumé scale

BEA below-elbow amputation; bioelectrical activity; bromoethylamine

BEAM brain electrical activity monitoring

BEAP bronchiectasis, eosinophilia, asthma, pneumonia

BEAR biological effects of atomic radiation

BEC bacterial endocarditis; blood ethyl alcohol; bromo-ergocryptine

BECF blood extracellular fluid

BEE basal energy expenditure

beg begin, beginning

beh behavior, behavioral

BEI back-scattered electron imaging; Biological Exposure Indexes; butanol-extractable iodine

BEIR biological effects of ionizing radiation

BEK bovine embryonic kidney [cells]

BEL blood ethanol level; bovine embryonic lung

BELIR beta-endorphin-like immunoreactivity

ben well [Lat. *bene*]

BENAR blood eosinophilic non-allergic rhinitis

Benz, benz benzene; benzidine; benzoate

BEP brain evoked potential; basic element of performance

B-EP β-endorphin

BER basic electrical rhythm

BERA brainstem evoked response audiometry

BES balanced electrolyte solution

BESM bovine embryonic skeletal muscle

BESP bovine embryonic spleen [cells]

BET benign epithelial tumor; bleeding esophageal varix; Brunauer-Emmet-Teller [method]

β [Greek letter beta] an anomer of a carbohydrate; buffer capacity; carbon separated from a carboxyl by one other carbon in aliphatic compounds; a constituent of a plasma protein fraction; probability of Type II error; a substituent group of a steroid that projects above the plane of the ring

1 − β power of statistical test

β₂m beta₂-microglobulin

BEV baboon endogenous virus

BeV, Bev billion electron volts

bev beverage

BF bentonite flocculation; bile flow; black

female; blastogenic factor; blister fluid; blood flow; body fat; bouillon filtrate [tuberculin] [Fr. *bouillon filtré*]; breakfast fed; breast feeding; buffered; burning feet [syndrome]; butter fat

bf bouillon filtrate [tuberculin]

B3F band 3 cytoplasmic fragment

B/F black female; bound/free [antigen ratio]

BFB biological feedback; bronchial foreign body

BFDI bronchodilation following deep inspiration

BFEC benign focal epilepsy of childhood

BFC benign febrile convulsion

BFE blood flow energy

BFH benign familial hematuria

BFL bird fancier's lung; Börjeson-Forssman-Lehman [syndrome]

BFLS Börjeson-Forssman-Lehmann syndrome

BFO balanced forearm orthosis; ball-bearing forearm orthosis; blood-forming organ

BFP biologic false-positive

BFPR biologic false-positive reaction

BFPSTS biologic false-positive serological test for syphilis

BFR biologic false reaction; blood flow rate; bone formation rate; buffered Ringer [solution]

BFS blood fasting sugar

BFT bentonite flocculation test; biofeedback training

BFU burst-forming unit

BFU-E burst-forming unit, erythroid

BFU-ME burst-forming unit, myeloid/erythroid

BFV bovine feces virus

BG basal ganglion; basic gastrin; Bender Gestalt [test]; beta-galactosidase; beta-glucuronidase; bicolor guaiac [test]; Birbeck granule; blood glucose; bone graft; brilliant green; buccogingival

B-G Bordet-Gengou [agar, bacillus, phenomenon]

BGA blue-green algae

BGAg blood group antigen

BGAV blue-green algae virus

BGC basal ganglion calcification; blood group class

BGCA bronchogenic carcinoma

BGD blood group degradation

BGE butyl glycidyl ether

BGG bovine gamma-globulin

bGH bovine growth hormone

Bg^J beige [mouse]

BGLB brilliant green lactose broth

BGlu blood glucose

BGMV bean golden mosaic virus

BGP beta-glycerophosphatase

BGS balance, gait, and station; blood group substance; British Geriatrics Society

BGSA blood granulocyte-specific activity

BGTT borderline glucose tolerance test

BH base hospital; benzalkonium and heparin; bill of health; birth history; Bishop-Harman [instruments]; board of health; Bolton-Hunter [reagent]; borderline hypertensive; both hands; brain hormone; breathholding; bronchial hyperreactivity; Bryan high titer; bundle of His

BH$_4$ tetrahydrobiopterin

BHA bound hepatitis antibody; butylated hydroxyanisole

BHAT Beta Blocker Heart Attack Trial

BHB beta-hydroxybutyrate

bHb bovine hemoglobin

BHBA beta-hydroxybutyric acid

BHC benzene hexachloride

BHCDA Bureau of Health Care Delivery and Assistance

BHF Bolivian hemorrhagic fever

BHI biosynthetic human insulin; brain-heart infusion [broth]; British Humanities Index; Bureau of Health Insurance

BHIA brain-heart infusion agar

BHI-ac brain-heart infusion broth with acetone

BHIB brain-heart infusion broth

BHIBA brain-heart infusion blood agar

BHIRS brain-heart infusion and rabbit serum

BHIS beef heart infusion supplemented [broth]

BHK baby hamster kidney [cells]; type-B Hong Kong [influenza virus]

BHL bilateral hilar lymphadenopathy; biological half-life

BHM Bureau of Health Manpower

BHN bephenium hydroxynaphthoate; Brinell hardness number

BHP basic health profile

BHR basal heart rate; benign hypertrophic prostatitis

BHS Bachelor of Health Science; beta-hemolytic streptococcus; breathholding spell

BHT beta-hydroxytheophylline; breath hydrogen test; butylated hydroxytoluene

BHU basic health unit

BHV bovine herpes virus

BH/VH body hematocrit-venous hematocrit [ratio]

BHyg Bachelor of Hygiene

BI background interval; bacterial or bactericidal index; base-in [prism]; basilar impression; Billroth I [operation]; biological indicator; bodily injury; bone injury; bowel impaction; brain injury; burn index

Bi bismuth

BIA biolectric impedance analysis; bioimmunoassay

BIAC Bioinstrumentation Advisory Council

BIB biliointestinal bypass; brought in by

bib drink [Lat. *bibe*]

biblio bibliography

BIBRA British Industrial Biological Research Association

B-IBS B-immunoblastic sarcoma

BIC blood isotope clearance

Bic biceps

BICAO bilateral internal carotid artery occlusion

bicarb bicarbonate

BID bibliographic information and documentation; brought in dead

bid twice a day [Lat. *bis in die*]

BIDLB block in posteroinferior division of left branch

BIDS brittle hair, intellectual impairment, decreased fertility, and short stature [syndrome]

BIG 6 analysis of 6 serum components

BIGGY bismuth glycine glucose yeast

BIH benign intracranial hypertension

bihor during two hours [Lat. *bihorium*]

BII Billroth II [operation]; butanol-insoluble iodine

BIL basal insulin level; bilirubin

Bil bilirubin

bil bilateral

BIL/ALB bilirubin/albumin [rate]

bilat bilateral

bili bilirubin

bili-c conjugated bilirubin

bilirub bilirubin

BIMA bilateral internal mammary artery

bin twice a night [Lat. *bis in noctus*]

biochem biochemistry, biochemical

BIOD bony intraorbital distance

bioeng bioengineering

BIOETHICSLINE Bioethical Information On-Line

biol biology, biological

bioLH biossay of luteinizing hormone

biophys biophysics, biophysical

BIOSIS BioScience Information Service

BIP bacterial intravenous protein; biparietal; bismuth iodoform paraffin; Blue Cross interim payment; brief infertility period

BIPLED bilateral, independent, periodic, lateralized epileptiform discharge

BIPM International Bureau of Weights and Measures [Fr. *Bureau International des Poids et Mesures*]

BIPP bismuth iodoform paraffin paste

BIR basic incidence rate; British Institute of Radiology

BIS bone cement implantation syndrome; Brain Information Service; building illness syndrome

bis twice [Lat.]

BiSP between ischial spines

bisp bispinous diameter

BIT bitrochanteric
BIU barrier isolation unit
BJ Bence Jones [protein, proteinuria]; biceps jerk; Bielschowsky-Jansky [syndrome]; bones and joints
B&J bones and joints
BJE bones, joints, and examination
BJM bones, joints, and muscles
BJP Bence Jones protein or proteinuria
BK below the knee; bovine kidney [cells]; bradykinin
B-K initials of two patients after whom a multiple cutaneous nevus [mole] was named
Bk berkelium
bk back
BKA below-knee amputation
BK-A basophil kallikrein of anaphylaxis
BK amp below-knee amputation
bkf breakfast
BKS beekeeper serum
BKTT below knee to toe
BKWP below knee walking plaster
BL Barré-Lieou [syndrome]; basal lamina; baseline; Bessey-Lowry [unit]; black light; bleeding; blind loop; blood loss; bone marrow lymphocyte; bronchial lavage; buccolingual; Burkitt's lymphoma
Bl black
B-l bursa-equivalent lymphocyte
bl bath [Lat. *balneum*]; black; blood, bleeding; blue
BLAD borderline left axis deviation
blad bladder
BLAT Blind Learning Aptitute Test
BLB Baker-Lima-Baker [mask]; Bessey-Lowry-Brock [method or unit]; black light bulb; Boothby-Lovelace-Bulbulian [oxygen mask]; bulb [syringe]
BL = BS bilateral equal breath sounds
BlC blood culture
BLCL Burkitt's lymphoma cell line
bl cult blood culture
BLD basal liquefactive degeneration; benign lymphoepithelial disease
bld blood
BLE both lower extremities
BLEL benign lympho-epithelial lesion

BLEO bleomycin
bleph blepharitis
BLFD buccolinguofacial dyskinesia
BLG beta-lactoglobulin
blH biologically active luteinizing hormone
BLI bombesin-like immunoreactivity
blk black
BLL below lower limit
BLLD British Library Lending Division
BLM bilayer lipid membrane; bimolecular liquid membrane; bleomycin; buccolinguomasticatory
BLN bronchial lymph node
BLOBS bladder obstruction
BLOT British Library of Tape
BLP beta-lipoprotein
BlP blood pressure
B-LPH beta-lipoprotein hormone
B-LPN beta-lipotropin
bl pr blood pressure
BLQ both lower quadrants
BLROA British Laryngological, Rhinological, and Otological Association
BLS bare lymphocyte syndrome; basic life support; blind loop syndrome; blood and lymphatic system; blood sugar; Bloom syndrome; Bureau of Labor Statistics
BlS blood sugar
BLSD bovine lumpy skin disease
BLT bleeding time; blood-clot lysis time; blood test
BlT bleeding time; blood test; blood type, blood typing
BLU Bessey-Lowry unit
BLV blood volume; bovine leukemia virus
BlV blood viscosity; blood volume
BLVR biliverdin reductase
Blx bleeding time
BM Bachelor of Medicine; basal medium; basal metabolism; basement membrane; basilar membrane; betamethasone; biomedical; black male; body mass; Bohr magneton; bone marrow; bowel movement; breast milk; buccal mass; buccomesial
B/M black male
bm salt-water bath [Lat. *balneum maris*]

B2M beta-2-microglobulin

BMA bone marrow arrest; British Medical Association

BmA Brugia malayi adult antigen

BMAP bone marrow acid phosphatase

BMB biomedical belt; bone marrow biopsy

BMBL benign monoclonal B cell lymphocytosis

BMC blood mononuclear cell; bone marrow cell; bone mineral content

BMD Becker's muscular dystrophy; Boehringer Mannheim Diagnostics; bone marrow depression; bone mineral density; bovine mucosal disease

BMDC Biomedical Documentation Center

BME basal medium Eagle; biundulant meningoencephalitis; brief maximal effort

BMed Bachelor of Medicine

BMedBiol Bachelor of Medical Biology

BMedSci Bachelor of Medical Science

BMET biomedical equipment technician

BMF bone marrow failure

BMG benign monoclonal gammopathy

BMI body mass index

BMic Bachelor of Microbiology

BMJ bones, muscles, joints; British Medical Journal

bmk birthmark

BML bone marrow lymphocytosis

BMLS billowing mitral leaflet syndrome

BMMP benign mucous membrane pemphigoid

BMN bone marrow necrosis

BMNC blood mononuclear cell

BMOC Brinster's medium for ovum culture

Bmod behavior modification

B-mode brightness modulation

BMP bone morphogenetic protein

BMPI bronchial mucous proteinase inhibitor

BMPP benign mucous membrane pemphigus

BMQA Board of Medical Quality Assurance

BMR basal metabolic rate

BMS Bachelor of Medical Science; betamethasone; biomedical monitoring system; bleomycin sulfate; Bureau of Medical Services; Bureau of Medicine and Surgery; burning mouth syndrome

BMSA British Medical Students Association

BMST Bruce maximum stress test

BMT Bachelor of Medical Technology; basement membrane thickening; benign mesenchymal tumor; bone marrow transplantation

BMU basic metabolic unit; basic multicellular unit

BMZ basement membrane zone

BN bladder neck; branchial neuritis; bronchial node; brown Norway [rat]

BNA Basle Nomina Anatomica

BND barely noticeable difference

BNDD Bureau of Narcotics and Dangerous Drugs

BNEd Bachelor of Nursing Education

BNF British National Formulary

BNIST National Bureau of Scientific Information [Fr. *Bureau National d'Information Scientifique*]

BNO bladder neck obstruction; bowels not opened

BNPA binasal pharyngeal airway

BNS benign nephrosclerosis

BNSc Bachelor of Nursing Science

BNT Boston Naming Test; brain neurotransmitter

BNYVV beet necrotic yellow vein virus

BO Bachelor of Osteopathy; base of prism out; behavior objective; belladonna and opium; body odor; bowel obstruction; bucco-occlusal

Bo Bolton point

bo bowels

B&O belladonna and opium

BOA born on arrival; British Orthopaedic Association

BOBA beta-oxybutyric acid

BOC blood oxygen capacity; Bureau of Census; butyloxycarbonyl

BOD biochemical oxygen demand

Bod Bodansky [unit]

BOEA ethyl biscoumacetate

BOH board of health

bol large pill [Lat. *bolus*]

BOLD bleomycin, Oncovin, lomustin, dacarbazine

BOM bilateral otitis media

BOMA bilateral otitis media, acute

BOOP bronchiolitis obliterans-organizing pneumonia

BOP buffalo orphan prototype [virus]

BOR basal optic root; before time of operation; bowels open regularly; branchio-oto-renal [syndrome]

BORR blood oxygen release rate

BoSM Bolivian squirrel monkey

BOT botulinum toxin

bot bottle

BOU branchio-oto-ureteral [syndrome]

BOW bag of waters

BP Bachelor of Pharmacy; back pressure; barometric pressure; basic protein; bathroom privileges; bed pan; before present; behavior pattern; Bell's palsy; benzpyrene; beta-protein; biotic potential; biparietal; biphenyl; bipolar; birth place; blood pressure; body plethysmography; boiling point; Bolton point; borderline personality; British Pharmacopoeia; bronchopleural; buccopulpal; bullous pemphigus; bypass

B/P blood pressure

bp base pair; bed pan; boiling point

BPA blood pressure assembly; bovine plasma albumin; British Paediatric Association; bronchopulmonary aspergillosis; burst-promoting activity

BPAEC bovine pulmonary artery endothelial cell

BPB bromphenol blue; biliopancreatic bypass

BPC Behavior Problem Checklist; bile phospholipid concentration; blood pressure cuff; British Pharmaceutical Codex

BPD biparietal diameter; blood pressure decrease; borderline personality disorder; bronchopulmonary dysplasia

BPE bacterial phosphatidylethanolamine

BPEC benign partial epilepsy of childhood; bipolar electrocardiogram

BPEI blepharophimosis, ptosis, epicanthus inversus

BPES blepharophimosis-ptosis-epicanthus inversus syndrome

BPF bradykinin-potentiating factor; bronchopulmonary fistula; burst-promoting factor

BPG benzathine penicillin G; blood pressure gauge; bypass graft

BPH Bachelor of Public Health; benign prostatic hypertrophy

BPh British Pharmacopoeia; buccopharyngeal

Bph bacteriopheophytin

BPharm Bachelor of Pharmacy

BPHEng Bachelor of Public Health Engineering

BPHN Bachelor of Public Health Nursing

BPI Basic Personality Inventory; beef-pork insulin; blood pressure increase

BPL benign proliferative lesion; benzyl penicilloyl-polylysine; beta-propiolactone

BPLA blood pressure, left arm

BPM beats per minute; biperidyl mustard; breaths per minute; brompheniramine maleate

BPMF British Postgraduate Medical Federation

BPMS blood plasma measuring system

BPN bacitracin, polymyxin B, neomycin sulfate; brachial plexus neuropathy

BPO basal pepsin output; benzyl penicilloyl

BPP biophysical profile; bovine pancreatic polypeptide; bradykinin potentiating peptide

BP&P blood pressure and pulse

BPPN benign paroxysmal positioning nystagmus

BPPV benign paroxysmal positional vertigo; bovine paragenital papilloma virus

BPQ Berne pain questionnaire

BPR blood pressure recorder; blood production rate

BPRA blood pressure, right arm

BPRS Brief Psychiatric Rating Scale; Brief Psychiatric Reacting Scale

BPS beats per second; Behavioral Pharmacological Society; bits per second; bovine papular stomatitis; brain protein solvent; breaths per second

BPSA bronchopulmonary segmental artery

BPsTh Bachelor of Psychotherapy

BPT benign paroxysmal torticollis

BPTI basic pancreatic trypsin inhibitor; basic polyvalent trypsin inhibitor

BPV benign paroxysmal vertigo; benign positional vertigo; bioprosthetic valve; bovine papilloma virus

BP(Vet) British Pharmacopoeia (Veterinary)

Bq becquerel

BQA Bureau of Quality Assurance

BR barrier reared [experimental animals]; baseline recovery; bathroom; bed rest; bedside rounds; bilirubin; biologic response; branchial; breathing rate; bronchial, bronchitis, bronchus; *Brucella,* brucellosis

Br breech; bregma; bridge; bromine; bronchitis; brown; *Brucella;* brucellosis

br boiling range; brachial; branch; branchial; breath; brother

BRA bilateral renal agenesis; bone-resorbing activity; brain-reactive antibody

BRAC basic rest-activity cycle

Brach brachial

Brady, brady bradycardia

BRAO branch retinal artery occlusion

BRAP burst of rapid atrial pacing

BrAP brachial artery pressure

BRAT Baylor rapid autologous transfusion [system]

BRATT bananas, rice, applesauce, tea and toast

BRB bright red blood

BRBC bovine red blood cell

BRBN blue rubber bleb nevus

BRBNS blue rubber bleb nevus syndrome

BRBPR bright red blood per rectum

BRbx breast biopsy

Brc bromocriptine

BRCM below right costal margin

BRCS British Red Cross Society

BRD bladder retraining drill; bovine respiratory disease

BrdU bromodeoxyuridine

BrdUrd bromodeoxyuridine

BRF bone-resorbing factor

BRH benign recurrent hematuria

BRIC benign recurrent intrahepatic cholestasis

BRIME brief repetitive isometric maximal exercise

Brkf breakfast

BRM biological response modifier; biuret reactive material

BRN Board of Registered Nursing

brn brown

BRO bronchoscopy

bro brother

brom bromide

Bron, Bronch bronchi, bronchial; bronchoscopy

BRP bathroom privileges; bilirubin production; bronchophony

Brph bronchophony

BRR baroreceptor reflex response; breathing reserve ratio

BRS battered root syndrome; Bibliographic Retrieval Services; British Roentgen Society

BrSM Brazilian squirrel monkey

BRT Brook reaction test

brth breath

BRU bone remodeling unit

BrU bromouracil

Bruc Brucella

BRVO branch retinal vein occlusion

BRW Brown-Robert-Wells [stereotactic system]

BS Bachelor of Science; Bachelor of Surgery; *Bacillus subtilis;* Bartter syndrome; base strap; bedside; before sleep;

Behçet syndrome; bilateral symmetrical; bile salt; Binet-Simon [test]; bismuth sulfite; blood sugar; Bloom syndrome; Blue Shield [plan]; borderline schizophrenia; bowel sound; breaking strength; breath sound; British Standard; buffered saline; Bureau of Standards

B&S Brown and Sharp [sutures]

bs bedside; bowel sound; breath sound

b x s brother x sister inbreeding

BSA benzenesulfonic acid; Biofeedback Society of America; bismuth-sulfite agar; bis-trimethylsilyl-acetamide; Blind Service Association; Blue Shield Association; body surface area; bovine serum albumin; bowel sounds active

bsa bovine serum albumin

BSAG Bristol Social Adjustment Guides

BSAM basic sequential access method

BSAP brief short-action potential; brief, small, abundant potentials

BSB body surface burned

BS = BL breath sounds equal bilaterally

BSC bedside commode; bedside care; bench scale calorimeter; bile salt concentration; Biological Stain Commission; Biomedical Science Corps

BSc Bachelor of Science

BSC-1, BS-C-1 *Cercopithecus* monkey kidney cells

BSCC British Society for Clinical Cytology

BSCP bovine spinal cord protein

BSD bedside drainage

BSDLB block in anterosuperior division of left branch

BSE behavior summarized evaluation; bilateral symmetrical and equal; breast self-examination

BSEP brain stem evoked potential

BSER brain stem evoked response [audiometry]

BSF back scatter factor; busulfan

BSG branchio-skeleto-genital [syndrome]

BSI Behavior Status Inventory; Borderline Syndrome Index; bound serum iron; British Standards Institution

BSID Bayley Scale of Infant Development

BSIF bile salt independent fraction

BSL benign symmetric lipomatosis; blood sugar level

BSM Bachelor of Science in Medicine

BSN Bachelor of Science in Nursing; bowel sounds normal

BSNA bowel sounds normal and active

BSO bilateral sagittal osteotomy; bilateral salpingo-oophorectomy; British School of Osteopathy

BSP bromsulphalein

BSp bronchospasm

BSPh Bachelor of Science in Pharmacy

BSQ Behavior Style Questionnaire

BSR basal skin resistance; blood sedimentation rate; bowel sounds regular; brain stimulation reinforcement

BSS Bachelor of Sanitary Science; balanced salt solution; Bernard-Soulier syndrome; black silk suture; buffered salt solution; buffered single substrate

B-SS Bernard-Soulier syndrome

BSSE bile salt–stimulated esterase

BSSG sitogluside

BSSL bile salt–stimulated lipase

BST bacteriuria screening test; blood serologic test; brief stimulus therapy

BSTFA bis-trimethylsilyltrifluoroacetamide

BSU Bartholin, Skene, urethral [glands]; basic structural unit; British standard unit

BSV binocular single vision

BT base of tongue; bedtime; bitemporal; bitrochanteric; bladder tumor; bleeding time; blood type, blood typing; blue tetrazolium; blue tongue; body temperature; bovine turbinate [cells]; brain tumor; breast tumor

BTA Blood Transfusion Association

BTB breakthrough bleeding; bromthymol blue

BTBL bromothymol blue lactose

BTC basal temperature chart; body temperature chart

BTDS benzoylthiamine disulfide

BTE bovine thymus extract

BTFS breast tumor frozen section
BTG beta-thromboglobulin
BTg bovine trypsinogen
BThU British thermal unit
BTL bilateral tubal ligation
BTLS basic trauma life support
BTM benign tertian malaria
BTMSA bis-trimethylsilacetylene
BTP biliary tract pain
BTPABA N-benzoyl-L-tyrosyl-p-aminobenzoic acid
BTPS at body temperature and ambient pressure, and saturated with water vapor [gas]
BTR Bezold-type reflex; biceps tendon reflex
BTr bovine trypsin
BTS blood transfusion service; blue toe syndrome; bradycardia-tachycardia syndrome
bTSH bovine thyroid-stimulating hormone
BTU British thermal unit
BTV blue tongue virus
BTX brevetoxin
BTX-B brevetoxin-B
BTZ benzothiazepine
BU base of prism up; Bethesda unit; blood urea; Bodansky unit; bromouracil; burn unit
Bu butyl
bu bushel
BUA blood uric acid; broadband ultrasonic attenuation
Buc, Bucc buccal
BUDR 5-bromodeoxyuridine
BUDS bilateral upper dorsal sympathectomy
BUE both upper extremities
BUF buffalo [rat]
BUG buccal ganglion
BUI brain uptake index
BULIT bulimia test
BULL buccal or upper lingual of lower
bull let it boil [Lat. *bulliat*]
BuMed Bureau of Medicine and Surgery
BUMP Behavioral Regression or Upset in Hospitalized Medical Patients [scale]

BUN blood urea nitrogen
bun br bundle branch
BUN/CR blood urea nitrogen/creatine ratio
BUO bleeding of undetermined origin, bruising of undetermined origin
BUQ both upper quadrants
BUR bilateral ureteral occlusion
Burd Burdick suction
BUS Bartholin, urethral, and Skene glands; busulfan
But, but butyrate, butyric
BV bacitracin V; biological value; blood vessel; blood volume; bronchovesicular
bv steam bath [Lat. *balneum vaporis*]
BVA Blind Veterans Association; British Veterinary Association
BVAD biventricular assist device
BVC British Veterinary Codex
BVD bovine viral diarrhea
BVDT brief vestibular disorientation test
BVDU bromovinyldeoxyuridine
BVE binocular visual efficiency; blood vessel endothelium; blood volume expander
BVH biventricular hypertrophy
BVI blood vessel invasion
BVL bilateral vas ligation
BVM bronchovascular markings; Bureau of Veterinary Medicine
BVMGT Bender Visual-Motor Gestalt Test
BVMOT Bender Visual-Motor Gestalt Test
BVMS Bachelor of Veterinary Medicine and Science
BVO branch vein occlusion
BVP blood vessel prosthesis; blood volume pulse; burst of ventricular pacing
BVR baboon virus replication
BVS blanked ventricular sense
BVSc Bachelor of Veterinary Science
BVU bromoisovalerylurea
BVV bovine vaginitis virus
BW bacteriological warfare; bed wetting; below waist; biological warfare; biological weapon; birth weight; bladder washout; blood Wasserman [reaction]; body water; body weight

B&W black and white [milk of magnesia and cascara extract]
bw body weight
BWD bacillary white diarrhea
BWFI bacteriostatic water for injection
BWS battered woman (or wife) syndrome; Beckwith-Wiedemann syndrome
BWST black widow spider toxin
BWSV black widow spider venom
BWt birth weight

BWYV beet western yellow virus
BX, bx bacitracin X; biopsy
BXD balanitis xerotica obliterans
BYDV barley yellow dwarf virus
BYE Barila-Yaguchi-Eveland [medium]
BZ benzodiazepine
Bz, Bzl benzoyl
BZD benzodiazepine
BZQ benzquinamide
BZS Bannayan-Zonana syndrome

C about [Lat. *circa*]; ascorbic acid; bruised [Lat. *contusus*]; calcitonin-forming [cell]; calculus; calorie [large]; *Campylobacter; Candida;* canine tooth; capacitance; carbohydrate; carbon; cardiac; cardiovascular disease; carrier; cast; cathode; Caucasian; cell; Celsius; centigrade; central; central electrode placement in electroencephalography; centromeric or constitutive heterochromatic chromosome [banding]; cerebrospinal; certified; cervical; cesarean [section]; chest (precordial) lead in electrocardiography; chicken; *Chlamydia;* chloramphenicol; cholesterol; class; clearance; clonus; *Clostridium;* closure; clubbing; coarse [bacterial colonies]; cocaine; coefficient; color sense; colored [guinea pig]; complement; complex; compliance; component; compound [Lat. *compositus*]; concentration; conditioned, conditioning; condyle; constant; consultation; contraction; control; conventionally reared [experimental animal]; convergence; correct; cortex; coulomb; *Cryptococcus*; cubic; cubitus; curie; cyanosis; cylinder; cysteine; cytidine; cytochrome; cytosine; gallon [Lat. *congius*]; horn [Lat. *cornu*]; hundred [Lat. *centum*]; large calorie; molar heat capacity; rib [Lat. *costa*]; velocity of light; with [Lat. *cum*]

C1 first cervical nerve; first cervical vertebra; first component of complement

C_1 first rib

$\bar{C}1$ activated first component of complement

C1 INH inhibitor of first component of complement

CI first cranial nerve

C2 second cervical nerve; second cervical vertebra; second component of complement

C_2 second rib

$\bar{C}2$ activated second component of complement

CII second cranial nerve

C3 third cervical nerve; third cervical vertebra; third component of complement

C_3 Collins' solution; third rib

$\bar{C}3$ activated third component of complement

CIII third cranial nerve

C4 fourth cervical nerve; fourth cervical vertebra; fourth component of complement

$\bar{C}4$ activated fourth component of complement

CIV fourth cranial nerve

C5 fifth cervical nerve; fifth cervical vertebra; fifth component of complement

$\bar{C}5$ activated fifth component of complement

CV fifth cranial nerve

C6 sixth cervical nerve; sixth cervical vertebra; sixth component of complement

$\bar{C}6$ activated sixth component of complement

CVI sixth cranial nerve

C7 seventh cervical nerve; seventh cervical vertebra; seventh component of complement

$\bar{C}7$ activated seventh component of complement

CVII seventh cranial nerve

C8 eighth component of complement

$\bar{C}8$ activated eighth component of complement

CVIII eighth cranial nerve

C9 ninth component of complement

$\bar{C}9$ activated ninth component of complement

CIX-CXII ninth to twelfth cranial nerves

°C degree Celsius

C' complement

c about [Lat. *circa*]; calorie [small]; candle; canine tooth; capacity; carat; centi-; complementary [strand]; concentration; contact; cup; curie; cyclic; meal [Lat. *cibus*]; specific heat capacity; with [Lat. *cum*]

c' coefficient of portage

CA anterior commissure [Lat. *commissura anterior*]; calcium antagonist; California [rabbit]; cancer; caproic acid; carbonic anhydrase; carcinoma; cardiac arrest; cardiac arrhythmia; carotid artery; cast; catecholamine, catecholaminergic; cathode; Caucasian adult; celiac axis; cerebral aqueduct; cerebral atrophy; cervicoaxial; Chemical Abstracts; chemotactic activity; chloroamphetamine; cholic acid; chromosomal aberration; chronic anovulation; chronological age; citric acid; clotting assay; coagglutination; coarctation of the aorta; coefficient of absorption; cold agglutinin; colloid antigen; common antigen; compressed air; conceptional age; coronary artery; corpora alata; corpora amylacea; corpus albicans; cortisone acetate; cricoid arch; croup-associated [virus]; cytosine arabinoside; cytotoxic antibody

Ca calcium; cancer, carcinoma; *Candida albicans;* cathode

ca about [Lat. *circa*]; candle; carcinoma

C&A Clinitest and Acetest

CA-2 second colloid antigen

CAA carotid audiofrequency analysis; cerebral amyloid angiopathy; circulating anodic antigen; Clean Air Act; computer-assisted assessment; constitutional aplastic anemia; coronary artery aneurysm; crystalline amino acids

CAAT computer-assisted axial tomography

CAB captive air bubble; cellulose acetate butyrate; coronary artery bypass

CABG coronary artery bypass grafting

CABGS coronary artery bypass graft surgery

CaBI calcium bone index

CaBP calcium-binding protein

CABS coronary artery bypass surgery

CAC cardiac-accelerator center; cardiac arrest code; circulating anticoagulant

CaCC cathodal closure contraction

CAC/CIC chronic active/inactive cirrhosis

CACP cisplatin

CaCTe cathodal closure tetanus

CaCV calicivirus

CaCX cancer of cervix

CAD cadaver, cadaveric; cold agglutinin disease; compressed air disease; computer-assisted design; computer-assisted diagnosis; congenital abduction deficiency; coronary artery disease; coronoradiographic documentation

Cad cadaver, cadaveric

CADL Communicative Abilities in Daily Living

CaDTe cathodal-duration tetanus

CAE caprine arthritis-encephalitis; cellulose acetate electrophoresis; contingent after-effects; coronary artery embolism

CaE calcium excretion

CaEDTA calcium disodium ethylenediaminetetraacetate

CAEP cortical auditory evoked potential

CAEV caprine arthritis-encephalitis virus

CAF cell adhesion factor; citric acid fermentation

Caf caffeine

CAG cholangiogram, cholangiography; chronic atrophic gastritis; coronary angiography

CAGE *c*ut down, *a*nnoyed by criticism, *g*uilty about drinking, *e*ye-opener drinks (a test for alcoholism)

CAH chronic active hepatitis; chronic aggressive hepatitis; combined atrial hypertrophy; congenital adrenal hyperplasia; cyanacetic acid hydrazide

CAHD coronary arteriosclerotic heart disease

CAHEA Committee on Allied Health Education and Accreditation

CAHS central alveolar hypoventilation syndrome

CAHV central alveolar hypoventilation

CAI complete androgen insensitivity; computer-assisted instruction

CAIS complete androgen insensitivity syndrome

CAL café au lait; calcium test; calculated average life; calories; chronic airflow limitation; computer-assisted learning; coracoacromial ligament

Cal caliber; large calorie

cal small calorie

C$_{alb}$ albumin clearance

Calc calcium

calc calculation

calcif calcification

CALD chronic active liver disease

calef make warm [Lat. *calefac*]; warmed [Lat. *calefactus*]

CALGB cancer and leukemia group B

CALH chronic active lupoid hepatitis

cALL common null cell acute lymphocytic leukemia

cALLA common acute lymphoblastic leukemia antigen

CALM café-au-lait macules

CAM calf aortic microsome; cell-associating molecule; chorioallantoic membrane; computer assisted myelography; contralateral axillary metastasis

C$_{am}$ amylase clearance

CAMAC computer automated measurement and control

CAMF cyclophosphamide, Adriamycin, methotrexate, fluorouracil

CAMP Christie-Atkins-Munch-Petersen [test]; computer-assisted menu planning; concentration of adenosine monophosphate; cyclophosphamide, Adriamycin, methotrexate, and procarbazine

cAMP cyclic adenosine monophosphate

CAMS computer-assisted monitoring system

CaMV cauliflower mosaic virus

Can cancer; Candida; *Cannabis*

CA/N child abuse and neglect

CANA circulating antineuronal antibody

canc cancelled

CANCERLIT Cancer Literature

CANCERPROJ Cancer Research Projects

CANP calcium-activated neutral protease

CANS central auditory nervous system

CAO chronic airway obstruction; coronary artery obstruction

CaOC cathodal opening contraction

CaOCL cathodal opening clonus

CAOD coronary artery occlusive disease

CAOM chronic adhesive otitis media

CaOTe cathodal opening tetanus

CAP camptodactyly-arthropathy-pericarditis [syndrome]; capsule; captopril; catabolite gene activator protein; cell attachment protein; cellular acetate propionate; cellulose acetate phthalate; central apical part; chloramphenicol; chronic alcoholic pancreatitis; College of American Pathologists; complement-activated plasma; compound action potential; coupled atrial pacing; cyclosphosphamide, Adriamycin, and Platino [cisplatin]; cystine aminopeptidase

cap capacity; capsule; let him take [Lat. *capiat*]

CAPA cancer-associated polypeptide antigen

CAPD continuous ambulatory peritoneal dialysis

CAPERS Computer Assisted Psychiatric Evaluation and Review System

capiend to be taken [Lat. *capiendus*]

cap moll soft capsule [Lat. *capsula mollis*]

CAPPS Current and Past Psychopathology Scale

cap quant vult to be taken as much as one wants to [Lat. *capiat quantum vult*]

CAPRCA chronic, acquired, pure red cell aplasia

CAPRI Cardiopulmonary Research Institute

caps capsule

CAPYA child and adolescent psychoanalysis

CAR Canadian Association of Radiologists; cancer-associated retinopathy;

cardiac ambulation routine; chronic articular rheumatism; computer-assisted research; conditioned avoidance response
car carotid
CARA chronic aspecific respiratory ailment
CARB carbohydrate; coronary artery bypass graft
carb carbohydrate; carbonate
carbo carbohydrate
CARD cardiac automatic resuscitative device
card cardiac
card insuff cardiac insufficiency
cardiol cardiology
CARE computerized adult and records evaluation [system]
CARF Commission on Accreditation and Rehabilitation Facilities
CARS Childhood Autism Rating Scale; Children's Affective Rating Scale
cart cartilage
CAS calcarine sulcus; calcific aortic stenosis; Cancer Attitude Survey; carbohydrate-active steroid; cardiac adjustment scale; cardiac surgery; Celite-activated normal serum; Center for Alcohol Studies; cerebral atherosclerosis; Chemical Abstract Service; cold agglutinin syndrome; congenital alcoholic syndrome; control adjustment strap; coronary artery spasm
Cas casualty
cas castration, castrated
CASA computer-assisted self assessment
CASH Commission for Administrative Services in Hospitals; corticoadrenal stimulating hormone; cruciform anterior spinal hyperextension
CASHD coronary arteriosclerotic heart disease
CASMD congenital atonic sclerotic muscular dystrophy
CAS-REGN Chemical Abstracts Service Registry Number
CASRT corrected adjusted sinus node recovery time

CASS Coronary Artery Surgery Study
CASSIS Classification and Search Support Information System [Patent Office]
CAST Cardiac Arrhythmia Suppression Trial; Children of Alcoholism Screening Test
CAT California Achievement Test; capillary agglutination test; catalase; cataract; catecholamine; Children's Apperception Test; chloramphenicol acetyltransferase; chlormerodrin accumulation test; choline acetyltransferase; chronic abdominal tympany; Cognitive Abilities Test; computed abdominal tomography; computed axial tomography; computer of average transients
cat catalysis, catalyst; cataract
CAT'ase catalase
CATCH Community Actions to Control High Blood Pressure
Cath cathartic; catheter, catheterize
CATLINE Catalog On-Line
CAT-S Children's Apperception Test, Supplemental
CAT scan computed axial tomography scan
CATT calcium tolerance test
Cauc Caucasian
caud caudal
caut cauterization
CAV congenital absence of vagina; congenital adrenal virilism; constant angular velocity; croup-associated virus
cav cavity
CAVB complete atrioventricular block
CAVD complete atrioventricular dissociation; completion, arithmetic problems, vocabulary, following directions [test]
CAVH continuous arteriovenous hemofiltration
CAVHD continuous arteriovenous hemodialysis
CAVLT Children's Auditory Verbal Learning Test
CAVO common atrioventricular orifice
CAVS Conformance Assessment to Voluntary Standards

CAVU continuous arteriovenous ultrafiltration

CAW central airways

C$_{AW}$ airway conductance

CB Bachelor of Surgery [Lat. *Chirurgiae Baccalaureus*]; calcium blocker; carbenicillin; carotid body; chocolate blood [agar]; chromatin body; chronic bronchitis; circumflex branch; code blue; color blind; compensated base; coracobrachial

Cb niobium [columbium]

CBA chronic bronchitis and asthma; cost-benefit analysis

CBAB complement-binding antibody

CBADAA Certifying Board of the American Dental Assistants Association

CBC carbenicillin; child behavior characteristics; complete blood cell count

cbc complete blood cell count

CBCL Child Behavior Checklist

CBCL/2-3 Child Behavior Checklist for ages 2-3

CBCN carbenicillin

CBD carotid body denervation; closed bladder drainage; common bile duct

CBDC chronic bullous disease of children

CBDE common bile duct exploration

CBET certified biomedical equipment technician

CBF capillary blood flow; cerebral blood flow; ciliary beat frequency; coronary blood flow; cortical blood flow

CBG capillary blood gases; coronary bypass graft; corticosteroid-binding globulin; cortisol-binding globulin

CBGv corticosteroid-binding globulin variant

CBH chronic benign hepatitis; cutaneous basophilic hypersensitivity

CBI continuous bladder irrigation

CBL circulating blood lymphocytes; cord blood leukocytes

Cbl cobalamin

cbl chronic blood loss

CBM capillary basement membrane

CBMMP chronic benign mucous membrane pemphigus

CBN cannabinol; central benign neoplasm; Commission on Biological Nomenclature

CBO Congressional Budget Office

CBOC completion bed occupancy care

CBP calcium-binding protein; carbohydrate-binding protein; chlorobiphenyl; cobalamin-binding protein

CBPA competitive protein-binding assay

CBR chemical, biological, and radiological [warfare]; chemically-bound residue; chronic bed rest; complete bed rest; crude birth rate

CBS cervicobrachial syndrome; chronic brain syndrome; conjugated bile salts; culture-bound syndrome; cystathionine beta-synthase

CBT carotid body tumor; computed body tomography

CBV capillary blood cell velocity; catheter balloon valvuloplasty; central blood volume; cerebral blood volume; circulating blood volume; cortical blood volume; corrected blood volume; Coxsackie B virus

CBVD cerebrovascular disease

CBW chemical and biological warfare

CBX computer-based examination

CBZ carbamazepine

CC calcaneal-cuboid; calcium cyclamate; cardiac catheterization; cardiac contusion; cardiac cycle; cardiovascular clinic; cell culture; central compartment; cerebral commissure; cerebral cortex; chest circumference; chief complaint; cholecalciferol; chondrocalcinosis; choriocarcinoma; chronic complainer; circulatory collapse; classical conditioning; clean catch [of urine]; Clinical Center [NIH]; clinical course; clomiphene citrate; closed cup; closing capacity; colony count; colorectal cancer; columnar cells; commission certified; common cold; compound cathartic; computer calculated; congenital cardiopathy; consumptive coagulopathy; contrast cystogram;

conversion complete; coracoclavicular; cord compression; corpus callosum; costochondral; Coulter counter; craniocervical; creatinine clearance; critical care; critical condition; Cronkhite-Canada [syndrome]; crus cerebri; cubic centimeter; current complaint; Current Contents

C-C convexo-concave

C&C cold and clammy

Cc concave

cc concave; corrected; cubic centimeter

CCA cephalin cholesterol antigen; chick cell agglutination; chimpanzee coryza agent; choriocarcinoma; circulating cathodic antigen; circumflex coronary artery; common carotid artery; congenital contractural arachnodactyly; constitutional chromosome abnormality

CCAT chick cell agglutination test; conglutinating complement absorption test

CCBV central circulating blood volume

CCC care-cure coordination; cathodal closure contraction; chronic calculous cholecystitis; chronic catarrhal colitis; comprehensive care clinic; consecutive case conference; critical care complex; cylindrical confronting cisternae

CC&C colony count and culture

CCCC centrifugal countercurrent chromatography

cccDNA covalently closed circular deoxyribonucleic acid

CCCl cathodal closure clonus

CCCP carbonyl cyanide *m*-chlorophenyl-hydrazone

CCCR closed chest cardiac resuscitation

CCCS condom catheter collecting system

CCCT closed craniocerebral trauma

CCCU comprehensive cardiac care unit

CCD calibration curve data; charge-coupled device; childhood celiac disease; countercurrent distribution; cumulative cardiotoxic dose

CCDC Canadian Communicable Disease Center

CCDN Central Council for District Nursing

ccDNA closed circle deoxyribonucleic acid

CCE carboline carboxylic acid ester; chamois contagious ecthyma; clear-cell endothelioma; clubbing, cyanosis, and edema; countercurrent electrophoresis

CCEI Crown-Crisp Experimental Index

CCF cancer coagulation factor; cardiolipin complement fixation; carotid-cavernous fistula; centrifuged culture fluid; cephalin-cholesterol flocculation; compound comminuted fracture; congestive heart failure; crystal-induced chemotactic factor

CCFA cefotoxin-cycloserine fructose agar

CCFAS compact colony-forming active substance

CCFE cyclophosphamide, cisplatin, fluorouracil, and extramustine

CCFMG Cooperating Committee on Foreign Medical Graduates

CCG cholecystogram, cholecystography

CCGC capillary column gas chromotography

CCH C-cell hyperplasia; chronic cholestatic hepatitis

CCHD cyanotic congenital heart disease

CCHE Central Council for Health Education

CCHMS Central Committee for Hospital Medical Services

CCHP Consumer Choice Health Plan

CCHS congenital central hypoventilation syndrome

CCI chronic coronary insufficiency; corrected count increment

CCK cholecystokinin

CCK-8 cholecystokinin octapeptide

CCKLI cholecystokinin-like immunoreactivity

CCK-OP cholecystokinin octapeptide

CCK-PZ cholecystokinin-pancreozymin

CCL carcinoma cell line; certified cell

line; Charcot-Leyden crystal; critical carbohydrate level

CCLI composite clinical and laboratory index

CCM cerebrocostomandibular [syndrome]; congestive cardiomyopathy; craniocervical malformation; critical care medicine

c cm cubic centimeter

CCMC Committee on the Costs of Medical Care

CCME Coordinating Council on Medical Education

CCMS cerebrocostomandibular syndrome; clean catch midstream [urine]; clinical care management system

CCMSU clean catch midstream urine

CCMT catechol methyltransferase

CCMU critical care medical unit

CCN caudal central nucleus; coronary care nursing; critical care nursing

CCNU N-(2-chloroethyl)-N'-cyclohexyl-N-nitrosourea

CCO cytochrome C oxidase

CCOT cervical compression overloading test

CCP ciliocytophthoria; chronic calcifying pancreatitis; cytidine cyclic phosphate

CCPD continuous cycling (cyclical) peritoneal dialysis

CCPDS Centralized Cancer Patient Data System

CCPR crypt cell production rate

CCR complete continuous remission

Ccr, C$_{cr}$ creatinine clearance

CCRIS Chemical Carcinogenesis Research Information System

CCRN Critical Care Registered Nurse

CCS casualty clearing station; cell cycle specific; cholecystosonography; chronic cerebellar stimulation; chronic compartment syndrome; cloudy cornea syndrome; concentration camp syndrome; costoclavicular syndrome

CCSCS central cervical spinal cord syndrome

CCSE Cognitive Capacity Screening Examination

CCSG Children's Cancer Study Group

CCT carotid compression tomography; central conduction time; cerebrocranial trauma; chocolate-coated tablet; coated compressed tablet; combined cortical thickness; composite cyclic therapy; computerized cranial tomography; controlled cord traction; coronary care team; cranial computed tomography; cyclocarbothiamine

CCTe cathodal closure tetanus

CCTP coronary care training program

CCTV closed circuit television

CCU cardiac care unit; Cherry-Crandall unit; coronary care unit; critical care unit

CCUP colpocystourethropexy

CCV channel catfish virus; conductivity cell volume

CCVD chronic cerebrovascular disease

CCVM congenital cardiovascular malformation

CCW chest wall compliance; counterclockwise

CD cadaver donor; canine distemper; canine dose; carbohydrate dehydratase; carbon dioxide; cardiac disease; cardiac dullness; cardiac dysrhythmia; cardiovascular disease; Carrel-Dakin [fluid]; Castleman's disease; caudad, caudal; celiac disease; cell dissociation; cervicodorsal; cesarean delivery; chemical dependency; circular dichroism; cluster of differentiation [antigens]; combination drug; common duct; communicable disease; completely denaturated; conduct disorder; conduction disorder; conjugata diagonalis; consanguineous donor; contact dermatitis; contagious disease; control diet; conventional dialysis; convulsive disorder; convulsive dose; corneal dystrophy; Cotrel-Dubousset [rod]; Crohn's disease; crossed diagonal; curative dose; cutdown; cystic duct; diagonal conjugate diameter of the pelvis [Lat. *conjugata diagonalis*]

C/D cigarettes per day; cup to disc ratio

C&D cystoscopy and dilatation

Cd cadmium; caudal; coccygeal; condylion

cd candela; caudal

c/d cigarettes per day

CD4 HIV helper cell count

CD8 HIV suppressor cell count

CD$_{50}$ median curative dose

CDA Canadian Dental Association; Certified Dental Assistant; chenodeoxycholic acid; ciliary dyskinesia activity; complement-dependent antibody; completely denatured alcohol; congenital dyserythropoietic anemia

C&DB cough and deep breath

CDC calculated date of confinement; cancer diagnosis center; capillary diffusion capacity; cell division cycle; Centers for Disease Control; chenodeoxycholate; Communicable Disease Center; complement-dependent cytotoxicity

CD-C controlled drinker-control

CDCA chenodeoxycholic acid

CDD certificate of disability for discharge; choledochoduodenostomy; chronic degenerative disease; chronic disabling dermatosis

CDDP cis-diaminedichloroplatinum

CDE canine distemper encephalitis; chlordiazepoxide; common duct exploration

CDEC Comprehensive Developmental Evaluation Chart

CDF chondrodystrophia foetalis

CDG central developmental groove

cDGS complete form of DiGeorge's syndrome

CDH ceramide dihexoside; congenital diaphragmatic hernia; congenital dislocation of hip; congenital dysplasia of hip

CDI cell-directed inhibitor; central or chronic diabetes insipidus; Children's Depression Inventory; cranial diabetes insipidus

CDILD chronic diffuse interstitial lung disease

CDK climatic droplet keratopathy

CDL chlordeoxylincomycin

CDLE chronic discoid lupus erythematosus

CDLS Cornelia de Lange syndrome

CDM chemically-defined medium; clinical decision making

cDNA circular deoxyribonucleic acid; complementary deoxyribonucleic acid

CDNB 1-chloro-2,4-dinitrobenzene

CDP chronic destructive periodontitis; collagenase-digestible protein; continuous distending pressure; coronary drug project; cytidine diphosphate; cytosine diphosphate

CDPC cytidine diphosphate choline

CDPX X-linked chondrodysplasia punctata

CDR calcium-dependent regulator; computerized digital radiography; cup/disk ratio

CDRS Children's Depression Rating Scale

CDS cardiovascular surgery; catechol-3, 5-disulfonate; caudal dysplasia syndrome; Chemical Data System; Christian Dental Society; cumulative duration of survival

CDSC Communicable Diseases Surveillance Centre [London]

CDSM Committee on Dental and Surgical Materials

cd-sr candela-steradian

CDSS clinical decision support system

CDT carbon dioxide therapy; Certified Dental Technician; *Clostridium difficile* toxin; combined diphtheria tetanus

CDTe cathode duration tetanus

CDV canine distemper virus

Cdyn, C$_{dyn}$ dynamic compliance

CDZ chlordiazepoxide; conduction delay zone

CE California encephalitis; cardiac enlargement; cardioesophageal; catamenial epilepsy; cell extract; chemical energy; chick embryo; chloroform ether; cholesterol esters; chorioepithelioma; chromatoelectrophoresis; ciliated epithelium; columnar epithelium; conjugated estrogens; constant error; continuing education; contractile element; converting enzyme; crude extract; cytopathic effect

Ce cerium

C-E chloroform-ether

CEA carcinoembryonic antigen; carotid endarterectomy; cholesterol-esterifying activity; cost-effectiveness analysis; crystalline egg albumin

CEARP Continuing Education Approval and Recognition Program

CEAT chronic ectopic atrial tachycardia

cEBV chronic Epstein-Barr virus [infection]

CEC ciliated epithelial cell

CECT contrast-enhanced computed tomography

CED chondroectodermal dysplasia

CEE Central European encephalitis; chick embryo extract

CEEA curved end-to-end anastomosis [stapler]

CEEG computer-analyzed electroencephalography

CEEV Central European encephalitis virus

CEF centrifugation extractable fluid; chick embryo fibroblast; constant electric field

CEFMG Council on Education for Foreign Medical Graduates

CEG chronic erosive gastritis

CEH cholesterol ester hydrolase

CEHC calf embryonic heart cell

CEI character education inquiry; converting enzyme inhibitor

CEID crossed electroimmunodiffusion

CEJ cement-enamel junction

CEK chick embryo kidney

Cell celluloid

CELO chick embryonal lethal orphan [virus]

Cels Celsius

CEM computerized electroencephalographic map; conventional transmission electron microscope

CEN Certificate for Emergency Nursing; Comité European de Normalisation (standards); continuous enteral nutrition

cen centromere; central

CENP centromere protein

cent centigrade; central

CEO chick embryo origin; Chief Executive Officer

CEOT calcifying epithelial odontogenic tumor

CEP chronic eosinophilic pneumonia; chronic erythropoietic porphyria; congenital erythropoietic porphyria; continuing education program; cortical evoked potential; counter-electrophoresis

CEPA chloroethane phosphoric acid

CEPH cephalic; cephalosporin

ceph cephalin

CEPH FLOC cephalin flocculation

CEQ Council on Environmental Quality

CER ceramide; conditioned emotional response; control electrical rhythm; cortical evoked response

CERCLA The Comprehensive Environmental Response, Compensation, and Liability Act

CERD chronic end-stage renal disease

CERP Continuing Education Recognition Program

Cert, cert certified

cerv cervix, cervical

CES cauda equina syndrome; cat's eye syndrome; central excitatory state; chronic electrophysiological study; conditioned escape response

CES-D Center for Epidemiologic Studies–Depression

CESD cholesterol ester storage disease

CET capital expenditure threshold; congenital eyelid tetrad

CETE Central European tick-borne encephalitis

CEU congenital ectropion uveae; continuing education unit

CEV California encephalitis virus; *Citrus exocortis* viroid

CEX clinical evaluation exercise

CEZ cefazolin

CF calcium leucovorin; calf blood flow;

calibration factor; cancer-free; carbolfuchsin; carbon filtered; cardiac failure; carotid foramen; carrier-free; cascade filtration; case file; Caucasian female; centrifugal force; characteristic frequency; chemotactic factor; chest and left leg [lead in electrocardiography]; Chiari-Frommel [syndrome]; chick fibroblast; Christmas factor; citrovorum factor; clotting factor; colicin factor; collected fluid; colonization factor; colony forming; complement fixation; computed fluoroscopy; constant frequency; contractile force; coronary flow; cough frequency; count fingers; counting finger; coupling factor; cycling fibroblast; cystic fibrosis

Cf californium

cf centrifugal force; bring together, compare [Lat. *confer*]

CFA colonization factor antigen; colony-forming assay; complement-fixing antibody; complete Freund's adjuvant; configuration frequency analysis; cryptogenic fibrosing alveolitis

CFB central fibrous body

CFC capillary filtration coefficient; colony-forming capacity; cardiofaciocutaneous [syndrome]; chlorofluorocarbon; colony-forming cell; continuous flow centrifugation

CFD cephalofacial deformity; craniofacial dysostosis

CFDS craniofacial dyssynostosis

CFF critical flicker fusion [test]; critical fusion frequency; cystic fibrosis factor; Cystic Fibrosis Foundation

cff critical flicker fusion; critical fusion frequency

CFFA cystic fibrosis factor activity

CFH Council on Family Health

CFI chemotactic-factor inactivator; complement fixation inhibition

CFM chlorofluoromethane; close-fitting mask; craniofacial microsomia

CFMA Council for Medical Affairs

CFMG Commission on Foreign Medical Graduates

CFND craniofrontonasal dysostosis

CFNS chills, fever, night sweats; craniofrontonasal syndrome

CFP chronic false positive; Clinical Fellowship Program; cyclophosphamide, fluorouracil, prednisone; cystic fibrosis of pancreas; cystic fibrosis protein

CFPP craniofacial pattern profile

CFPR Canadian Familial Polyposis Registry

CFR case-fatality ratio; citrovorum-factor rescue; Code of Federal Regulations; complement-fixation reaction; correct fast reaction; cyclic flow reduction

CFS cancer family syndrome; Chiari-Frommel syndrome; chronic fatigue syndrome; craniofacial stenosis; crush fracture syndrome; culture fluid supernatant; Cystic Fibrosis Society

CFSE crystal field stabilization energy

CFSTI Clearinghouse for Federal Scientific and Technical Information

CFT cardiolipin flocculation test; clinical full time; complement-fixation test

CFU colony-forming unit

CFU-C colony-forming unit-culture

CFU-E, CFU$_E$ colony-forming unit-erythrocyte

CFU$_{EOS}$ colony-forming unit-eosinophil

CFU-F, CFU$_F$ colony-forming unit-fibroblastoid

CFU$_{GM}$ colony-forming unit-granulocyte macrophage

CFU$_L$ colony-forming unit-lymphoid

CFU$_M$ colony-forming unit-megakaryocyte

CFU$_{MEG}$ colony-forming unit-megakaryocyte

CFU$_{NM}$ colony-forming unit-neutrophil-monocyte

CFU$_S$ colony-forming unit-spleen

CFV continuous flow ventilation

CFW Carworth farm [mouse], Webster strain

CFWM cancer-free white mouse

CFX cefoxitin; circumflex coronary artery

CFZ capillary free zone

CFZC continuous-flow zonal centrifugation

CG cardiography; cardiogreen; choking gas; choriogenic gynecomastia; chorionic gonadotropin; chromogranin; chronic glomerulonephritis; cingulate gyrus; colloidal gold; control group; cryoglobulin; cystine guanine; phosgene [choking gas]
cg center of gravity; centigram; chemoglobulin
CGA catabolite gene activator
CGAS Children's Global Assessment Scale
CGB chronic gonadotropin, beta-unit
CGD chronic granulomatous disease
CGDE contact glow discharge electrolysis
CGFH congenital fibrous histiocytoma
CGFNS Commission on Graduates of Foreign Nursing Schools
CGH chorionic gonadotropic hormone
CGI chronic granulomatous inflammation; Clinical Global Impression [scale]; computer-generated imagery
CGKD complex glycerol kinase deficiency
CGL chronic granulocytic leukemia
c gl correction with glasses
CGM central gray matter
cgm centigram
CGMMV cucumber green mottle mosaic virus
cGMP cyclic guanosine monophosphate
CGN chronic glomerulonephritis
CGNB composite ganglioneuroblastoma
CG/OQ cerebral glucose-oxygen quotient
CGP N-carbobenzoxy-glycyl-L-phenylalanine; chorionic growth hormone-prolactin; choline glycerophosphatide; circulating granulocyte pool
CGRP calcitonin gene-related peptide
CGS cardiogenic shock; catgut suture
CGS, cgs centimeter-gram-second [system]
CGT chorionic gonadotropin; cyclodextrin glucanotransferase
CGTT cortisone glucose tolerance test
cGy centigray (1 rad)
CH case history; Chediak-Higashi [syndrome]; chiasma; Chinese hamster; chloral hydrate; cholesterol; Christchurch chromosome; chronic hepatitis; chronic hypertension; common hepatic [duct]; communicating hydrocele; community health; completely healed; Conradi-Hünermann [syndrome]; continuous heparin [infusion]; crown-heel [length]; cycloheximide; cystic hygroma; wheelchair
C′H₅₀ $C'H_{50}$ 50% hemolyzing dose of complement
C_H C_H constant domain of H chain
C&H cocaine and heroin; coarse and harsh [breathing]
Ch chest; Chido [antibody]; chief; child; choline; Christchurch [syndrome]; chromosome
cH⁺ cH^+ hydrogen ion concentration
ch chest; child; chronic
CHA Catholic Hospital Association; Chinese hamster; chronic hemolytic anemia; common hepatic artery; congenital hypoplasia of adrenal glands; congenital hypoplastic anemia; continuously heated aerosol; cyclohexyladenosine; cyclohexylamine
ChA choline acetylase
ChAC choline acetyltransferase
CHAD cyclophosphamide, hexamethylmelamine, Adriamycin (doxorubicin), and cisplatin
CHAMP Children's Hospital Automated Medical Program
CHAMPUS Civilian Health and Medical Program of Uniformed Services
CHAMPVA Civilian Health and Medical Program of Veterans Administration
CHANDS curly hair–ankyblepharon–nail dysplasia syndrome
Chang C Chang conjunctiva cells
Chang L Chang liver cells
CHAP Certified Hospital Admission Program
CHARGE coloboma, heart disease, atresia choanae, retarded growth and retarded development and/or CNS anomalies, genital hypoplasia, and ear anomalies and/or deafness [syndrome]

chart paper [Lat. *charta*]

CHAS Center for Health Administration Studies

ChAT choline acetyltransferase

CHB chronic hepatitis B; complete heart block; congenital heart block

ChB Bachelor of Surgery [Lat. *Chirurgiae Baccalaureus*]

CHBHA congenital Heinz body hemolytic anemia

CHC community health center; community health computing; community health council

CH_3CCNU semustine

CHCP correctional health care program

CHD Chediak-Higashi disease; childhood disease; chronic hemodialysis; congenital or congestive heart disease; congenital hip dislocation; constitutional hepatic dysfunction; coronary heart disease; cyanotic heart disease

ChD Doctor of Surgery [Lat. *Chirurgiae Doctor*]

CHDM comprehensive hospital drug monitoring

ChE cholinesterase

che a gene involved in chemotaxis

CHEC community hypertension evaluation clinic

CHEF Chinese hamster embryo fibroblast

chem chemistry, chemical; chemotherapy

ChemID Chemical Identification

CHEMLINE Chemical Dictionary On-Line

CHEMTREC Chemical Transportation Emergency Center

CHERSS continuous high-amplitude EEG rhythmical synchronous slowing

CHF chick embryo fibroblast; chronic heart failure; congenital hepatic fibrosis; congestive heart failure; Crimean hemorrhagic fever

CHFD controlled high flux dialysis

CHFV combined high-frequency ventilation

chg change, changed

CHH cartilage-hair hypoplasia

CHI closed head injury

chi chimera

χ Greek letter *chi*

$χ^2$ chi-squared statistic; chi-squared [test, measure goodness of fit]

$χ_m$ magnetic susceptibility

$χ_s$ electric susceptibility

Chi-A chimpanzee leukocyte antigen

CHILD congenital hemidysplasia with ichthyosiform erythroderma and limb defects [syndrome]

CHIME coloboma, heart anomaly, ichthyosis, mental retardation, ear abnormality

CHINA chronic infectious neurotropic agent

CHIP comprehensive health insurance plan

CHIPASAT Children's Paced Auditory Serial Addition Task

CHIPS catastrophic health insurance plans

Chir Doct Doctor of Surgery [Lat. *Chirurgiae Doctor*]

chirug surgical [Lat. *chirurgicalis*]

CHL Chinese hamster lung; chlorambucil; chloramphenicol

Chl chloroform; chlorophyll

CHLA cyclohexyl linoleic acid

Chlb chlorobutanol

CHLD chronic hypoxic lung disease

chlor chloride

ChM Master of Surgery [Lat. *Chirurgiae Magister*]

CHMD clinical hyaline membrane disease

CHN carbon, hydrogen, and nitrogen; child neurology; Chinese [hamster]; community health nurse

CHO carbohydrate; Chinese hamster ovary; chorea

Cho choline

C_{H_2O} water clearance

choc chocolate

CHOL, chol cholesterol

c hold withhold

CHOP cyclophosphamide, hydroxydaunomycin, Oncovin, and prednisone

CHP capillary hydrostatic pressure; charcoal hemoperfusion; Chemical Hygiene Plan; child psychiatry; comprehensive health planning; coordinating hospital physician; cutaneous hepatic porphyria

ChP chest physician

chpx chickenpox

CHQ chloroquinol

CHR cerebrohepatorenal [syndrome]

Chr *Chromobacterium*

chr chromosome; chronic

c hr candle hour

c-hr curie-hour

ChRBC chicken red blood cell

CHRIS Cancer Hazards Ranking and Information System

chron chronic

CHRPE congenital hypertrophy of the retinal pigment epithelium

CHRS cerebrohepatorenal syndrome

CHS central hypoventilation syndrome; Chediak-Higashi syndrome; cholinesterase; chondroitin sulfate; compression hip screw; congenital hypoventilation syndrome; contact hypersensitivity

CHSD Children's Health Services Division

CHSO total hemolytic serum C activity

CHSS cooperative health statistics system

CHT combined hormone therapy; contralateral head turning

ChTg chymotrypsinogen

ChTK chicken thymidine kinase

CHU closed head unit

CHV canine herpes virus; centigrade heat unit

CI cardiac index; cardiac insufficiency; cell immunity; cell inhibition; cephalic index; cerebral infarction; chemotactic index; chemotherapeutic index; chromatid interchange; chronic infection; clinical investigator; clomipramine; clonus index; coefficient of intelligence; colloidal iron; color index; confidence interval; contamination index; continued insomnia; continuous infusion; convergence insufficiency; coronary insufficiency; corrected count increment; crystalline insulin; cumulative incidence; cytotoxic index

Ci curie

CIA chemiluminescent immunoassay; chymotrypsin inhibitor activity; colony-inhibiting activity; congenital intestinal aganglionosis

cib food [Lat. *cibus*]

CIBD chronic inflammatory bowel disease

CIBHA congenital inclusion-body hemolytic anemia

CIBP chronic intractable benign pain

CIBPS chronic intractable benign pain syndrome

CIC cardioinhibitor center; circulating immune complex; constant initial concentration; crisis intervention center

CICA cervical internal carotid artery

CICU cardiac intensive care unit; cardiovascular inpatient care unit; coronary intensive care unit

CID cellular immunodeficiency; chick infective dose; combined immunodeficiency disease; cytomegalic inclusion disease

CIDEP chemically induced dynamic electron polarization

CIDNP chemically induced dynamic nuclear polarization

CIDP chronic idiopathic polyradiculopathy; chronic inflammatory demyelinating polyradiculoneuropathy

CIDS cellular immunity deficiency syndrome; circular intensity differential scattering; continuous insulin delivery system

CIE cellulose ion exchange; countercurrent immunoelectrophoresis; counterimmunoelectrophoresis

CIEP counterimmunoelectrophoresis

CIF cloning inhibitory factor

CIFC Council for the Investigation of Fertility Control

CIG cold-insoluble globulin
CIg intracytoplasmic immunoglobulin
cIgM cytoplasmic immunoglobulin M
CIH carbohydrate-induced hyperglycer-idemia; Certificate in Industrial Health; children in hospital
ci-hr curie-hour
CIHS central infantile hypotonic syndrome
CII Carnegie Interest Inventory
CIIA common internal iliac artery
CIIP chronic idiopathic intestinal pseudo-obstruction
CIM cimetidine; cortically induced movement; Cumulated Index Medicus
Ci/ml curies per milliliter
CIMS chemical ionization mass spectrometry
CIN central inhibition; cervical intraepithelial neoplasia; chronic interstitial nephritis
CIN1, CIN I cervical intraepithelial neoplasia, grade 1 (mild dysplasia)
CIN 2, CIN II cervical intraepithelial neoplasia, grade 2 (moderate-severe)
CIN 3, CIN III cervical intraepithelial neoplasia, grade 3 (severe dysplasia and carcinoma in situ)
C_{in} insulin clearance
CINCA chronic infantile neurological cutaneous and auricular [syndrome]
CINE chemotherapy-induced nausea and emesis
CIOMS Council for International Organizations of Medical Sciences
CIP chronic idiopathic polyradiculoneu-ropathy; chronic intestinal pseudo-obstruction; Collection de l'Institut Pasteur
CIPD chronic inflammatory demyelin-ating polyneuropathy
CIPF clinical illness promoting factor
CIPN chronic inflammatory polyneuro-pathy
CIPSO chronic intestinal pseudo-obstruction
cir circular

circ circuit; circular; circumcision; circumference
circ & sens circulation and sensation
CIS carcinoma in situ; catheter-induced spasm; central inhibitory state; Chemical Information Service; clinical information system
CI-S calculus index, simplified
CiS cingulate sulcus
cis-DPP cisplatin
CISP chronic intractable shoulder pain
CIT citrate; combined intermittent therapy; conjugated-immunoglobulin technique
cit citrate
cit disp dispense quickly [Lat. *cito dispensetur*]
CIVII continuous intravenous insulin infusion
CIXA constant infusion excretory urogram
CJ conjunctivitis
CJD Creutzfeldt-Jakob disease
CJS Creutzfeldt-Jakob syndrome
CK calf kidney; chicken kidney; cholecystokinin; choline kinase; contralateral knee; creatine kinase; cyanogen chloride; cytokinin
ck check, checked
CKC cold-knife conization
CKG cardiokymography
CK-PZ cholecystokinin-pancreozymin
CKS classic form of Kaposi's sarcoma
CL capillary lumen; cardiolipin; cell line; centralis lateralis; chemiluminescence; chest and left arm [lead in electrocardiography]; cholelithiasis; cholesterol-lecithin; chronic leukemia; cirrhosis of liver; clavicle; clear liquid; clearance; cleft lip; clinical laboratory; clomipramine; complex loading; confidence limit or level; contact lens; corpus luteum; cricoid lamina; criterion level; critical list; cycle length; cytotoxic lymphocyte
C_L constant domain of L chain
Cl chloride; chlorine; clavicle; clear; clinic; *Clostridium*; closure; colistin

cl centiliter; clarified; clean; clear; cleft; clinic; clinical; clonus; clotting; cloudy

CLA Certified Laboratory Assistant; cervicolinguoaxial; contralateral local anesthesia; cyclic lysine anhydride

ClAc chloroacetyl

CLAH congenital lipoid adrenal hyperplasia

CLam cervical laminectomy

CLAS congenital localized absence of skin

class, classif classification

clav clavicle

CLB chlorambucil; curvilinear body

CLBBB complete left bundle branch block

CLBP chronic low back pain

CLC Charcot-Leyden crystal; Clerc-Levy-Cristesco [syndrome]

CL/CP cleft lip/cleft palate

CLD chronic liver disease; chronic lung disease; congenital limb deficiency; crystal ligand field

CLDH choline dehydrogenase

cldy cloudy

CLE centrilobular emphysema; continuous lumbar epidural [anesthesia]

CLED cystine-lactose-electrolyte-deficient [agar]

CLF cardiolipin fluorescent [antibody]; cholesterol-lecithin flocculation

CLH chronic lobular hepatitis; corpus luteum hormone; cutaneous lymphoid hyperplasia

CLI corpus luteum insufficiency

CLIA Clinical Laboratories Improvement Act

CLIF cloning inhibitory factor; *Crithidia luciliae* immunofluorescence

clin clinic, clinical

CLINPROT Clinical Cancer Protocols

CLIP corticotropin-like intermediate lobe peptide

CLL cholesterol-lowering lipid; chronic lymphatic leukemia; chronic lymphocytic leukemia; cow lung lavage

CLMA Clinical Laboratory Management Association

CLML Current List of Medical Literature

CLMV cauliflower mosaic virus

CLO cod liver oil

clo "clothing"–a unit of thermal insulation

CLOF clofibrate

CLON clonidine

Clon *Clonorchis*

Clostr *Clostridium*

CLP chymotrypsin-like protein; cleft lip with cleft palate; paced cycle length

CL(P) cleft lip without cleft palate

ClP clinical pathology

CLS Clinical Laboratory Scientist; Coffin-Lowry syndrome; Cornelia de Lange syndrome

CLSE calf lung surfactant extract

CLSH corpus luteum stimulating hormone

CLSL chronic lymphosarcoma (cell) leukemia

CLT Certified Laboratory Technician; chronic lymphocytic thyroiditis; Clinical Laboratory Technician; clot lysis time; clotting time

CL$_{TB}$ total body clearance

CLT(NCA) Laboratory Technician Certified by the National Certification Agency for Medical Laboratory Personnel

CLV cassava latent virus; constant linear velocity

CL VOID clean voided specimen [urine]

CLZ clozapine

CM California mastitis [test]; calmodulin; capreomycin; carboxymethyl; cardiac muscle; cardiomyopathy; carpometacarpal; Caucasian male; cause of death [Lat. *causa mortis*]; cell membrane; center of mass; cerebral malaria; cerebral mantle; cervical mucosa or mucus; Chick-Martin [coefficient]; chloroquinemepacrine; chondromalacia; chopped meat [medium]; circular muscle; circulating monocyte; circumferential measurement; clindamycin; clinical medicine; clinical modification; coccidioidal meningitis; cochlear microphonic; common migraine; complete medium; complications; conditioned medium; congenital malformation; congestive myocardiopathy; continuous murmur; contrast medium; copulatory mechanism; costal margin; cow's milk; cytometry; cytoplasmic membrane; Master of Surgery [Lat. *Chirurgiae Magister*]; narrow-diameter endosseous screw implant [Fr. *crête manche*]

C/M counts per minute

C&M cocaine and morphine

Cm curium

C$_m$ maximum clearance

cM *centi-morgan*

cm centimeter; costal margin; tomorrow morning [Lat. *cras mane*]

cm^2 square centimeter

cm^3 cubic centimeter

CMA Canadian Medical Association; Certified Medical Assistant; chronic metabolic acidosis; cow's milk allergy; cultured macrophages

CMAP compound muscle (or motor) action potential

Cmax, C$_{max}$ maximum concentration

CMB carbolic methylene blue; Central Midwives' Board; chloromercuribenzoate

CMC carboxymethylcellulose; care management continuity; carpometacarpal; cell-mediated cytolysis or cytotoxicity; chloramphenicol; chronic mucocutaneous candidiasis; critical micellar concentration

CMCC chronic mucocutaneous candidiasis

CMCt care management continuity across settings

CMD cartilage matrix deficiency; childhood muscular dystrophy; comparative mean dose; congenital muscular dystrophy; count median diameter

CME cervical mediastinal exploration; continuing medical education; Council on Medical Education; crude marijuana extract; cystoid macular edema

CMF calcium-magnesium free; catabolite modular factor; chondromyxoid fibroma; Christian Medical Fellowship; cold mitten fraction; cortical magnification factor; craniomandibulofacial; cyclophosphamide, methotrexate, and fluorouracil

CMFT cardiolipin microflocculation test

CMFV cyclophosphamide, methotrexate, fluorouracil, and vincristine

CMFVP cyclophosphamide, methotrexate, fluorouracil, vincristine, prednisone

CMG canine or congenital myasthenia gravis; chopped meat glucose [medium]; cystometrography, cystometrogram

CMGN chronic membranous glomerulonephritis

CMGS chopped meat-glucose-starch [medium]

CMGT chromosome-mediated gene transfer

CMH congenital malformation of the heart

CMHC community mental health center

cmH$_2$O centimeters of water

CMI carbohydrate metabolism index; care management integration; cell-mediated immunity; cell multiplication inhibition; chronic mesenteric ischemia; circulating microemboli index; colonic motility index; Commonwealth Mycological Institute; Cornell Medical Index

CMID cytomegalic inclusion disease

c/min cycles per minute

CMIR cell-mediated immune response

CMIT Current Medical Information and Terminology

CMJ carpometacarpal joint

CMK chloromethyl ketone; congenital multicystic kidney

CML cell-mediated lymphocytotoxicity; chronic myelocytic leukemia; chronic myelogenous leukemia

CMM cell-mediated mutagenesis; cutaneous malignant melanoma

cmm cubic millimeter

CMME chloromethyl methyl ether

CMML chronic myelomonocytic leukemia

CMMoL chronic myelomonocytic leukemia

CMMS Columbia Mental Maturity Scale

CMN caudal mediastinal node; cystic medial necrosis

CMNA complement-mediated neutrophil activation

CMN-AA cystic medial necrosis of ascending aorta

CMO cardiac minute output; Chief Medical Officer; comfort measures only; corticosterone methyloxidase

cMO centimorgan

CMOL chronic monocytic leukemia

CMOS complementary metal-oxide semiconductor

CMP cardiomyopathy; chondromalacia patellae; competitive medical plan; comprehensive medical plan; cytidine monophosphate

CMPD chronic myeloproliferative disorder

CMPGN chronic membranoproliferative glomerulonephritis

cmps centimeters per second

CMR cerebral metabolic rate; chief medical resident; common mode rejection; crude mortality ratio

CMRG cerebral metabolic rate of glucose

CMRglu cerebral metabolic rate of glucose

CMRL cerebral metabolic rate of lactate

CMRO, CMRO₂ cerebral metabolic rate of oxygen

CMRR common mode rejection ratio

CMS Christian Medical Society; chronic myelodysplastic syndrome; chromosome modification site; circulation, motion, sensation; clofibrate-induced muscular syndrome; Clyde Mood Scale; complement-mediated solubility

cms to be taken tomorrow morning [Lat. *cras mane sumendus*]

cm/s centimeters per second

cm/sec centimeters per second

CMSS circulation, motor ability, sensation, and swelling; Council of Medical Specialty Societies

CMT California mastitis test; cancer multistep therapy; catechol methyltransferase; cervical motion tenderness; Charcot-Marie-Tooth [syndrome]; circus movement tachycardia; complex motor unit; continuous memory test; Council on Medical Television; Current Medical Terminology

CMTC cutis marmorata telangiectatica congenita

CMTD Charcot-Marie-Tooth disease

CMTS Charcot-Marie-Tooth syndrome

CMU chlorophenyldimethylurea

CMUA continuous motor unit activity

CMV continuous mandatory ventilation; controlled mechanical ventilation; conventional mechanical ventilation; cool mist vaporizer; cucumber mosaic virus; cytomegalovirus

CMV-MN cytomegalovirus mononucleosis

CMX cefmenoxime

CN caudate nucleus; cellulose nitrate; charge nurse; child nutrition; chloroacetophenone; clinical nursing; cochlear nucleus; congenital nystagmus; cranial nerve; Crigler-Najjar [syndrome]; cyanogen; cyanosis neonatorum

C/N carbon/nitrogen [ratio]; carrier/ noise [ratio]

CN⁻ cyanide anion

cn tomorrow night [Lat. *cras nocte*]

CNA calcium nutrient agar; Canadian Nurses Association

CNAF chronic nonvalvular atrial fibrillation

CNAG chronic narrow angle glaucoma

CNAP compound nerve action potential

CNB cutting needle biopsy

CNCbl cyanocobalamin

CNDC chronic nonspecific diarrhea of childhood; chronic nonsuppurative destructive cholangitis

CNE chronic nervous exhaustion; concentric needle electrode

CNES chronic nervous exhaustion syndrome

CNF chronic nodular fibrositis; congenital nephrotic syndrome of the Finnish [type]

CNH central neurogenic hyperpnea; community nursing home

CNHD congenital nonspherocytic hemolytic disease

CNI center of nuclear image; chronic nerve irritation

CNK cortical necrosis of kidneys

CNL cardiolipin natural lecithin; chronic neutrophilic leukemia

CNM Certified Nurse-Midwife; computerized nuclear morphometry

CNMT Certified Nuclear Medicine Technologist

CNP community nurse practitioner; continuous negative pressure; cranial nerve palsy; 2',3'-cyclic nucleotide 3'-phosphodiesterase

CNPase 2',3'-cyclic nucleotide 3'-phosphohydrolase

CNPV continuous negative pressure ventilation

CNRT corrected sinus node recovery time

CNS central nervous system; clinical nurse specialist; coagulase-negative staphylococci; congenital nephrotic syndrome; sulfocyanate

cns to be taken tomorrow night [Lat. *cras nocte sumendus*]

CNSHA congenital nonspherocytic hemolytic anemia

CNS-L central nervous system leukemia

CNSLD chronic nonspecific lung disease

CNV choroidal neovascularization; contingent negative variation; cutaneous necrotizing vasculitis

CO carbon monoxide; cardiac output; castor oil; casualty officer; centric occlusion; cervicoaxial; choline oxidase; coccygeal; coenzyme; compound; control; corneal opacity; cross over

C/O check out; complains of; in care of

CO₂ carbon dioxide

Co cobalt

co compounded, a compound [Lat. *compositus*]

Co I coenzyme I

Co II coenzyme II

COA Canadian Ophthalmological Association; Canadian Orthopaedic Association; cervico-oculo-acusticus [syndrome]; condition on admission

CoA coenzyme A

COAD chronic obstructive airway disease

COAG chronic open angle glaucoma

coag coagulation, coagulated

CoASH uncombined coenzyme A

CoA-SPC coenzyme A-synthetizing protein complex

COAT Children's Orientation and Amnesia Test

COB chronic obstructive bronchitis; coordination of benefits

coban cohesive bandage

COBOL common business oriented language

COBRA Consolidated Omnibus Reconciliation Act

COBS cesarean-obtained barrier-sustained; chronic organic brain syndrome

COBT chronic obstruction of the biliary tract

COC cathodal opening contraction; coccygeal; combination oral contraceptive

cochl a spoonful [Lat. *cochleare*]

cochl amp a heaping spoonful [Lat. *cochleare amplum*]

cochl mag a tablespoonful [Lat. *cochleare magnum*]

cochl med a dessertspoonful [Lat. *cochleare medium*]

cochl mod a dessertspoonful [Lat. *Cochleare modicum*]

cochl parv a teaspoonful [Lat. *cochleare parvum*]

COCI Consortium on Chemical Information

COCl cathodal opening clonus

COCM congestive cardiomyopathy

coct boiling [Lat. *coctio*]

COD cause of death; chemical oxygen demand; codeine; condition on discharge
cod codeine
COD-MD cerebro-ocular dysplasia-muscular dystrophy [syndrome]
CODATA Committee on Data for Science and Technology
coeff coefficient
COEPS cortical originating extrapyramidal system
COF cutoff frequency
CoF cobra factor; cofactor
COFS cerebro-oculo-facial-skeletal [syndrome]
COG cognitive function tests
CoGME Council on Graduate Medical Education
COGTT cortisone oral glucose tolerance test
COH carbohydrate
CoHb carboxyhemoglobin
COHSE Confederation of Health Service Employees
COI Central Obesity Index
COIF congenital onychodysplasia of the index finger
col collection; colicin; collagen; colony; colored; column; strain [Lat. *cola*]
colat strained [Lat. *colatus*]
COLD chronic obstructive lung disease
COLD A cold agglutinin titer
colet let it be strained [Lat. *coletur*]
coll collateral; collection, collective; college; colloidal
collat collateral
collun nosewash [Lat. *collunarium*]
collut mouthwash [Lat. *collutorium*]
collyr eyewash [Lat. *collyrium*]
color colorimetry; let it be colored [Lat. *coloretur*]
COM chronic otitis media; College of Osteopathic Medicine; computer-output microfilm
com comminuted; commitment
comb combination, combine
COMC carboxymethylcellulose
comf comfortable
comm, commun communicable

COMP complication
comp comparative; compensation, compensated; complaint; complete; composition; compound, compounded; comprehension; compress; computer
compd compound, compounded
compl complaint; complete, completed, completion; complication, complicated
complic complication, complicated
compn composition
compr compression
COMS cerebrooculomuscular syndrome
COMT catechol-O-methyltransferase
COMTRAC computer-based case tracing
COMUL complement fixation murine leukosis [test]
CON certificate of need
Con concanavalin
con against [Lat. *contra*]
Con A concanavalin A
Con A-HRP concanavalin A-horseradish peroxidase
C-onc cellular oncogene
conc, concentr concentrate, concentrated, concentration
concis cut [Lat. *concisus*]
cond condensation, condensed; condition, conditioned; conductivity; conductor
conf conference; confined; confinement; confusion
cong congested, congestion; gallon [Lat. *congius*]
congen congenital
coniz conization
conj conjunctiva, conjunctival
conjug conjugated, conjugation
CONPA-DRI I vincristine, doxorubicin, and melphalan
CONPA-DRI III conpa-dri I plus intensified doxorubicin
CONS consultation; consultant
cons conservation; conservative; consultation; keep [Lat. *conserva*]
consperg dust, sprinkle [Lat. *consperge*]
const constant

constit constituent

consult consultant, consultation

cont against [Lat. *contra*]; bruised [Lat. *contusus*]; contains, contents; continue, continuation

contag contagion, contagious

conter rub together [Lat. *contere*]

contin let it be continued [Lat. *continuetur*]

contr contracted, contraction

contra contraindicated

contralat contralateral

cont rem let the medicine be continued [Lat. *continuetur remedium*]

contrib contributory

contrit broken down [Lat. *contritus*]

contus bruised [Lat. *contusus*]

conv convalescence, convalescent, convalescing; convergence, convergent; convulsions, convulsive

converg convergence, convergent

COOD chronic obstruction outflow disease

COOP cooperative

coord coordination, coordinated

COP capillary osmotic pressure; change of plaster; coefficient of performance; colloid oncotic pressure; colloid osmotic pressure; cyclophosphamide, Oncovin, and prednisone

COPA Council on Postsecondary Accreditation

COPC community oriented primary care

COPD chronic obstructive pulmonary disease

COPE chronic obstructive pulmonary emphysema

COP$_i$ colloid osmotic pressure in interstitial fluid

COPP cyclophosphamide, vincristine, procarbazine, and prednisone

COP$_p$ colloid osmotic pressure in plasma

COPRO coproporphyrin

CoQ coenzyme Q

coq boil [Lat. *coque*]

coq in s a boil in sufficient water [Lat. *coque in sufficiente aqua*]

coq s a boil properly [Lat. *coque secundum artem*]

COR body [Lat. *corpus*]; cardiac output recorder; comprehensive outpatient rehabilitation; conditioned orientation reflex; consensual ophthalmotonic reaction; corrosion, corrosive; cortisone; cortex; custodian of records

CoR Congo red

cor body [Lat. *corpus*]; coronary; correction, corrected;

CORA conditioned orientation reflex audiometry

CORD Commissioned Officer Residency Deferment

corr correspondence, corresponding

CORT corticosterone

cort bark [Lat. *cortex*]; cortex

COS cheiro-oral syndrome; chief of staff; Clinical Orthopaedic Society; clinically observed seizures

COSATI Committee on Scientific and Technical Information

COSMIS Computer System for Medical Information Systems

COSTAR Computer-Stored Ambulatory Record

COSTEP Commissioned Officer Student Training and Extern Program

COT colony overlay test; content of thought; contralateral optic tectum; critical off-time

COTA Certified Occupational Therapy Assistant

COTD cardiac output by thermodilution

COTe cathodal opening tetanus

COTRANS Coordinated Transfer Application System

coul coulomb

COV cross-over value

COVESDEM costovertebral segmentation defect with mesomelia [syndrome]

CoVF cobra venom factor

COWS cold to opposite and warm to same side

COX cytochrome c oxidase

CP candle power; capillary pressure; cardiac pacing; cardiac performance;

cardiopulmonary; caudate putamen; cell passage; central pit; cerebellopontine; cerebral palsy; ceruloplasmin; chemically pure; chest pain; child psychiatry; child psychology; chloropurine; chloroquine-primaquine; chondrodysplasia punctata; chronic pain; chronic pancreatitis; chronic polyarthritis; chronic pyelonephritis; cicatricial pemphigoid; cleft palate; clinical pathology; clock pulse; closing pressure; cochlear potential; code of practice; cold pressor; color perception; combining power; compound; compressed; congenital porphyria; constant pressure; coproporphyrin; cor pulmonale; coracoid process; C peptide; creatine phosphate; creatine phosphokinase; crosslinked protein; crude protein; current practice; cyclophosphamide; cyclophosphamide and prednisone; cytosol protein

C&P compensation and pension; complete and pain free [joint movement]; cystoscopy and pyelography

C/P cholesterol-phospholipid [ratio]

Cp ceruloplasmin; chickenpox; *Corynebacterium parvum;* peak concentration

C$_p$ constant pressure; phosphate clearance

cP centipoise

cp candle power; chemically pure; centipoise; compare

c$_p$ constant pressure

CPA Canadian Psychiatric Association; cardiopulmonary arrest; carotid phonoangiography; cerebellopontine angle; chlorophenylalanine; circulating platelet aggregate; complement proactivator; costophrenic angle; cyclophosphamide; cyproterone acetate

C3PA complement-3 proactivator

CPAF chlorpropamide-alcohol flushing

C$_{pah}$ para-aminohippurate clearance

CPAP continuous positive airway pressure

CPB cardiopulmonary bypass; cetylpyridinium bromide; competitive protein binding

CPBA competitive protein-binding analysis

CPBV cardiopulmonary blood volume

CPC central posterior curve; cerebellar Purkinje cell; cerebral palsy clinic; cetylpyridinium chloride; chronic passive congestion; circumferential pneumatic compression; clinicopathological conference

CPCL congenital pulmonary cystic lymphangiectasia

CPCP chronic progressive coccidioidal pneumonitis

CPCR cardiopulmonary cerebral resuscitation

CPCS circumferential pneumatic compression suit

CPD calcium pyrophosphate deposition; cephalopelvic disproportion; childhood or congenital polycystic disease; chorioretinopathy and pituitary dysfunction; chronic peritoneal dialysis; chronic protein deprivation; citrate-phosphate-dextrose; contact potential difference; contagious pustular dermatitis; critical point drying; cyclopentadiene

cpd compound; cycles per degree

CPDA citrate-phosphate-dextrose-adenine

CPDD calcium pyrophosphate deposition disease; cis-platinum-diamine dichloride

cpd E compound E

cpd F compound F

CPDL cumulative population doubling level

CPDX cefpodoxime

CPDX-PR cefpodoxime proxetil

CPE cardiac pulmonary edema; chronic pulmonary emphysema; compensation, pension, and education; complete physical examination; corona-penetrating enzyme; cytopathogenic effect

CPEO chronic progressive external ophthalmoplegia

CPF clot-promoting factor; contraction peak force

CPG capillary blood gases; cardiopneumographic recording; carotid phonoangiogram

CPGN chronic proliferative glomerulonephritis

CPH Certificate in Public Health; chronic paroxysmal hemicrania; chronic persistent hepatitis; chronic primary headache; corticotropin-releasing hormone

CPHA Commission on Professional and Hospital Activities

CPHA-PAS Commission on Professional and Hospital Activities–Professional Activity Study

CPI California Personality Inventory; Cancer Potential Index; congenital palatopharyngeal incompetence; constitutional psychopathic inferiority; coronary prognosis index; cysteine proteinase inhibitor

CPIB chlorophenoxyisobutyrate

CPIP chronic pulmonary insufficiency of prematurity

CPIR cephalic-phase insulin release

CPK creatine phosphokinase

CPKD childhood polycystic kidney disease

CPL caprine placental lactogen; conditioned pitch level; congenital pulmonary lymphangiectasia

C/PL cholesterol/phospholipid [ratio]

cpl complete, completed

CPLM cysteine-peptone-liver infusion medium

CPM central pontine myelinosis; chlorpheniramine maleate; continuous passive motion; cyclophosphamide

cpm counts per minute; cycles per minute

CPMP complete patient management problems

CPMS chronic progressive multiple sclerosis

CPMV cowpea mosaic virus

CPN chronic polyneuropathy; chronic pyelonephritis

CPNM corrected perinatal mortality

CPP cancer proneness phenotype; canine pancreatic polypeptide; cerebral perfu-

sion pressure; dl-2[3-(2'-chlorophenoxy)phenyl] propionic [acid]; chronic pigmented purpura; cyclopentenophenanthrene

CPPB continuous positive pressure breathing

CPPD calcium pyrophosphate dihydrate deposition [syndrome]; cisplatin

CPPV continuous positive pressure ventilation

CPR cardiopulmonary reserve; cardiopulmonary resuscitation; centripetal rub; cerebral cortex perfusion rate; chlorophenyl red; cortisol production rate; cumulative patency rate; customary, prevailing and reasonable [rate]

c-PR cyclopropyl

CPRAM controlled partial rebreathing anesthesia method

CPRCA constitutional pure red cell aplasia

CPRD Committee on Prosthetics Research and Development

CPRS Children's Psychiatric Rating Scale; Comprehensive Psychopathological Rating Scale

CPS carbamyl phosphate synthetase; cardioplegic perfusion solution; centipoise; cervical pain syndrome; characters per second; chest pain syndrome; Child Personality Scale; Child Protective Services; chloroquine, pyrimethamine, and sulfisoxazole; chronic prostatitis syndrome; clinical performance score; Clinical Pharmacy Services; coagulase-positive *Staphylococcus*; complex partial seizures; constitutional psychopathic state; contagious pustular stomatitis; C-polysaccharide; cumulative probability of success; current population survey

cps counts per second; cycles per second

CPSC congenital paucity of secondary synaptic clefts [syndrome]; Consumer Products Safety Commission

CPSP central poststroke pain

CPT carnitine palmityl transferase; carotid pulse tracing; chest physiotherapy; ciliary particle transport; cold pressor test; combining power test; continuous performance test; Current Procedural Terminology

CPTH chronic post-traumatic headache

CPTN culture-positive toxin-negative

CPTP culture-positive toxin-positive

CPTX chronic parathyroidectomy

CPU caudate putamen; central processing unit

CPUE chest pain of unknown etiology

CPV canine parvovirus; cytoplasmic polyhedrosis virus

CPVD congenital polyvalvular disease

CPX complete physical examination

CPZ cefoperazone; chlorpromazine; Compazine

CQ chloroquine; chloroquine-quinine; circadian quotient; conceptual quotient

CQI continuous quality improvement

CQM chloroquine mustard

CR calculation rate; calculus removed; calorie-restricted; cardiac rehabilitation; cardiac resuscitation; cardiac rhythm; cardiorespiratory; cardiorrhexis; caries-resistant; cathode ray; centric relation; chest and right arm [lead in electrocardiography]; chest roentgenogram, chest roentgenography; chief resident; child-resistant [bottle top]; choice reaction; chromium; chronic rejection; clinical record; clinical research; clot retraction; coefficient of fat retention; colon resection; colonization resistance; colony reared [animal]; colorectal; complement receptor; complete remission; complete response; conditioned reflex, conditioned response; congenital rubella; Congo red; controlled release; controlled respiration; conversion rate; cooling rate; cortico-resistant; creatinine; cremaster reflex; cresyl red; critical ratio; crown-rump [measurement]

C&R convalescence and rehabilitation

Cr chromium; cranium, cranial; creatinine; crown

CRA central retinal artery; Chinese restaurant asthma; chronic rheumatoid arthritis; constant relative alkalinity

CRABP cellular retinoic acid-binding protein

cran cranium, cranial

CRAO central retinal artery occlusion

crast for tomorrow [Lat. *crastinus*]

CRB chemical, radiological, and biological

CRBBB complete right bundle branch block

CRBC chicken red blood cell

CRBP cellular retinol-binding protein

CRC cardiovascular reflex conditioning; clinical research center; colorectal carcinoma; concentrated red blood cells; cross-reacting cannabinoids

CrCl creatinine clearance

CRCS cardiovascular reflex conditioning system

CRD chronic renal disease; chronic respiratory disease; child restraint device; childhood rheumatic disease; chorioretinal degeneration; chronic renal disease; chronic respiratory disease; complete reaction of degeneration; congenital rubella deafness; cone-rod dystrophy; crown-rump distance

CR-DIP chronic relapsing demyelinating inflammatory polyneuropathy

CRE cumulative radiation effect

creat creatinine

crem cremaster

crep crepitation; crepitus

CREST calcinosis, Raynaud's phenomenon, esophageal involvement, sclerodactyly, and telangiectasia [syndrome]

CRF case report form; chronic renal failure; chronic respiratory failure; coagulase-reacting factor; continuous reinforcement; corticotropin-releasing factor

CRFK Crandell feline kidney cells

CRG cardiorespirogram

CRH corticotropin-releasing hormone

CRHL Collaborative Radiological Health Laboratory

CRHV cottontail rabbit herpes virus

CRI Cardiac Risk Index; catheter-related infection; chronic renal insufficiency; chronic respiratory insufficiency; Composite Risk Index; congenital rubella infection; cross-reaction idiotype

CRIE crossed radioimmunoelectrophoresis

CRISP Computer Retrieval of Information on Scientific Projects

Crit, crit critical; hematocrit

CRL cell repository line; Certified Record Librarian; complement receptor location; complement receptor lymphocyte; crown-rump length

CRM Certified Reference Materials; counting rate meter; cross-reacting material; crown-rump measurement

CRMO chronic recurrent multifocal osteomyelitis

CRN complement requiring neutralization

CRNA Certified Registered Nurse Anesthetist

cRNA chromosomal ribonucleic acid

CRNF chronic rheumatoid nodular fibrositis

Cr Nn, cr nn cranial nerves

CRO cathode ray oscilloscope; centric relation occlusion

CROM cervical range of motion

CROS contralateral routing of signal

CRP chronic relapsing pancreatitis; corneal-retinal potential; coronary rehabilitation program; C-reactive protein; cross-reacting protein; cyclic AMP receptor protein

CrP creatine phosphate

CRPA C-reactive protein antiserum

CRPD chronic restrictive pulmonary disease

CRPF chloroquine-resistant *Plasmodium falciparum;* contralateral renal plasma flow

CRS catheter-related sepsis; caudal regression syndrome; Chinese restaurant syndrome; colon and rectum surgery; compliance of the respiratory system; congenital rubella syndrome

CRSM cherry red spot myoclonus

CRSP comprehensive renal scintillation procedure

CRST calcinosis, Raynaud's phenomenon, sclerodactyly, telangiectasia [syndrome]; corrected sinus recovery time

CRT cardiac resuscitation team; cathode-ray tube; certified; Certified Record Techniques; choice reaction time; chromium release test; complex reaction time; computerized renal tomography; copper reduction test; corrected; corrected retention time; cortisone resistant thymocyte; cranial radiation therapy

crt hematocrit

CRTP Consciousness Research and Training Project

CRTT Certified Respiratory Therapy Technician

CRU cardiac rehabilitation unit; clinical research unit

CRV central retinal vein

CRVF congestive right ventricular failure

CRVO central retinal vein occlusion

cryo cryogenic; cryoglobulin; cryoprecipitate; cryosurgery; cryotherapy

crys, cryst crystal, crystalline

CS calf serum; campomelic syndrome; carcinoid syndrome; cardiogenic shock; caries-susceptible; carotid sheath; carotid sinus; cat scratch; celiac sprue; central service; central supply; cerebrospinal; cervical spine; cervical stimulation; cesarean section; chest strap; chief of staff; cholesterol stone; chondroitin sulfate; chorionic somatomammotropin; chronic schizophrenia; cigarette smoker; citrate synthase; climacteric syndrome; clinical laboratory scientist; clinical stage; Cockayne syndrome; complete stroke; compression syndrome; concentrated strength; conditioned stimulus; congenital syphilis; conjunctival secretion; conscious, consciousness; constant spring; contact sensitivity; continue same; contrast sensitivity; control serum; convalescence, convalescent; coronary sclerosis; coronary sinus; corpus striatum; corticoid-sensitive; corticosteroid; crush syndrome; current smoker; current strength;

Cushing's syndrome; cycloserine; cyclosporine

C/S cesarean section; cycles per second

C&S calvarium and scalp; conjunctiva and sclera; culture and sensitivity

CS IV clinical stage 4

C4S chondroitin-4-sulfate

Cs case; cell surface; cesium; cyclosporine

C$_s$ standard clearance; static respiratory compliance

cS centistoke

cs chromosome; consciousness

CSA canavaninosuccinic acid; carbonyl salicylamide; cell surface antigen; chondroitin sulfate A; colony-stimulating activity; compressed spectral assay; computerized spectral analysis; cross section area; cyclosporine A

CsA cyclosporine A

CSAA Child Study Association of America

CSAVP cerebral subarachnoid venous pressure

CSB contaminated small bowel

csb chromosome break

CSBF coronary sinus blood flow

CSBS contaminated small bowel syndrome

CSC blow on blow (administration of small amounts of drugs at short intervals) [Fr. *coup sur coup*]; collagen sponge contraceptive; corticostriatocerebellar; cryogenic storage container

CSCD Center for Sickle Cell Disease

CSCR Central Society for Clinical Research

CSD carotid sinus denervation; cat scratch disease; combined system disease; conditionally streptomycin dependent; conduction system disease; cortical spreading depression; craniospinal defect; critical stimulus duration

CSDB cat scratch disease bacillus

CSE clinical-symptom/self-evaluation [questionnaire]; cone-shaped epiphysis; cross-sectional echocardiography

C sect, C-section cesarean section

CSEP cortical somatosensory evoked potential

CSER cortical somatosensory evoked response

CSF cancer family syndrome; cerebrospinal fluid; cold stability factor; colony-stimulating factor; coronary sinus flow

CSFH cerebrospinal fluid hypotension

CSFP cerebrospinal fluid pressure

CSFV cerebrospinal fluid volume

CSF-WR cerebrospinal fluid-Wassermann reaction

csg chromosome gap

CSGBI Cardiac Society of Great Britain and Ireland

CSGBM collagenase soluble glomerular basement membrane

CSH carotid sinus hypersensitivity; chronic subdural hematoma; cortical stromal hyperplasia

CSHH congenital self-healing histiocytosis

CSI calculus surface index; cancer serum index; cavernous sinus infiltration; cholesterol saturation index; computerized severity of illness [index]; coronary sinus intervention

CSICU cardiac surgical intensive care unit

CSII continuous subcutaneous insulin infusion

CSIIP continuous subcutaneous insulin infusion pump

CSIN Chemical Substances Information Network

CSIS clinical supplies and inventory system

CSL cardiolipin synthetic lecithin; corticosteroid liposome

CSLM confocal scanning microscopy

CSLU chronic stasis leg ulcer

CSM carotid sinus massage; cerebrospinal meningitis; circulation, sensation, motion; Committee on Safety of Medicines; corn-soy milk

CSMA chronic spinal muscular atrophy

CSMB Center for the Study of Multiple Births

CSMMG Chartered Society of Massage and Medical Gymnastics

CSMP chloramphenicol-sensitive microsomal protein

CSMT chorionic somatomammotropin

CSN cardiac sympathetic nerve; carotid sinus nerve

CSNA congenital sensory neuropathy with anhidrosis [syndrome]

CSNB congenital stationary night blindness

CS(NCA) Clinical Laboratory Scientist Certified by the National Certification Agency for Medical Laboratory Personnel

CSNRT, cSNRT corrected sinus node recovery time

CSNS carotid sinus nerve stimulation

CSO claims services only; common source outbreak

CSOM chronic suppurative otitis media

CSOP coronary sinus occlusion pressure

CSP carotid sinus pressure; cavum septi pellucidi; cell surface protein; cerebrospinal protein; Chartered Society of Physiotherapy; chemistry screening panel; chondroitin sulfate protein; Cooperative Statistical Program; criminal sexual psychopath; cyclosporin

Csp, C-spine cervical spine

CSPS continual skin peeling syndrome

CSR central supply room; Cheyne-Stokes respiration; continued stay review; corrected sedimentation rate; corrected survival rate; cortisol secretion rate; cumulative survival rate

CSRT corrected sinus recovery time

CSS Cancer Surveillance System; carotid sinus stimulation; carotid sinus syndrome; cavernous sinus syndrome; central sterile supply; chewing, sucking, swallowing; chronic subclinical scurvy; Churg-Strauss syndrome; cranial sector scan

CSSD central sterile supply department

CST cardiac stress test; cavernous sinus thrombosis; Christ-Siemens Touraine [syndrome]; compliance, static; computer scatter tomography; contraction stress test; convulsive shock therapy; corticospinal tract; cosyntropin stimulation test

C_{st} static compliance

cSt centistoke

C_{stat} static compliance

CSTI Clearinghouse for Scientific and Technical Information

CSTT cold-stimulation time test

CSU casualty staging unit; catheter specimen of urine; central statistical unit; clinical specialty unit

CSUF continuous slow ultrafiltration

CSV chick syncytial virus

CSW Certified Social Worker; current sleep walker

CT calcitonin; calf testis; cardiac tamponade; cardiothoracic [ratio]; carotid tracing; carpal tunnel; cell therapy; cerebral thrombosis; cerebral tumor; cervical traction; cervicothoracic; chemotherapy; chest tube; chicken tumor; *Chlamydia trachomatis*; chlorothiazide; cholera toxin; cholesterol, total; chordae tendineae; chronic thyroiditis; chymotrypsin; circulation time; classic technique; closed thoracotomy; clotting time; coagulation time; coated tablet; cobra toxin; cognitive therapy; coil test; collecting tubule; colon, transverse; combined tumor; compressed tablet; computed tomography; connective tissue; continue treatment; continuous-flow tub; contraceptive technique; contraction time; controlled temperature; Coombs' test; corneal transplant; coronary thrombosis; corrected transposition; corrective therapy; cortical thickness; cough threshold; crest time; cystine-tellurite; cytotechnologist; cytotoxic therapy; unit of attenuation [number]

C/T compression/traction [ratio]

C&T color and temperature

Ct carboxyl terminal

ct carat; chromatid; count

C_{T-1824} T-1824 (Evans blue) clearance

CTA Canadian Tuberculosis Association; chemotactic activity; chromotropic acid; Committee on Thrombolytic Agents; congenital trigeminal anesthesia; cyano-trimethyl-androsterone; cystine trypti-case agar; cytoplasmic tubular aggre-gate; cytotoxic assay

Cta menses [Lat. *catamenia*]

CTAB cetyltrimethyl-ammonium bro-mide

CTAC Cancer Treatment Advisory Committee

cTAL cortical thick ascending limb

c tant with the same amount [Lat. *cum tanto*]

CTAP connective tissue activating pep-tide

CTAT computerized transaxial tomog-raphy

CTB ceased to breathe

ctb chromated break

CTC chlortetracycline; Clinical Trial Certificate; computer-aided tomographic cisternography; cultured T cells

CTCL cutaneous T-cell lymphoma

ctCO₂ carbon dioxide concentration

CTD carpal tunnel decompression; chest tube drainage; congenital thymic dyspla-sia; connective tissue disease

CT&DB cough, turn, and deep breathe

ctDNA chloroplast deoxyribonucleic acid

CTE calf thymus extract; cultured thy-mic epithelium

CTEM conventional transmission elec-tron microscopy

CTF cancer therapy facility; certificate; Colorado tick fever; cytotoxic factor

ctf certificate

CTFE chlorotrifluoroethylene

CTFS complete testicular feminization syndrome

CTG cardiotocography; cervicothoracic ganglion; chymotrypsinogen

C/TG cholesterol-triglyceride [ratio]

ctg chromated gap

CTGA complete transposition of great arteries

CTH ceramide trihexoside; chronic ten-sion headache

CTh carrier-specific T-helper [cell]

CTHD chlorthalidone

CTL cervico-thoraco-lumbar; cytotoxic T-lymphocyte

CTLL cytotoxic lymphoid line

CTM cardiotachometer; Chlortrimeton; cricothyroid muscle

CTMM computed tomographic metri-zamide myelography

CTMM-SF California Test of Mental Maturity–Short Form

CTN calcitonin; computer tomography number; continuous noise

cTNM TNM (*q.v.*) staging of tumors as determined by clinical noninvasive examination

CTP California Test of Personality; comprehensive treatment plan; cytidine triphosphate; cytosine triphosphate

C-TPN cyclic total parenteral nutrition

CTPP cerebral tissue perfusion pressure

CTPVO chronic thrombotic pulmonary vascular obstruction

CTR cardiothoracic ratio; carpal tunnel release; central tumor registry

ctr central; center; centric

CTRB chymotrypsinogen B

CTRX ceftriaxone

CTS carpal tunnel syndrome; composite treatment score; computed tomographic scan; contralateral threshold shift; cor-ticosteroid

CTSNFR corrected time of sinoatrial node function recovery

CTT cefotetan; central tegmental tract; central transmission time; compressed tablet triturate; computerized transaxial tomography; critical tracking time

CTU cardiac-thoracic unit; centigrade thermal unit; constitutive transcription unit

CTV cervical and thoracic vertebrae

CTW central terminal of Wilson; com-bined testicular weight

CTX cefotaxime; cerebrotendinous xan-thomatosis; chemotaxis; costotendinous xanthomatosis; cyclophosphamide

CTx cardiac transplantation; conotoxin

CTZ chemoreceptor trigger zone; chlorothiazide

CU cardiac unit; casein unit; cause unknown or undetermined; chymotrypsin unit; clinical unit; color unit; contact urticaria; convalescent unit

Cu copper [Lat. *cuprum*]

C_u urea clearance

cu cubic

CuB copper band

CUC chronic ulcerative colitis

cu cm cubic centimeter

CUD cause undetermined; congenital urinary deformity

CuD copper deficiency

CUE cumulative urinary excretion

CUG cystidine, uridine, and guanidine; cystourethrogram, cystourethrography

CUI Cox-Uphoff International [tissue expander]

cu in cubic inch

cuj of which [Lat. *cujus*]

cuj lib of whatever you please [Lat. *cujus libet*]

cult culture

cum cumulative

cu m cubic meter

CUMITECH Cumulative Techniques and Procedures in Clinical Microbiology

cu mm cubic millimeter

CUP carcinoma unknown primary

CUR cystourethrorectal

cur cure, curative; current

CURN Conduct and Utilization of Research in Nursing

CUS carotid ultrasound examination; catheterized urine specimen; contact urticaria syndrome

CuS copper supplement

CUSA Cavitron ultrasonic aspirator

CuTS cubital tunnel syndrome

CV cardiac volume; cardiovascular; carotenoid vesicle; cell volume; central venous; cerebrovascular; cervical vertebra; Chikungunya virus; closing volume; coefficient of variation; color vision; concentrated volume; conducting vein; conduction velocity; contrast ventricu-

lography; conventional ventilation; corpuscular volume; costovertebral; cresyl violet; crystal violet; cutaneous vasculitis; tomorrow evening [Lat. *cras vespere*]; true conjugate [diameter of the pelvic inlet] [Lat. *conjugata vera*]

C/V coulomb per volt

Cv specific heat at constant volume

C_v constant volume

cv cultivar

CVA cardiovascular accident; cerebrovascular accident; chronic villous arthritis; costovertebral angle; cyclophosphamide, vincristine, and Adriamycin

CVAH congenital virilizing adrenal hyperplasia

CVAP cerebrovascular amyloid peptide

CVAT costovertebral angle tenderness

CVB chorionic villi biopsy

CVC central venous catheter

CV cath central venous catheter

CVCT cardiovascular computed tomography

CVD cardiovascular disease; cerebrovascular disease; color-vision-deviant

CVF cardiovascular failure; central visual field; cervicovaginal fluid; cobra venom factor

CVG contrast ventriculography; coronary venous graft

CVH cerebroventricular hemorrhage; cervicovaginal hood; combined ventricular hypertrophy; common variable hypogammaglobulinemia

CVHD chronic valvular heart disease

CVI cardiovascular incident; cardiovascular insufficiency; cerebrovascular incident; cerebrovascular insufficiency; chronic venous insufficiency; common variable immunodeficiency

CVID common variable immunodeficiency

CVLT California Verbal Learning Test; clinical vascular laboratory

CVM cardiovascular monitor; cerebral venous malformation; cyclophosphamide, vincristine, and methotrexate

CVMP Committee on Veterans Medical Problems

CVO central vein occlusion; central venous oxygen; Chief Veterinary Officer; obstetric conjugate [of the pelvic inlet] [Lat. *conjugata vera obstetrica*]

CVOD cerebrovascular obstructive disease

CVP cardioventricular pacing; cell volume profile; central venous pressure; cyclophosphamide, vincristine, and prednisone

cvPO$_2$, cvP$_{O_2}$ cerebral venous partial pressure of oxygen

CVR cardiovascular-renal; cardiovascular-respiratory; cephalic vasomotor response; cerebrovascular resistance

CVRD cardiovascular-renal disease

CVRR cardiovascular recovery room

CVS cardiovascular surgery; cardiovascular system; challenge virus strain; chorionic villi sampling; clean voided specimen; current vital signs

CVT central venous temperature; congenital vertical talus

CVTR charcoal viral transport medium

CW cardiac work; case work; cell wall; chemical warfare; chemical weapon; chest wall; children's ward; clockwise; continuous wave; crutch walking

C/W compare with; consistent with

CWBTS capillary whole blood true sugar

CWD cell wall defect; continuous-wave Doppler

CWDF cell wall-deficient form [bacteria]

CWF Cornell Word Form

CWH cardiomyopathy and wooly haircoat [syndrome]

CWHB citrated whole human blood

CWI cardiac work index

CWL cutaneous water loss

CWMS color, warmth, movement sensation

CWOP childbirth without pain

CWP childbirth without pain; coal worker's pneumoconiosis

CWPEA Childbirth Without Pain Education Association

CWS cell wall skeleton; chest wall stimulation; child welfare service; cold water-soluble; cotton wool spots

CWT cold water treatment

Cwt, cwt hundredweight

CWXSP Coal Workers' X-ray Surveillance Program

CX cervix; chest x-ray; critical experiment

Cx cervix; circumflex; clearance; complaint; complex; convex

cx complex; cylinder axis

CXR chest x-ray

CY casein-yest autolysate [medium]; cyclophosphamide

Cy cyanogen; cyclophosphamide; cyst; cytarabine

cy, cyan cyanosis

CyA cyclosporine A

cyath a glassful [Lat. *cyathus*]

CYC cyclophosphamide

cyc cyclazocine; cycle; cyclotron

CYCLO, Cyclo cyclophosphamide; cyclopropane

Cyclo C cyclocytidine hydrochloride

Cyd cytidine

CYE charcoal yeast extract [agar]

CYL casein yeast lactate

cyl cylinder; cylindrical lens

CYN cyanide

CYP cyproheptadine

CYS cystoscopy

Cys cyclosporine; cysteine

Cys-Cys cystine

CYSTO cystogram

cysto cystoscopy

CYT cytochrome

Cyt cytoplasm; cytosine

cyt cytology, cytological; cytoplasm, cytoplasmic

cytol cytology, cytological

CY-VA-DIC cyclophosphamide, vincristine, Adriamycin, and dacarbazine

CZ cefazolin

Cz central midline placement of electrodes in electroencephalography

CZI crystalline zinc insulin

C$_{Zn}$ zinc clearance

CZP clonazepam

D

D absorbed dose aspartic acid; cholecalciferol; coefficient of diffusion; dacryon; date; daughter; day; dead; dead air space; debye; deceased; deciduous; decimal reduction time; degree; density; dental; dermatology, dermatologist, dermatologic; deuterium; deuteron; development; deviation; dextro; dextrose; diagnosis; diagonal; diameter; diarrhea; diastole; diathermy; died; difference; diffusion, diffusing; dihydrouridine; dilution [rate]; diopter; diplomate; disease; dispense; displacement [loop]; distal; diuresis; diurnal; divergence; diverticulum; divorced; doctor; dog; donor; dorsal; dose [Lat. *dosis*]; drive; drug; dual; duct; duodenum, duodenal; duration; dwarf; electric displacement; give [Lat. *da*]; let it be given [Lat. *detur*]; mean dose; right [Lat. *dexter*]; unit of vitamin D potency

D̄ mean dose

D₁ diagonal one; first dorsal vertebra

1-D one-dimensional

D₂ diagonal two; second dorsal vertebra

2-D two-dimensional

2,4-D 2,4-dichlorophenoxyacetic acid

D/3 distal third

3-D three-dimensional

D₃₋₁₂ third to twelfth dorsal vertebrae

D4 fourth digit

D₁₀ decimal reduction time

d atomic orbital with angular momentum quantum number 2; day [Lat. *dies*]; dead; deceased; deci-; decrease, decreased; degree; density; deoxy.; deoxyribose; dextro-; dextrorotatory; diameter; died; diopter; distal; diurnal; dorsal; dose; doubtful; duration; dyne; give [Lat. *dentur*]; right [Lat. *dexter*]

Δ see *delta*

δ see *delta*

1/d once a day

2/d twice a day

DA dark adaptation; dark agouti [rat]; daunomycin; degenerative arthritis; delayed action; Dental Assistant; deoxyadenosine; developmental age; diabetic acidosis; differential analyzer; differentiation antigen; diphenylchlorarsine; Diploma in Anesthetics; direct agglutination; disability assistance; disaggregated; dopamine; drug addict, drug addiction; ductus arteriosus

D/A date of accident; date of admission; digital-to-analog [converter]; discharge and advise

D-A donor-acceptor

D&A dilatation and aspiration

Da dalton

da daughter; day; deca-; give [Lat. *da*]

DAA decompensated autonomous adenoma; dementia associated with alcoholism; dialysis-associated amyloidosis; diaminoanisole

DAAO diaminoacid oxidase

DAB days after birth; 3,3'-diaminobenzidine; dysrhythmic aggressive behavior

DABA 2,4-diaminobutyric acid

DAC digital-to-analog converter; disaster assistance center; Division of Ambulatory Care

dac dacryon

DACL Depression Adjective Check List

DACM N-(7-diamethylamino-4-methyl-3-coumarinyl) maleimide

DACS data acquisition and control system

DACT dactinomycin

DAD delayed after depolarization; diffuse alveolar damage; dispense as directed

DADA dichloroacetic acid diisopropylammonium salt

DADDS diacetyldiaminodiphenylsulfone

DADS Director Army Dental Service

75

DAE diphenylanthracene endoperoxide; diving air embolism

DAF decay-accelerating factor; delayed auditory feedback; drug-adulterated food

DAG diacylglycerol; dianhydrogalactitol

DAGT direct antiglobulin test

DAH disordered action of the heart

DAHEA Department of Allied Health Education and Accreditation

DAHM Division of Allied Health Manpower

DALA delta-aminolevulinic acid

DALE Drug Abuse Law Enforcement

DAM data-associated message; degraded amyloid; diacetyl monoxime; diacetylmorphine

dam decameter

DAMA discharged against medical advice

dAMP deoxyadenosine monophosphate; deoxyadenylate adenosine monophosphate

D and C dilatation and curettage

dand to be given [Lat. *dandus*]

DANS 1-dimethylaminonaphthalene-5-sulfonyl chloride

DAO diamine oxidase

DAo descending aorta

DAP data acquisition processor; depolarizing afterpotential; diaminopimelic acid; diastolic aortic pressure; dihydroxyacetone phosphate; dipeptidylaminopeptidase; direct latex agglutination pregnancy [test]; Draw-a-Person [test]

DAP&E Diploma of Applied Parasitology and Entomology

DAPRE daily adjustable progressive resistive exercise

DAPRU Drug Abuse Prevention Resource Unit

DAPT diaminophenylthiazole; direct agglutination pregnancy test

DAQ Diagnostic Assessment Questionnaire

DAR death after resuscitation; diacereine; differential absorption ratio

DARP drug abuse rehabilitation program

DARTS Drug and Alcohol Rehabilitation Testing System

DAS dead air space; Death Anxiety Scale; delayed anovulatory syndrome; dextroamphetamine sulfate

DASD direct access storage device

DASH Distress Alarm for the Severely Handicapped

DAT delayed-action tablet; dementia Alzheimer's type; dental aptitude test; diacetylthiamine; diet as tolerated; differential agglutination titer; Differential Aptitude Test; diphtheria antitoxin; direct agglutination test; direct antiglobulin test; Disaster Action Team

DATE dental auxiliary teacher education

DATP deoxyadenosine triphosphate

DATTA diagnostic and therapeutic technology assessment

DAU 3-deazauridine; Dental Auxiliary Utilization

dau daughter

DAV data valid; Disabled American Veterans; duck adenovirus

DAVIT Danish Verapamil Infarction Trial

DAvMED Diploma in Aviation Medicine

DAVP deamino-arginine vasopressin

DAW dispense as written

DB data base; date of birth; deep breath; dense body; dextran blue; diabetes, diabetic; diagonal band; diet beverage; direct bilirubin; disability; distobuccal; double-blind [study]; Dutch belted [rabbit]; duodenal bulb

Db diabetes, diabetic

dB, db decibel

db date of birth; diabetes, diabetic

DBA Diamond-Blackfan anemia; dibenzanthracene; *Dolichos biflorus* agglutinin

DBAE dihydroxyborylaminoethyl

DBC dibencozide; dye-binding capacity

DB&C deep breathing and coughing

DBCL dilute blood clot lysis [method]

DBD definite brain damage; dibromodulcitol

DBDG distobuccal developmental groove

DBE deep breathing exercise; dibromoethane

DBED penicillin G benzathine

DBH dopamine beta-hydroxylase

DBI development at birth index; phenformin hydrochloride

DBIOC data base input/output control

DBIR Directory of Biotechnology Information Resources

dBk decibels above 1 kilowatt

DBM data base management; dibromomannitol; dobutamine

dBm decibels above 1 milliwatt

DBMS data base management systems

DBO distobucco-occlusal

db/ob diabetic obese [mouse]

DBP diastolic blood pressure; dibutylphthalate; distobuccopulpal; Döhle body panmyelopathy; vitamin D-binding protein

DBR distorted breathing rate

DBS deep brain stimulation; Denis Browne splint; despeciated bovine serum; Diamond-Blackfan syndrome; dibromosalicil; diminished breath sounds; direct bonding system; Division of Biological Standards

DBT dry bulb temperature

DBW desirable body weight

dBW decibels above 1 watt

DC daily census; data communication; data conversion; decrease; deep compartment; Dental Corps; deoxycholate; descending colon; dextran charcoal; diagonal conjugate; diagnostic center; diagnostic code; differentiated cell; digit copying; digital computer; dilatation and curettage; dilation catheter; diphenylcyanoarsine; direct Coombs' [test]; direct current; discharge; discharged; discontinue, discontinued; distal colon; distocervical; Doctor of Chiropractic; donor cells; dressing change; duodenal cap; Dupuytren contracture; dyskeratosis

congenita; electric defibrillator using DC discharge

Dc critical dilution rate

D/C discontinue

DC65 Darvon compound 65

D&C dilatation and curettage; drugs and cosmetics

dC deoxycytidine

dc decrease; direct current; discharge; discontinue

DCA deoxycholate-citrate agar; deoxycholic acid; desoxycorticosterone acetate; dichloroacetate

DCABG double coronary artery bypass graft

DCB dichlorobenzidine

DCBE double contrast barium enema

DCBF dyamic cardiac blood flow

DCC day care center; detected in colon cancer; dextran-coated charcoal; N,N'-dicyclohexylcarbodiimide; disaster control center; dorsal cell column; double concave

DCCMP daunomycin, cyclocytidine, 6-mercaptopurine, and prednisolone

DC$_{CO_2}$ diffusing capacity for carbon dioxide

DCD Diploma in Chest Diseases

D/c'd, dc'd discontinued

DCET dicarboxyethoxythiamine

DCF 2'-deoxycoformycin; direct centrifugal flotation; dopachrome conversion factor

DCG deoxycorticosterone glucoside; disodium cromoglycate; dynamic electrocardiography

DCH delayed cutaneous hypersensitivity; Diploma in Child Health

DCh Doctor of Surgery [Lat. *Doctor Chirurgiae*]

DCHEB dichlorohexafluorobutane

DCHN dicyclohexylamine nitrite

DChO Doctor of Ophthalmic Surgery

DCI dichloroisoprenaline; dichloroisoproterenol

DCIS ductal carcinoma in situ

DCL dicloxacillin; diffuse or disseminated cutaneous leishmaniasis

DCLS deoxycholate citrate lactose saccharose

DCM dichloromethane; dichloromethotrexate; dilated cardiomyopathy; Doctor of Comparative Medicine; dyssynergia cerebellaris myoclonica

DCML dorsal column medial lemniscus

DCMP daunomycin, cytosine arabinoside, 6-mercaptopurine, and prednisolone

dCMP deoxycytidine monophosphate

DCMT Doctor of Clinical Medicine of the Tropics

DCMX 2,4-dichloro-m-xylenol

DCN data collection network; deep cerebral nucleus; delayed conditioned necrosis; depressed, cognitively normal; dorsal column nucleus; dorsal cutaneous nerve

DCNU chlorozotocin

DCO Diploma of the College of Optics

D_{CO} diffusing capacity for carbon monoxide

DCOG Diploma of the College of Obstetricians and Gynaecologists

DCP dicalcium phosphate; Diploma in Clinical Pathology; Diploma in Clinical Psychology; District Community Physician; dynamic compression plate

DCR dacryocystorhinostomy; data conversion receiver; direct cortical response

DCS decompression sickness; dense canalicular system; diffuse cortical sclerosis; dorsal column stimulation, dorsal column stimulator; dynamic condylar screw; dyskinetic cilia syndrome

DCT direct Coombs' test; distal convoluted tubule; diurnal cortisol test; dynamic computed tomography

dct boiled down [Lat. *decoctum*]

DCTMA desoxycorticosterone trimethylacetate

dCTP deoxycytidine triphosphate

DCTPA desoxycorticosterone triphenylacetate

DCX double charge exchange

DCx double convex

DD dangerous drug; data definition; day

of delivery; degenerated disc; degenerative disease; delusional disorder; detrusor dyssynergia; developmental disability; died of the disease; differential diagnosis; digestive disorder; Di Guglielmo's disease; disc diameter; discharge diagnosis; discharged dead; dog dander; double diffusion; drug dependence; dry dressing; Duchenne's dystrophy; Dupuytren's disease

dd daily [Lat. *de die*]; disc diameter; let it be given to [Lat. *detur ad*]

D6D delta-6-desaturase

DDA Dangerous Drugs Act; dideoxyadenosine

ddA 2',3'-dideoxyadenosine

DDAVP, dDAVP 1-deamino-8-D-arginine vasopressin

DDC dangerous drug cabinet; dideoxycytidine; diethyl-dithiocarbamate; direct display console; diverticular disease of the colon

DDc double concave

ddC dideoxycytidine

DDD AV universal [pacemaker]; defined daily dose; degenerative disc disease; dehydroxydinaphthyl disulfide; dense deposit disease; Denver dialysis disease; dichlorodiphenyl-dichloroethane; dihydroxydinaphthyl disulfide; Dowling-Degos disease

DDD CT double-dose-delay computed tomography

DDE dichlorodiphenyldichloroethylene

DDG deoxy-D-glucose

DDH Diploma in Dental Health; dissociated double hypertropia

DDI, ddI dideoxyinosine

DDIB Disease Detection Information Bureau

dd in d from day to day [Lat. *de die in diem*]

DDM Diploma in Dermatological Medicine; Doctor in Dental Medicine; Dyke-Davidoff-Masson [syndrome]

dDNA denatured deoxyribonucleic acid

DDNTP dideoxynucleoside triphosphate

DDO Diploma in Dental Orthopaedics

DDP cisplatin; density-dependent phosphoprotein; difficult denture patient; digital data processing; distributed data processing

DDPA Delta Dental Plans Association

DDR diastolic descent rate; Diploma in Diagnostic Radiology

DDRB Doctors' and Dentists' Review Body

DDS damaged disc syndrome; dendrodendritic synaptosome; dental distress syndrome; depressed DNA synthesis; dialysis disequilibrium syndrome; diaminodiphenylsulfone; directional Doppler sonography; Director of Dental Services; disability determination service; Disease-Disability Scale; Doctor of Dental Surgery; dodecyl sulfate; double decidual sac; dystrophy-dystocia syndrome

DDSc Doctor of Dental Science

DDSI digital damage severity index

DDSO diaminodiphenylsulfoxide

DDST Denver Developmental Screening Test

DDT dichlorodiphenyltrichloroethane; ductus deferens tumor

DDTN dideoxy-didehydrothymidine

ddTTP dideoxythymidine triphosphate

DDU dermo-distortive urticaria

D/DW dextrose in distilled water

D 5% DW 5% dextrose in distilled water

DDx differential diagnosis

DE deprived eye; diagnostic error; dialysis encephalopathy; digestive energy; dose equivalent; dream elements; drug evaluation; duration of ejection

D&E diet and elimination; dilatation and evacuation

2DE two-dimensional echocardiography

DEA dehydroepiandrosterone; diethanolamine; Drug Enforcement Agency

DEAE diethylaminoethyl [cellulose]

DEAE-D diethylaminoethyl dextran

DEB diepoxybutane; diethylbutanediol; Division of Environmental Biology; dystrophic epidermolysis bullosa

deb debridement

DEBA diethylbarbituric acid

debil debilitation

DEBRA Dystrophic Epidermolysis Bullosa Research Association

DEBS dominant epidermolysis bullosa simplex

deb spis of the proper consistency [Lat. *debita spissutudine*]

DEC decrease; deoxycholate citrate; diethylcarbamazine; dynamic environmental conditioning

Dec, dec decant

dec deceased; deciduous; decimal; decompose, decomposition; decrease, decreased

decd deceased

decoct decoction

decomp decompensation; decomposition, decompose

decr decrease, decreased

decub lying down [Lat. *decubitus*]

DED date of expected delivery; defined exposure dose; delayed erythema dose

DEEG depth electroencephalogram, depth electroencephalography

de d in d from day to day [Lat. *de die in diem*]

DEF decayed primary teeth requiring filling, decayed primary teeth requiring extraction, and primary teeth successfully filled

def defecation; deficiency, deficient; deferred

defib defibrillation

defic deficiency, deficient

deform deformed, deformity

DEFT direct epifluorescent filter technique

DEG diethylene glycol

Deg, deg degeneration, degenerative; degree

degen degeneration, degenerative

deglut let it be swallowed [Lat. *deglutiatur*]

DEH dysplasia epiphysealis hemimelica

DEHP di(2-ethylhexyl)phthalate

DEHS Division of Emergency Health Services

DEHT developmental hand function test

dehyd dehydration, dehydrated

DEJ, dej dentino-enamel junction

del deletion; delivery; delusion

deliq deliquescence, deliquescent

Delt deltoid

Δ Greek capital letter *delta*

δ Greek lower case letter *delta*; immunoglobulin D

DEM demerol; diethylmaleate

Dem Demerol

DEN denervation; dengue; dermatitis exfoliativa neonatorum; diethylnitrosamine

denat denatured

DENT Dental Exposure Normalization Technique

Dent, dent dentistry, dentist, dental, dentition; let it be given [Lat. *dentur*]

dent tal dos give of such doses [Lat. *dentur tales doses*]

DENTALPROJ Dental Research Projects

DEP diethylpropanediol; dilution end point

dep dependent; deposit; purified [Lat. *depuratus*]

DEPA diethylene phosphoramide

DEPC diethyl pyrocarbonate

depr depression, depressed

DEPS distal effective potassium secretion

DEP ST SEG depressed ST segment

dept department

DEQ Depression Experiences Questionnaire

DER disulfiram-ethanol reaction; dual energy radiography

DeR degeneration reaction

der derivative chromosome

deriv derivative, derived

Derm, derm dermatitis, dermatology, dermatologist, dermatological; dermatome

DES dermal-epidermal separation; dialysis encephalopathy syndrome; diethylstilbestrol; diffuse esophageal spasm; disequilibrium syndrome; doctor's emergency service

desat desaturated

desc descendant; descending

Desc Ao descending aorta

DESI drug efficacy study implementation

desq desquamation

DEST Denver Eye Screening Test; dichotic environmental sounds test

dest distill, distilled [Lat. *destilla, destillatus*]

DET diethyltryptamine; dipyridamole echocardiography test

det let it be given [Lat. *detur*]

Det-6 detroid-6 [human sternal marrow cells]

determ determination, determined

det in dup, det in 2 plo let twice as much be given [Lat. *detur in duplo*]

detn detention

detox detoxification

det s let it be given and labeled [Lat. *detur et signetur*]

DEUV direct electronic urethrocystometry

DEV deviant, deviation; duck embryo vaccine or virus

dev development; deviation

devel development

DevPd developmental pediatrics

DEX dexamethasone

dex dexterity; dextrorotatory; right [Lat. *dexter*]

DEXA dual-energy x-ray absorptiometry

DF decapacitation factor; decontamination factor; deferoxamine; deficiency factor; defined flora [animal]; degree of freedom; diabetic father; dietary fibers; digital fluoroscopy; discriminant function; disseminated foci; distribution factor, dorsiflexion

Df *Dermatophagoides farinae*

df degrees of freedom

DFA direct fluorescent antibody; dorsiflexion assistance

DFB dinitrofluorobenzene; dysfunctional bleeding
DFC developmental field complex; dry-filled capsule
DFD defined formula diets; diisopropyl phosphorofluoridate
DFDT difluoro-diphenyl-trichloroethane
DFE diffuse fasciitis with eosinophilia; distal femoral epiphysis
DFECT dense fibroelastic connective tissue
DFG direct forward gaze
DFHom Diploma of the Faculty of Homeopathy
DFI disease-free interval
DFM decreased fetal movement
DFMC daily fetal movement count
DFMO difluoromethylornithine
DFMR daily fetal movement record
DFO, DFOM deferoxamine
DFP diastolic filling period; diisopropylfluorophosphate
DF^{32}P radiolabeled diisopropylfluorophosphate
DFPP double filtration plasmapheresis
DFR diabetic floor routine
DFS disease-free survival
DFSP dermatofibrosarcoma protuberans
DFT diagnostic function test; defibrillation threshold
DFT$_3$ dialyzable fraction of triiodothyronine
DFT$_4$ dialyzable fraction of thryoxine
DFU dead fetus in utero; dideoxyfluorouridine
DFV diarrhea with fever and vomiting
DG dentate gyrus; deoxyglucose; diagnosis; diastolic gallop; diglyceride; distogingival
2DG 2-deoxy-*D*-glucose
dg decigram; diagnosis
DGAVP desglycinamide-9-[Arg-8]-vasopressin
DGBG dimethylglyoxal bisguanylhydrazone
DGE delayed gastric emptying
dge drainage

DGF duct growth factor
DGI disseminated gonococcal infection
DGLA dihomogamma-linolenic acid
dGMP deoxyguanosine monophosphate
DGMS Division of General Medical Sciences
DGN diffuse glomerulonephritis
DGO Diploma in Gynaecology and Obstetrics
DGP 2,3-diglycerophosphate
DGPG diffuse proliferative glomerulonephritis
DGS developmental Gerstmann's syndrome; diabetic glomerulosclerosis; Di George's syndrome
dGTP deoxyguanosine triphosphate
DGV dextrose-gelatin-Veronal [buffer]
DH daily habits; day hospital; dehydrocholate; dehydrogenase; delayed hypersensitivity; dermatitis herpetiformis; developmental history; diaphragmatic hernia; disseminated histoplasmosis; dominant hand; dorsal horn; ductal hyperplasia; Dunkin-Hartley [guinea pig]
D/H deuterium/hydrogen [ratio]
DHA dehydroacetic acid; dehydroascorbic acid; dehydroepiandrosterone; dihydroacetic acid; dihydroxyacetone; district health authority
DHAD mitoxantrone hydrochloride
DHAP dihydroxyacetone phosphate
DHAP-AT dihydroxyacetone phosphate acyltransferase
DHAS dehydroandrostenedione
DHB duck hepatitis B
DHBE dihydroxybutyl ether
DHBG dihydroxybutyl guanine
DHBS dihydrobiopterin synthetase
DHBV duck hepatitis B virus
DHC dehydrocholesterol; dehydrocholate
DHCA deep hypothermia and circulatory arrest
DHD district health department
DHE dihematoporphirin ether; dihydroergotamine
DHEA dehydroepiandrosterone
DHEAS dehydroepiandrosterone sulfate

DHEC dihydroergocryptine

DHES Division of Health Examination Statistics

DHESN dihydroergosine

DHEW Department of Health, Education, and Welfare

DHF dengue hemorrhagic fever; dorsihyperflexion

DHF/DSS dengue hemorrhagic fever/dengue shock syndrome

DHFR dihydrofolate reductase

DHg Doctor of Hygiene

DHGG deaggregated human gammaglobulin

DHHS Department of Health and Human Services

DHI Dental Health International; dihydroxyindole

DHIA dehydroisoandrosterol

DHIC dihydroisocodeine

DHL diffuse histiocytic lymphoma

DHM dihydromorphine

DHMA 3,4-dihydroxymandelic acid

DHP dehydrogenated polymer; dihydropyridines; dihydroprogesterone

DHPA dihydroxypropyl adenine

DHPG dihydroxyphenylglycol; dihydroxyproproxymethylguanine

DHPR dihydropteridine reductase

DHR delayed hypersensitivity reaction

DHS delayed hypersensitivity; diabetic hyperosmolar state; duration of hospital stay

D-5-HS 5% dextrose in Harman's solution

DHSM dihydrostreptomycin

DHSS Department of Health and Social Security; dihydrostreptomycin sulfate

DHT dehydrotestosterone; dihydroergotoxine; dihydrotachysterol; dihydrotestosterone; dihydrothymine; dihydroxytryptamine

5,7-DHT 5,7-dihydroxytryptamine

DHTP dihydrotestosterone propionate

DHTR dihydrotestosterone receptor

DHy, DHyg Doctor of Hygiene

DHZ dihydralazine

DI date of injury; defective interfering

[particle]; dentinogenesis imperfecta; deoxyribonucleic acid index; deterioration index; detrusor instability; diabetes insipidus; diagnostic imaging; dialyzed iron; disability insurance; disto-incisal; dorso-iliac; double indemnity; drug information; drug interactions; dyskaryosis index

DIA depolarization-induced automaticity; diabetes; diazepam; Drug Information Association

DiA Diego antigen

dia diakinesis; diathermy

diab diabetes, diabetic

diag diagonal; diagnosis; diagram

diam diameter

diaph diaphragm

dias diastole, diastolic

diath diathermy

DIB diagnostic interview for borderlines; disability insurance benefits; dot immunobinding; duodenoileal bypass

diBr-HQ 5,7-dibromo-8-hydroxy-quinidine

DIC dicarbazine; differential interference contrast microscopy; diffuse intravascular coagulation; disseminated intravascular coagulation; drug information center

dic dicentric

DICD dispersion-induced circular dichroism

DID dead of intercurrent disease; double immunodiffusion

DIDD dense intramembranous deposit disease

DIDMOA diabetes insipidus-diabetes mellitus-optic atrophy [syndrome]

DIDMOAD diabetes insipidus, diabetes mellitus, optic atrophy, deafness [syndrome]

DIE died in emergency department

dieb alt on alternate days [Lat. *diebus alternis*]

dieb secund every second day [Lat. *diebus secundis*]

dieb tert every third day [Lat. *diebus tertiis*]

DIF diffuse interstitial fibrosis; direct immunofluorescence; dose increase factor

DIFF, diff difference, differential; diffusion

diff diagn differential diagnosis

DIFP diffuse interstitial fibrosing pneumonitis; diisopropyl fluorophosphonate

DIG digitalis; digoxin; drug-induced galactorrhea

dig digitalis; digoxin; let it be digested [Lat. *digeretur*]

DIH Diploma in Industrial Health

DIHE drug-induced hepatic encephalopathy

diHETE dihydroxyeicosatetraenoic acid

DIHPPA di-iodohydroxyphenylpyruvic acid

DIL, Dil Dilantin

dil dilute, dilution, diluted

dilat dilatation

DILD diffuse infiltrative lung disease; diffuse interstitial lung disease

DILE drug-induced lupus erythematosus

Diluc at daybreak [Lat. *diluculo*]

dilut dilute, dilution, diluted

DIM divalent ion metabolism; medium infective dose [Lat. *dosis infectionis media*]

dim dimension; diminished; one half [Lat. *dimidius*]

DIMIT 3,5-dimethyl-3'-isopropyl-L-thyronine

DIMOAD diabetes insipidus, diabetes mellitus, optic atrophy, deafness

DIMS disorders of initiating and maintaining sleep

din damage inducible [gene]

d in p aeq divide into equal parts [Lat. *dividetur in partes aequales*]

DIP desquamative interstitial pneumonitis; diisopropyl phosphate; diisopropylamine; diphtheria; distal interphalangeal; drip infusion pyelogram; dual-in-line package

Dip diplomate

dip diploid; diplotene

DIPA diisopropylamine

DipBact Diploma in Bacteriology

DIPC diffuse interstitial pulmonary calcification

DipChem Diploma in Chemistry

DipClinPath Diploma in Clinical Pathology

diph diphtheria

diph-tet diphtheria-tetanus [toxoid]

diph-tox AP alum precipitated diphtheria toxoid

DIPJ distal interphalangeal joint

DipMicrobiol Diploma in Microbiology

DipSocMed Diploma in Social Medicine

DIR double isomorphous replacement

Dir, dir director; direction, directions [Lat. *directione*]

DIRD drug-induced renal disease

dir direct; direction

DIRLINE Directory of Information Resources On-Line

dir prop with proper direction [Lat. *directione propria*]

DIS Diagnostic Interview Schedule

DI-S debris index, simplified

dis disability, disabled; disease; dislocation; distal; distance

DISC Diagnostic Interview Schedule for Children

disc discontinue

disch discharge, discharged

DISH diffuse idiopathic skeletal hyperostosis

DISI dorsal intercalated segmental instability

disinfect disinfection

disl, disloc dislocation, dislocated

disod disodium

disp dispensary, dispense

diss dissolve, dissolved

dissem disseminated, dissemination

dist distal; distill, distillation, distilled; distance; distribution; disturbance, disturbed

DIT deferoxamine infusion test; diet-induced thermogenesis; diiodotyrosine; drug-induced thrombocytopenia

dITP deoxyinosine triphosphate
div divergence, divergent; divide, divided, division
DIVBC disseminated intravascular blood coagulation
DIVC disseminated intravascular coagulation
div in par aeq divide into equal parts [Lat. *dividetur in partes aequales*]
DJD degenerative joint disease
DJOA dominant juvenile optic atrophy
DJS Dubin-Johnson syndrome
DK dark; decay; diabetic ketoacidosis; diet kitchen; diseased kidney; dog kidney [cells]
dk deka
DKA diabetic ketoacidosis
DKB deep knee bends
dkg dekagram
dkl decaliter
dkm dekameter
DKP dikalium phosphate
DKTC dog kidney tissue culture
DKV deer kidney virus
DL danger list; De Lee [catheter]; deep lobe; developmental level; difference limen; diffusion lung [capacity]; direct laryngoscopy; disabled list; distolingual; equimolecular mixture of the dextrorotatory and levorotatory enantiomorphs; lethal dose [Lar. *dosis lethalis*]
DL, D-L Donath-Landsteiner [antibody]
D_L diffusing capacity of the lungs
dl deciliter
DLa distolabial
DLaI distolabioincisal
DLaP distolabiopulpal
DL&B direct larygoscopy and bronchoscopy
DLBD diffuse Lewy body disease
DLC Dental Laboratory Conference; differential leukocyte count; dual-lumen catheter
DLCO carbon monoxide diffusion in the lung; single-breath diffusing capacity
DL_{CO2} carbon dioxide diffusion in the lungs

$DL_{CO}{}^{SB}$ single-breath carbon monoxide diffusing capacity of the lungs
$DL_{CO}{}^{SS}$ steady-state carbon monoxide diffusing capacity of the lungs
DLE delayed light emission; dialyzable leukocyte extract; discoid lupus erythematosus; disseminated lupus erythematosus
D_1LE diagonal 1 lower extremity
D_2LE diagonal 2 lower extremity
DLF Disabled Living Foundation; dorsolateral funiculus
DLG distolingual groove
DLI distolinguoincisal; double label index
DLIS digoxin-like immunoreactive substance
DLL dihomo-gammalinoleic acid
DLLI dulcitol lysine lactose iron
DLMP date of last menstrual period
DLNMP date of last normal menstrual period
DLO Diploma in Laryngology and Otology; distolinguo-occlusal
D_{LO2} diffusing capacity of the lungs for oxygen
DLP delipidized serum protein; direct linear plotting; dislocation of patella; distolinguopulpal; dysharmonic luteal phase
D_5LR dextrose in 5% lactated Ringer's solution
DLT dihydroepiandrosterone loading test
DLTS digoxin-like immunoreactive substance
DLV defective leukemia virus
DLW dry lung weight
DM dermatomyositis; Descemet's membrane; dextromaltose; dextromethorphan; diabetes mellitus; diabetic mother; diastolic murmur; distal metastases; dopamine; dorsomedial; double minute [chromosome]; duodenal mucosa; dry matter
D_M membrane component of diffusion
dm decimeter; diabetes mellitus; dorsomedial
dm^2 square decimeter
dm^3 cubic decimeter

DMA dimethylamine; dimethylaniline; dimethylarginine; direct memory access

DMAB dimethylaminobenzaldehyde

DMAC N,N-dimethylacetamide

DMAE dimethylaminoethanol

DMARD disease-modifying anti-rheumatic drug

DMBA 7,12-dimethylbenz[a]anthracene

DMC demeclocycline; di(p-chlorophenyl)methylcarbinol; direct microscopic count; duration of muscle contraction

DMCC direct microscopic clump count

DMCL dimethylclomipramine

DMCT, DMCTC dimethylchlortetracycline

DMD disease-modifying drug; Doctor of Dental Medicine; Duchenne's muscular dystrophy; dystonia musculorum deformans

DMDC dimethyldithiocarbamate

DMDT dimethoxydiphenyl trichloroethane

DMDZ desmethyldiazepam

DME degenerative myoclonus epilepsy; dimethyl diester; dimethyl ether; diphasic meningoencephalitis; director of medical education; dropping mercury electrode; drug-metabolizing enzyme; Dulbecco's modified Eagle's [medium]; durable medical equipment

DMEM Dulbecco's modified Eagle's medium

DMF decayed, missing, and filled [teeth]; N,N-dimethylformamide; diphasic milk fever

DMG dimethylglycine

DMGBL dimethyl-gammabutyrolactone

DMH diffuse mesangial hypercellularity

DMI Defense Mechanism Inventory; Diagnostic Medical Instruments; diaphragmatic myocardial infarction; direct migration inhibition

dmin double minute

DMJ Diploma in Medical Jurisprudence

DMKA diabetes mellitus ketoacidosis

DML distal motor latency

DMM dimethylmyleran; disproportionate micromelia

DMN dimethylnitrosamine; dorsal motor nucleus; dysplastic melanocytic nevus

DMNA dimethylnitrosamine

DMNL dorsomedial hypothalamic nucleus lesion

DMO 5,5-dimethyl-2,4-oxazolidinedione (dimethadione)

D_{mo2} membrane diffusing capacity for oxygen

DMOA diabetes mellitus–optic atrophy [syndrome]

DMOOC diabetes mellitus out of control

DMP diffuse mesangial proliferation; dimercaprol; dimethylphthalate

DMPA depot medroxyprogesterone acetate

DMPE, DMPEA 3,4-dimethoxyphenylethylamine

DMPP dimethylphenylpiperazinium

DMPS dysmyelopoietic syndrome

DMR Diploma in Medical Radiology

DMRD Diploma in Medical Radio-Diagnosis

DMRE Diploma in Medical Radiology and Electrology

DMRF dorsal medullary reticular formation

DMRT Diploma in Medical Radio-Therapy

DMS delayed match-to-sample; delayed microembolism syndrome; demarcation membrane system; department of medicine and surgery; dermatomyositis; diffuse mesangial sclerosis; dimethylsulfate; dimethylsulfoxide; District Management Team; Doctor of Medical Science; dysmyelopoietic syndrome

DMSA dimercaptosuccinic acid; disodium monomethanearsonate

DMSO dimethyl sulfoxide

DMT dermatophytosis; N,N-dimethyltryptamine; Doctor of Medical Technology

DMTU dimethylthiourea

DMU dimethanolurea

DMV Doctor of Veterinary Medicine

DMWP distal mean wave pressure

DN Deiter's nucleus; dextrose-nitrogen; diabetic neuropathy; dibucaine number; dicrotic notch; dinitrocresol; Diploma in Nursing; Diploma in Nutrition; District Nurse; Doctor of Nursing

D/N dextrose/nitrogen [ratio]

D&N distance and near [vision]

Dn dekanem

dn decinem

DNA deoxyribonucleic acid; did not answer

DNAP deoxyribonucleic acid phosphorus

DNAse, DNase deoxyribonuclease

DNB dinitrobenzene; Diplomate of the National Board [of Medical Examiners]; dorsal nonadrenergic bundle

DNBP dinitrobutylphenol

DNC did not come; dinitrocarbanilide; dinitrocresol; Disaster Nursing Chairman

DNCB dinitrochlorobenzene

DND died a natural death

DNE Director of Nursing Education; Doctor of Nursing Education

DNFB dinitrofluorobenzene

DNK did not keep [appointment]

DNKA did not keep appointment

DNLL dorsal nucleus of lateral lemniscus

DNMS Director of Naval Medical Services

DNO District Nursing Officer

DNOC dinitroorthocresol

DNP deoxyribonucleoprotein; dinitrophenol

DNPH dinitrophenylhydrazine

DNPM dinitrophenol-morphine

DNR daunorubicin; do not resuscitate; dorsal nerve root

DNS deviated nasal septum; diaphragmatic nerve stimulation; did not show [for appointment]; Doctor of Nursing Services; dysplastic nevus syndrome

D$_5$NSS 5% dextrose in normal saline solution

DNT did not test

DNTM disseminated nontuberculous mycobacterial [infection]

dNTP deoxyribonucleoside triphosphate

DNV dorsal nucleus of vagus nerve

DO diamine oxidase; digoxin; Diploma in Ophthalmology; Diploma in Osteopathy; dissolved oxygen; disto-occlusal; Doctor of Ophthalmology; Doctor of Optometry; Doctor of Osteopathy; doctor's orders; drugs only

D$_O$ oxygen diffusion

D$_{O2}$ oxygen delivery

do the same, as before [Lat. *dictum*]

DOA date of admission; dead on arrival; Department of Agriculture; differential optical absorption; dominant optic atrophy

DOAC Dubois oleic albumin complex

DOB date of birth; doctor's order book

DObstRCOG Diploma of the Royal College of Obstetricians and Gynaecologists

DOC date of conception; deoxycholate; deoxycorticosterone; died of other causes; disorders of cornification; dissolved organic carbon

doc doctor; document, documentation

DOCA deoxycorticosterone acetate

DOCG deoxycorticosterone glucoside

DOCLINE Documents On-Line

DOCS deoxycorticosteroids

DOcSc Doctor of Ocular Science

DOD date of death; dementia syndrome of depression; died of disease; dissolved oxygen deficit

DOE date of examination; desoxyephedrine; direct observation evaluation; dyspnea on exertion

DOES disorders of excessive sleepiness

DOFOS disturbance of function occlusion syndrome

DOH department of health

DOHyg Diploma in Occupational Hygiene

DOI date of injury; died of injuries

dol pain [Lat. *dolor*]

DOLLS [Lee's] double-loop locking suture

DOM deaminated O-methyl metabolite; department of medicine; dimethoxyme-thylamphetamine; dissolved organic matter; dominance, dominant

dom dominant

DOMA dihydromandelic acid

DOMF 2'7'-dibromo-4'-(hydroxymer-curi)fluorescein

DOMS Diploma in Ophthalmic Medicine and Surgery

DON Director of Nursing; diazooxonor-leucine

don until [Lat. *donec*]

donec alv sol fuerit until the bowels are opened (until a bowel movement takes place) [Lat. *donec alvus soluta fuerit*]

DOOR deafness, onycho-osteodystro-phy, mental retardation [syndrome]

DOPA, dopa dihydroxyphenylalanine

DOPAC dihydrophenylacetic acid

dopase dihydroxyphenylalanine oxidase

DOPC determined osteogenic precursor cell

DOph Doctor of Ophthalmology

DOPP dihydroxyphenylpyruvate

DOPS diffuse obstructive pulmonary syndrome; dihydroxyphenylserine

dor dorsal

DORNA desoxyribonucleic acid

Dors dorsal

DOrth Diploma in Orthodontics; Diploma in Orthoptics

DORV double outlet right ventricle

DOS day of surgery; deoxystreptamine; disk operating system; Doctor of Ocular Science; Doctor of Optical Science

dos dosage, dose

DOSC Dubois oleic serum complex

DOSS distal over-shoulder strap; dioctyl sodium sulfosuccinate; docusate sodium

DOT date of transfer; Dictionary of Occupational Titles

DOTC Dameshek's oval target cell

Dox doxorubicin

DP data processing; deep pulse; definitive procedure; degradation product; degree of polymerization; dementia praecox; dementia pugillistica; dental prosthodontics, dental prosthesis; dexamethasone pretreatment; diastolic pressure; diffuse precipitation; diffusion pressure; digestible protein; diphosgene; diphosphate; dipropionate; directional preponderance; disability pension; discrimination power; distal pancreatec-tomy; distal phalanx; distal pit; disto-pulpal; Doctor of Pharmacy; Doctor of Podiatry; donor's plasma; dorsalis pedis; with proper direction [Lat. *directione propria*]

Dp dyspnea

D$_p$ pattern difference

DPA D-penicillamine; Department of Public Assistance; diphenylalanine; dipicolinic acid; dipropylacetic acid; dual photoabsorptiometry; dynamic physical activity

DPB days post-burn; diffuse panbron-chiolitis

DPBP diphenylbutylpiperidine

DPC delayed primary closure; desaturated phosphatidylcholine; diethylpyro-carbonate; direct patient care; discharge planning coordinator; distal palmar crease

DPCRT double-blind placebo-controlled randomized clinical trial

DPD Department of Public Dispensary; depression pure disease; desoxypyridox-ine; diffuse pulmonary disease; diphen-amid; Diploma in Public Dentistry

DPDL diffuse poorly differentiated lymphocytic lymphoma

dpdt double-pole double-throw [switch]

DPE dipiperidinoethane

DPF Dental Practitioners' Formulary; dilsopropyl fluorophosphate

DPFC distal flexion palmar crease

DPFR diastolic pressure-flow relationship

DPG 2,3-diphosphoglycerate; displacement placentogram

2,3-DPG 2,3-diphosphoglycerate

2,3-DPGM 2,3-diphosphoglycerate mutase

DPGN diffuse proliferative glomerulonephritis

DPGP diphosphoglycerate phosphatase

DPH Department of Public Health; diphenhydramine; diphenylhexatriene; diphenylhydantoin; Diploma in Public Health; Doctor of Public Health; Doctor of Public Hygiene; dopamine beta-hydrolase

DPhC Doctor of Pharmaceutical Chemistry

DPhc Doctor of Pharmacology

DPHN Doctor of Public Health Nursing

DPhys Diploma in Physiotherapy

DPhysMed Diploma in Physical Medicine

DPI daily permissible intake; days post inoculation; dietary protein intake; diphtheria-pertussis immunization; disposable personal income; drug prescription index; Dynamic Personality Inventory

Dpi *Dermatophagoides pteronyssinus*

DPJ dementia paralytica juvenilis

DPL dipalmitoyl lecithin; distopulpolingual

DPLa distopulpolabial

DPLN diffuse proliferative lupus nephritis

DPM Diploma in Psychological Medicine; discontinue previous medication; Doctor of Physical Medicine; Doctor of Podiatric Medicine; Doctor of Preventive Medicine; Doctor of Psychiatric Medicine; dopamine

dpm disintegrations per minute

DPN dermatosis papulosa nigra; diabetic polyneuropathy; diphosphopyridine nucleotide; disabling pansclerotic morphea

DPNB dorsal penile nerve block

DPNH reduced diphosphopyridine nucleotide

DPO dimethoxyphenyl penicillin

DPP differential pulse polarography; dimethylphenylpenicillin

DPPC dipalmitoylphosphatidylcholine; double-blind placebo-controlled trial

DPS descending perineum syndrome; dimethylpolysiloxane; dysesthetic pain syndrome

dps disintegrations per second

dpst double-pole single-throw [switch]

DPT Demerol, Phenergan, and Thorazine; dichotic pitch discrimination test; diphtheria-pertussis-tetanus [vaccine]; diphtheritic pseudotabes; dipropyltryptamine; dumping provocation test

Dpt house dust mite

DPTA diethylenetriamine penta-acetic acid

DPTI diastolic pressure time index

DPTPM diphtheria-pertussis-tetanus-poliomyelitis-measles [vaccine]

Dptr diopter

DPV disabling positional vertigo

DPVS Denver peritoneovenous shunt

DPW distal phalangeal width

DQ deterioration quotient; developmental quotient

DQE detective quantum efficiency

DR degeneration reaction; delivery room; deoxyribose; diabetic retinopathy; diagnostic radiology; direct repeat; distribution ratio; doctor; dorsal raphe; dorsal root; dose ratio; drug receptor

Dr doctor

dr dorsal root; drain; dram; dressing

DRA dextran-reactive antibody

DRACOG Diploma of Royal Australian College of Obstetricians and Gynaecologists

DRACR Diploma of Royal Australasian College of Radiologists

DRAM dynamic random access memory

dr ap dram, apothecary

DRAT differential rheumatoid agglutination test

DRB daunorubicin

DRBC denaturated red blood cell; dog red blood cell; donkey red blood cell

DRC damage risk criterion; dendritic reticulum cell; digitorenocerebral [syndrome]; dorsal root, cervical

DRCOG Diploma of Royal College of Obstetricians and Gynaecologists

DRCPath Diploma of Royal College of Pathologists
DRD dorsal root dilator
DREF dose rate effectiveness factor
DREZ dorsal root entry zone
DRF Daily Rating Form; daily replacement factor; Deafness Research Foundation; dose reduction factor
DRG diagnosis-related group; Division of Research Grants [NIH]; dorsal respiratory group; dorsal root ganglion; duodenal-gastric reflux gastropathy
drg drainage
DrHyg Doctor of Hygiene
DRI discharge readiness inventory
dRib deoxyribose
DRID double radial immunodiffusion; double radioisotope derivative
DRL dorsal root, lumbar; drug-related lupus
D5RL 5% dextrose in Ringer's lactate [solution]
DRME Division of Research in Medical Education
Dr Med Doctor of Medicine
DRMS drug reaction monitoring system
DrMT Doctor of Mechanotherapy
DRN dorsal raphe nucleus
DRNDP diribonucleoside-3',3'-diphosphate
DRnt diagnostic roentgenology
DRO differential reinforcement of other behavior; Disablement Resettlement Officer
DRP digoxin reduction product; dorsal root potential
dRp deoxyribose-phosphate
DrPH Doctor of Public Health; Doctor of Public Hygiene
DRQ discomfort relief quotient
DRR Division of Research Resources [NIH]; dorsal root reflex
DRS descending rectal septum; Division of Research Services [NIH]; drowsiness; Duane retraction syndrome; dynamic renal scintigraphy; Dyskinesia Rating Scale
drsg dressing
DRUJ distal radioulnar joint

DRT dorsal root, thoracic
DS dead air space; dead space; deep sedative; deep sleep; defined substrate; dehydroepiandrosterone sulfate; delayed sensitivity; dendritic spine; density standard; dental surgery; dermatan sulfate; dermatology and syphilology; desynchronized sleep; Devic's syndrome; dextran sulfate; dextrose-saline; diaphragm stimulation; diastolic murmur; differential stimulus; diffuse scleroderma; dilute strength; dioptric strength; disaster services; discrimination score; disoriented; disseminated sclerosis; dissolved solids; Doctor of Science; donor's serum; Doppler sonography; double-stranded; double strength; Down's syndrome; drug store; dry swallow; dumping syndrome; duration of systole
D/S dextrose/saline
D&S dermatology and syphilology
D-5-S 5% dextrose in saline solution
ds double-stranded
DSA digital subtraction angiography
DSACT, D-SACT direct sinoatrial conduction time
DSAP disseminated superficial actinic porokeratosis
DSAS discrete subaortic stenosis
Dsb single-breath diffusion capacity
DSBL disabled
DSBT donor-specific blood transfusion
DSC de Sanctis-Cacchione [syndrome]; disodium chromoglycate; Doctor of Surgical Chiropody; Down's syndrome child
DSc Doctor of Science
DSCF Doppler-shifted constant frequency
DSCG disodium chromoglycate
DSCT dorsal spinocerebellar tract
DSD depression spectrum disease; discharge summary dictated; dry sterile dressing
DSDDT double sampling dye dilution technique
dsDNA double-stranded deoxyribonucleic acid
DSE Doctor of Sanitary Engineering

DSG dry sterile gauze

DSH deliberate self harm; dexamethasone suppressible hyperaldosteronism

DSHR delayed skin hypersensitivity reaction

DSI deep shock insulin; Depression Status Inventory; Down Syndrome International

DSIM Doctor of Science in Industrial Medicine

DSIP delta sleep-inducing peptide

DSL distal sensory latency

DSL M-U distal sensory latency—median-ulnar

dslv dissolve

DSM dextrose solution mixture; Diagnostic and Statistical Manual [of Mental Disorders]; Diploma in Social Medicine; drink skim milk

DSO distal subungual onychomycosis

DSP decreased sensory perception; delayed sleep phase; dibasic sodium phosphate; digital subtraction phlebography

DSPC disaturated phosphatidylcholine

DSPN distal sensory polyneuropathy; distal symmetrical polyneuropathy

DSR distal spleno-renal; double simultaneous recording

dsRNA double-stranded ribonucleic acid

DSRS distal splenorenal shunt

DSS dengue shock syndrome; dioctyl sodium sulfosuccinate; Disability Status Scale; docusate sodium; double simultaneous stimulation

DSSc Diploma in Sanitary Science

DSSEP dermatomal somatosensory evoked potential

DSST Digit Symbol Substitution Task

DST desensitization test; dexamethasone suppression test; dihydrostreptomycin; disproportionate septal thickening; donor-specific transfusion

DSUH directed suggestion under hypnosis

DSur Doctor of Surgery

DSVP downstream venous pressure

DSWI deep surgical wound infection

DT defibillation threshold; delirium tremens; dental technician; depression of transmission; digitoxin; diphtheria-tetanus [toxoid]; discharge tomorrow; dispensing tablet; distance test; dorsalis tibialis; double tachycardia; duration of tetany; dye test

D/T date of treatment; total ratio of deaths

dT deoxythymidine; due to

dt dystonic

DTA differential thermal analysis

DTB dedicated time block

DTBC d-tubocurarine

DTBN di-t-butyl nitroxide

DTC day treatment center; differential thyroid carcinoma

dTc d-tubocurarine

DTCD Diploma in Tuberculosis and Chest Diseases

DTCH Diploma in Tropical Child Health

dtd give such a dose [Lat. *datur talis dosis*]

dTDP deoxythymidine diphosphate

DTE desiccated thyroid extract

DTF detector transfer function

DTH delayed-type hypersensitivity; Diploma in Tropical Hygiene

DTI dipyridamole-thallium imaging

DTIC dacarbazine; dimethyltriazenyl imidazole carboxamide

DTICH delayed traumatic intracerebral hemorrhage

D time dream time

DTLA Detroit Test of Learning Aptitudes

DTM dermatophyte test medium; Diploma in Tropical Medicine

DTM&H Diplomate of Tropical Medicine and Hygiene

DTMP deoxythymidine monophosphate

DTN diphtheria toxin, normal

DTNB 5,5'-dithiobis-(2-nitrobenzoic) acid

DTO deodorized tincture of opium

d tox toxic dose [Lat. *dosis toxica*]

DTP diphtheria-tetanus-pertussis [vaccine]; distal tingling on percussion; Tinel's sign

DTPA diethylenetriaminepentaacetic acid
DTPH Diploma in Tropical Public Health
dTPM deoxythymidine monophosphate
DTR deep tendon reflex
DTRTT digital temperature recovery time test
DTS dense tubular system; diphtheria toxin sensitivity; donor transfusion, specific
DT's delirium tremens
DTT diagnostic and therapeutic team; diphtheria tetanus toxoid; direct transverse traction
dTTP deoxythymidine triphosphate
DTUS diathermy, traction, and ultrasound
DT-VAC diphtheria-tetanus vaccine
DTVM Diploma in Tropical Veterinary Medicine
DTVMI developmental test of visual motor integration
DTVP developmental test of visual perception
DTX detoxification
DTZ diatrizoate
DU decubitus ulcer; density unknown; deoxyuridine; dermal ulcer; diagnosis undetermined; diazouracil; dog unit; duodenal ulcer; duroxide uptake; Dutch [rabbit]
dU deoxyuridine
du dial unit
DUA dorsal uterine artery
DUB dysfunctional uterine bleeding
dUDP deoxyuridine dephosphate
D₁UE diagonal 1 upper extremity
D₂UE diagonal 2 upper extremity
DUF Doppler ultrasonic flowmeter; drug use forecast
DUI driving under the influence
DUL diffuse undifferentiated lymphoma
dulc sweet [Lat. *dulcis*]
dUMP deoxyuridine monophosphate
duod duodenum, duodenal
dup duplication
DUR drug use review
dur during; hard [Lat. *duris*]

dur dolor while pain lasts [Lat. *durante dolore*]
DUSN diffuse unilateral subacute neuroretinitis
DUV damaging ultraviolet [radiation]
DV dependent variable; difference in volume; digital vibration; dilute volume; distemper virus; domiciliary visit; dorsoventral; double vibration; double vision
D&V diarrhea and vomiting
dv double vibrations
DVA developmental venous anomaly; distance visual acuity; duration of voluntary apnea; vindesine
DVB divinylbenzene
DVC divanillylcyclohexane
DVCC Disease Vector Control Center
DVD dissociated vertical deviation
DV&D Diploma in Venereology and Dermatology
dVDAVP 1-deamine-4-valine-D-arginine vasopressin
DVE duck virus enteritis
DVH Diploma in Veterinary Hygiene; Division for the Visually Handicapped
DVI digital vascular imaging; Doppler velocity index; AV sequential [pacemaker]
DVIS digital vascular imaging system
DVIU direct-vision internal urethrotomy
DVL deep vastus lateralis
DVM digital voltmeter; Doctor of Veterinary Medicine
DVMS Doctor of Veterinary Medicine and Surgery
DVN dorsal vagal nucleus
DVR digital vascular reactivity; Doctor of Veterinary Radiology; double valve replacement; double ventricular response
DVS Doctor of Veterinary Science; Doctor of Veterinary Surgery
DVSc Doctor of Veterinary Science
DVT deep venous thrombosis
DW daily weight; deionized water; dextrose in water; distilled water; doing well; dry weight
D/W dextrose in water
D₅W 5% dextrose in water

D10W 10% aqueous dextrose solution
dw dwarf [mouse]
DWA died from wounds by the action of the enemy
DWD died with disease
DWDL diffuse well-differentiated lymphocytic lymphoma
DWI driving while impaired; driving while intoxicated
DWS Dandy-Walker syndrome; disaster warning system
DWT dichotic word test
dwt pennyweight
DX dextran; dicloxacillin
Dx, dx diagnosis

DXD discontinued
DXM dexamethasone
DXR deep x-ray
DXRT deep x-ray therapy
DXT deep x-ray therapy; dextrose
dXTP deoxyxanthine triphosphate
DY dense parenchyma
Dy dysprosium
dy dystrophia muscularis [mouse]
dyn dynamic; dynamometer; dyne
dysp dyspnea
DZ diazepam; dizygotic; dizziness
dz disease; dozen
DZM dorsal zone of membranelle
DZP diazepam

E air dose; cortisone [compound E]; each; edema; elastance; electric charge; electric field vector; electrode potential; electromotive force; electron; embryo; emmetropia; encephalitis; endangered [animal]; endogenous; endoplasm; enema; energy; *Entamoeba*; enterococcus; enzyme; eosinophil; epicondyle; epinephrine; error; erythrocyte; erythroid; erythromycin; *Escherichia;* esophagus; ester; estradiol; ethanol; ethyl; examination; expectancy [wave]; expected frequency in a cell of a contingency table; experiment, experimenter; expiration; expired air; extract, extracted, extraction; extraction fraction; extralymphatic; eye; glutamic acid; internal energy; kinetic energy; mathematical expectation; redox potential; stereodescriptor to indicate the configuration at a double bond [Ger. *entgegen* opposite]; unit [Ger. *Einheit*]

E* lesion on the erythrocyte cell membrane at the site of complement fixation

Ē average beta energy

E$_0$ electric affinity

E$_1$ estrone

E$_2$ 17β-estradiol

E$_3$ estriol

E$_4$ estetrol

4E four-plus edema

E° standard electrode potential

e base of natural logarithms, approximately 2.7182818285; egg transfer; electric charge; electron; elementary charge; exchange

e$^-$ negative electron

e$^+$ positron

ε see *epsilon*

η see *eta*

EA early antigen; educational age; egg albumin; electric affinity; electroacupuncture; electroanesthesia; electrophysiological abnormality; embryonic antibody; endocardiographic amplifier; Endometriosis Association; enteral alimentation; enteroanastomosis; enzymatically active; epiandrosterone; erythrocyte antibody; erythrocyte antiserum; esophageal atresia; estivo-autumnal; ethacrynic acid

E&A evaluate and advise

ea each

Eα kinetic energy of alpha particles

EAA electroacupuncture analgesia; Epilepsy Association of America; essential amino acid; extrinsic allergic alveolitis

EAB elective abortion; Ethics Advisory Board

EABV effective arterial blood volume

EAC Ehrlich ascites carcinoma; electroacupuncture; epithelioma adenoides cysticum; erythema annulare centrifugum; erythrocyte, antibody, complement; external auditory canal

EACA epsilon-aminocaproic acid

EACD eczematous allergic contact dermatitis

EAD early afterdepolarization; extracranial arterial disease

ead the same [Lat. *eadem*]

EA-D early antigen diffuse [component]

E-ADD epileptic attentional deficit disorder

EADS early amnion deficit spectrum or syndrome

EAE experimental allergic encephalomyelitis; experimental autoimmune encephalitis

EAEC enteroadherent *Escherichia coli*

EAG electroarteriography

EAHF eczema, asthma, and hay fever

EAHLG equine antihuman lymphoblast globulin

EAHLS equine antihuman lymphoblast serum

EAI Emphysema Anonymous, Inc.; erythrocyte antibody inhibition

EAK ethyl amyl ketone

EAM external acoustic meatus

EAMG experimental autoimmune myasthenia gravis

EAN experimental allergic neuritis

EAO experimental allergic orchiitis

EAP electric acupuncture; epiallopregnanolone; erythrocyte acid phosphatase; evoked action potential

EAQ eudismic affinity quotient

Ea R reaction of degeneration [Ger. *Entartungs-Reaktion*]

EARR extended aortic root replacement

EAST elevated-arm stress test; Emory angioplasty vs. surgery trial; external rotation, abduction stress test

EAT Eating Attitudes Test; Ehrlich ascites tumor; electro-aerosol therapy; epidermolysis acuta toxica; experimental autoimmune thymitis; experimental autoimmune thyroiditis

EATC Ehrlich ascites tumor cell

EAV equine abortion virus

EAVC enhanced atrioventricular conduction

EAVM extramedullary arteriovenous malformation

EAVN enhanced atrioventricular nodal [conduction]

EB elective abortion; elementary body; endometrial biopsy; epidermolysis bullosa; Epstein-Barr [virus]; esophageal body; estradiol benzoate; Evans blue

EBA epidermolysis bullosa acquisita; epidermolysis bullosa atrophicans; orthoethoxybenzoic acid

EBC esophageal balloon catheter

EBCDIC Extended Binary Coded Decimal Interchange Code

EBD epidermolysis bullosa dystrophica

EBDD epidermolysis bullosa dystrophica dominant

EBDR epidermolysis bullosa dystrophica recessiva

EBF erythroblastosis fetalis

EBG electroblepharogram, electroblepharography

EBI emetine bismuth iodide; erythroblastic island; estradiol binding index

EBK embryonic bovine kidney

EBL erythroblastic leukemia; estimated blood loss

eBL endemic Burkitt's lymphoma

EBL/S estimated blood loss during surgery

EBM electrophysiologic behavior modification; expressed breast milk

EBNA Epstein-Barr virus-associated nuclear antigen

E/BOD electrolyte biochemical oxygen demand

EBP estradiol-binding protein

EBRT electron beam radiotherapy

EBS elastic back strap; electric brain stimulation; Emergency Bed Service; epidermolysis bullosa simplex

EBSS Earle's balanced salt solution

EBT external beam therapy

EBV effective blood volume; Epstein-Barr virus

EBZ epidermal basement zone

EC effective concentration; ejection click; electrochemical; electron capture; embryonal carcinoma; endemic cretinism; endocrine cells; endothelial cell; energy charge; enteric coating; entering complaint; enterochromaffin; entorhinal cortex; Enzyme Commission; epidermal cell; epithelial cell; equalization-cancellation; error correction; *Escherichia coli*; esophageal carcinoma; excitation-contraction; experimental control; expiratory center; external carotid [artery]; external conjugate; extracellular; extracellular concentration; extracranial; eye care; eyes closed

E-C ether-chloroform [mixture]

E/C endocystoscopy; estrogen/creatinine ratio

Ec ectoconchion

EC$_{50}$ median effective concentration

ECA electrical control activity; electrocardioanalyzer; endothelial cytotoxic activity; enterobacterial common antigen; epidemiological catchment area; ethacrynic acid; ethylcarboxylate adenosine; external carotid artery

E-CABG endarterectomy and coronary artery bypass graft

ECAO enteric cytopathogenic avian orphan [virus]

ECBD exploration of common bile duct

ECBO enteric cytopathogenic bovine orphan [virus]

ECBV effective circulating blood volume

ECC electrocorticogram, electrocorticography; embryonal cell carcinoma; emergency cardiac care; endocervical cone; endocervical curettage; estimated creatinine clearance; external cardiac compression; extracorporeal circulation

ECCE extracapsular cataract extraction

ECCLS European Committee for Clinical Laboratory Standards

ECCO enteric cytopathogenic cat orphan [virus]

ECCO₂R extracorporeal carbon dioxide removal

ECD electrochemical detector; electron capture detector; endocardial cushion defect; enzymatic cell dispersion

ECDO enteric cytopathic dog orphan [virus]

ECE equine conjugated estrogen

ECEO enteric cytopathogenic equine orphan [virus]

ECF effective capillary flow; eosinophilic chemotactic factor; erythroid colony formation; extended care facility; extracellular fluid

ECFA eosinophilic chemotactic factor of anaphylaxis

ECFC eosinophilic chemotactic factor complement

ECFMG Educational Commission on Foreign Medical Graduates; Educational Council for Foreign Medical Graduates

ECFMS Educational Council for Foreign Medical Students

ECFV extracellular fluid volume

ECG electrocardiogram, electrocardiography

ECGF endothelial cell growth factor

ECGS endothelial cell growth supplement

ECHO echocardiography; enteric cytopathic human orphan [virus]; Etoposide, cyclophosphamide, Adriamycin, and vincristine

EchoCG echocardiography

Echo-Eg echoencephalography

Echo-VM echoventriculometry

ECHSCP Exeter Community Health Services Computer Project

ECI electrocerebral inactivity; eosinophilic cytoplasmic inclusions; extracorporeal irradiation

ECIB extracorporeal irradiation of blood

EC-IC extracranial-intracranial

ECIL extracorporeal irradiation of lymph

ECIS equipment control information system

ECK extracellular potassium

ECL emitter-coupled logic; enterochromaffin-like [type]; euglobin clot lysis

ECLT euglobulin clot lysis time

ECM embryonic chick muscle; erythema chronicum migrans; experimental cerebral malaria; external cardiac massage; extracellular material; extracellular matrix

ECMO enteric cytopathic monkey orphan [virus]; extracorporeal membrane oxygenation

E co *Escherichia coli*

ECochG electrocochleography

ECOG Eastern Cooperative Oncology Group

ECoG electrocorticogram, electrocorticography

E coli *Escherichia coli*

ECP ectrodactyly-cleft palate [syndrome]; effector cell precursor; endocardial potential; eosinophil cationic protein; erythrocyte coproporphyrin; erythroid committed precursor; *Escherichia coli* polypeptide; estradiol cyclopentane propionate; external cardiac pressure; external counterpulsation; free cytoporphyrin of erythrocytes

ECPO enteric cytopathic porcine orphan [virus]

ECPOG electrochemical potential gradient

ECPR external cardiopulmonary resuscitation

ECR effectiveness-cost ratio; electrocardiographic response; emergency chemical restraint

ECRB extensor carpi radialis brevis

ECRL extensor carpi radialis longus

ECRO enteric cytopathogenic rodent orphan [virus]

ECS elective cosmetic surgery; electrocerebral silence; electroconvulsive shock, electroshock; extracellular space

ECSO enteric cytopathic swine orphan [virus]

ECSP epidermal cell surface protein

ECT electroconvulsive therapy; emission computed tomography; enteric coated tablet; euglobulin clot test; European compression technique

ect ectopic, ectopy

ECTA Everyman's Contingency Table Analysis

ECU environmental control unit; extended care unit; extensor carpi ulnaris

ECV epithelial cell vacuolization; extracellular volume; extracorporeal volume

ECVD extracellular volume of distribution

ECW extracellular water

ED early differentiation; ectodermal dysplasia; ectopic depolarization; effective dose; Ehlers-Danlos [syndrome]; elbow disarticulation; electrodialysis; electron diffraction; embryonic death; emergency department; emotional disorder, emotionally disturbed; entering diagnosis; Entner-Doudoroff [pathway]; enzyme deficiency; epidural; epileptiform discharge; equine dermis [cells]; erythema dose; ethyl dichlorarsine; ethynodiol; evidence of disease; exertional dyspnea; extensive disease; extensor digitorum; external diameter; extra-low dispersion

E-D ego-defense

ED_{50} median effective dose

E_d depth dose

ed edema

EDA electrodermal activity; electrodermal audiometry; electrolyte-deficient agar; electron donor acceptor

EDAM electron-dense amorphous material

EDAX energy dispersive x-ray analysis

EDB early dry breakfast; electron-dense body; extensor digitorum brevis

EDBP erect diastolic blood pressure

EDC emergency decontamination center; end-diastolic count; estimated date of conception; expected date of confinement; expected delivery, cesarean; extensor digitorum communis

ED&C electrodesiccation and curettage

EDCF endothelium-derived contracting factor

EDCI energetic dynamic cardiac insufficiency

EDCS end-diastolic chamber stiffness; end-diastolic circumferential stress

EDD effective drug duration; electron dense deposit; end-diastolic dimension; estimated due date; expected date of delivery

EDDA expanded duty dental auxiliary

edent edentia, edentulous

EDF extradural fluid

EDG electrodermography

EDH extradural hematoma

EDIM epizootic diarrhea of infant mice

E-diol estradiol

EDL end-diastolic length; end-diastolic load; estimated date of labor; extensor digitorum longus

ED/LD emotionally disturbed and learning disabled

EDM early diastolic murmur; extramucosal duodenal myotomy

EDMA ethylene glycol dimethacrylate

EDMD Emery-Dreifuss muscular dystrophy

EDN electrodesiccation; eosinophil-derived neurotoxin

EDNA Emergency Department Nurses Association

EDNF endogenous digitalis-like natriuretic factor

EDOC estimated date of confinement

EDP electron dense particle; electronic data processing; end-diastolic pressure

EDQ extensor digiti quinti

EDR early diastolic relaxation; effective direct radiation; electrodermal response

EDRF endothelium-derived relaxing factor

EDS edema disease of swine; egg drop syndrome; Ehlers-Danlos syndrome; Emery-Dreifus syndrome; energy-dispersive spectrometry; epigastric distress syndrome; excessive daytime sleepiness; extradimensional shift

EDSS expanded disability status scale

EDT end-diastolic thickness; erythrocyte density test

EDTA ethylenediamine tetraacetic acid

Educ education

EDV end-diastolic volume

EDVI end-diastolic volume index

EDWTH end-diastolic wall thickness

EDX, EDx electrodiagnosis

EDXA energy-dispersive x-ray analysis

EE embryo extract; end-to-end; end expiration; energy expenditure; *Enterobacteriaceae* enrichment [broth]; equine encephalitis; ethinyl estradiol; external ear; eye and ear

E&E eye and ear

E-E erythema-edema [reaction]

EEA electroencephalic audiometry; end-to-end anastomosis

EEC ectrodactyly–ectodermal dysplasia–clefting [syndrome]; enteropathogenic *Escherichia coli*

EECD endothelial-epithelial corneal dystrophy

EECG electroencephalography

EEE eastern equine encephalitis; eastern equine encephalomyelitis; experimental enterococcal endocarditis; external eye examination

EEEP end-expiratory esophageal pressure

EEEV eastern equine encephalomyelitis virus

EEG electroencephalogram, electroencephalography

EEGA electroencephalographic audiometry

EEG-CSA electroencephalography with computerized spectral analysis

EELS elecron energy loss spectroscopy

EEM ectodermal dysplasia, ectrodactyly, macular dystrophy [syndrome]; erythema exudativum multiforme

EEME, EE3ME ethinylestradiol-3-methyl ether

EEMG evoked electromyogram

EENT eye, ear, nose, and throat

EEP end-expiratory pressure; equivalent effective photon

EEPI extraretinal eye position information

EER electroencephalographic response

EES erythromycin ethylsuccinate; ethyl ethanesulfate

EESG evoked electrospinogram

EF ectopic focus; edema factor; ejection fraction; elastic fibril; electric field; elongation factor; embryo-fetal; embryo fibroblasts; emergency facility; encephalitogenic factor; endothoracic fascia; endurance factor; eosinophilic fasciitis; epithelial focus; equivalent focus; erythroblastosis fetalis; erythrocyte fragmentation; exposure factor; extrafine; extended field [radiotherapy]; extrinsic factor

EFA Epilepsy Foundation of America; essential fatty acid; extrafamily adoptee

EFAD essential fatty acid deficiency

EFAS embryofetal alcohol syndrome

EFC elastin fragment concentration; endogenous fecal calcium; ephemeral fever of cattle

EFDA expanded function dental assistant

EFE endocardial fibroelastosis

eff effect; efferent; efficiency; effusion

effect effective

effer efferent
EFFU epithelial focus-forming unit
EFH explosive follicular hyperplasia
EFL effective focal length
EFM elderly fibromyalgia; electronic fetal monitoring; external fetal monitor
EFP early follicular phase; effective filtration pressure; endoneural fluid pressure
EFR effective filtration rate
EFS electric field stimulation; event-free survival
EFT Embedded Figures Test
EFV extracellular fluid volume
EFVC expiratory flow-volume curve
EFW estimated fetal weight
EG enteroglucagon; external genitalia; esophagogastrectomy
eg for example [Lat. *exempli gratia*]
EGA estimated gestational age
EGBUS external genitalia, Bartholin, urethral, Skene's glands
EGC early gastric cancer; epithelioid-globoid cell
EGD esophagogastroduodenoscopy
EGDF embryonic growth and development factor
EGF epidermal growth factor
EGF-R epidermal growth factor, receptor
EGF-URO epidermal growth factor, urogastrone
EGG electrogastrogram
EGH equine growth hormone
EGL eosinophilic granuloma of the lung
EGLT euglobin lysis time
EGM electrogram; extracellular granular material
EGME ethylene glycol monomethyl ether
EGN experimental glomerulonephritis
EGOT erythrocytic glutamic oxaloacetic transaminase
EGR erythema gyratum repens
E-GR erythrocyte glutathione reductase
EGRA equilibrium-gated radionuclide angiography
EGRAC erythrocyte glutathione reductase activity coefficient

EGS electrogalvanic stimulation; external guide sequence
EGT ethanol gelation test
EGTA esophageal gastric tube airway; ethyleneglycol-bis-(ß-aminoethylether)-N,N,N',N'-tetraacetic acid
EH enlarged heart; external hyperalimentation; epidermolytic hyperkeratosis; epoxide hydratase; essential hypertension
E/H environment and heredity
E&H environment and heredity
E$_h$ redox potential
eh enlarged heart
EHA Emotional Health Anonymous; Environmental Health Agency
EHAA epidemic hepatitis-associated antigen
EHB elevate head of bed
EHBA extrahepatic biliary atresia
EHBD extrahepatic bile duct
EHBF estimated hepatic blood flow; exercise hyperemia blood flow; extrahepatic blood flow
EHC enterohepatic circulation; enterohepatic clearance; essential hypercholesterolemia; ethylhydrocupreine hydrochloride; extended health care; extrahepatic cholestasis
EHD electrohemodynamics; epizootic hemorrhagic disease
EHDP ethane-1-hydroxy-1,1-diphosphate
EHDV epizootic hemorrhagic disease virus
EHF epidemic hemorrhagic fever; exophthalmos-hyperthyroid factor; extreme high frequency
EHH esophageal hiatal hernia
EHL effective half-life; endogenous hyperlipidemia; Environmental Health Laboratory; essential hyperlipemia; extensor hallucis longus
EHME employee health maintenance examination
EHMS electrohemodynamic ionization mass spectometry

EHNA 9-erythro-2-(hydroxy-3-nonyl) adenine

EHO extrahepatic obstruction

EHP di-(20-ethylhexyl) hydrogen phosphate; Environmental Health Perspectives; excessive heat production; extra-high potency

EHPAC Emergency Health Preparedness Advisory Committee

EHPH extrahepatic portal hypertension

EHPT Eddy hot plate test

EHSDS experimental health services delivery system

EHT electrohydrothermoelectrode; essential hypertension

EHV electric heart vector; equine herpes virus

EI electrolyte imbalance; electron impact; electron ionization; emotionally impaired; enzyme inhibitor; eosinophilic index; excretory index

E/I expiration/inspiration [ratio]

EIA electroimmunoassay; enzyme immunoassay; enzyme-linked immunosorbent assay; equine infectious anemia; erythroimmunoassay; exercise-induced asthma; an interface between a computer and a system for transmitting digital information

EIAB extracranial-intracranial arterial bypass

EIAV equine infectious anemia virus

EIB electrophoretic immunoblotting; exercise-induced bronchospasm

EIC elastase inhibition capacity; enzyme inhibition complex

EID egg infectious dose; electroimmunodiffusion; emergency infusion device

EIEC enteroinvasive *Escherichia coli*

EIEE early infantile epileptic encephalopathy

EIF erythrocyte initiation factor; eukaryotic initiation factor

eIF erythrocyte initiation factor

EIM excitability-inducing material

EIMS electron ionization mass spectrometry

EIP end-expiratory pause; extensor indicis proprius

EIPS endogenous inhibitor of prostaglandin synthase

EIRnv extra incidence rate of non-vaccinated groups

EIRP effective isotropic radiated power

EIRv extra incidence in vaccinated groups

EIS Environmental Impact Statement; Epidemic Intelligence Service

EIT erythroid iron turnover

EIV external iliac vein

EIVA equine infectious anemia virus

EJ elbow jerk; external jugular

EJB ectopic junctional beat

EJP excitation junction potential

ejusd of the same [Lat. *ejusdem*]

EK enterokinase; erythrokinase

EKC epidemic keratoconjunctivitis

EKG electrocardiogram, electrocardiography

EKS epidemic Kaposi sarcoma

EKV erythrokeratodermia variabilis

EKY electrokymogram, electrokymography

EL early latent; elbow; electroluminescence; erythroleukemia; exercise limit; external lamina

El elastase

el elixir

ELA elastomer-lubricating agent; endotoxin-like activity

ELAS extended lymphadenopathy syndrome

ELB early light breakfast; elbow

elb elbow

ELBW extremely low birth weight

ELD egg lethal dose

elec electricity, electric

elect elective; electuary

ELEM equine leukoencephalomalacia

elem elementary

elev elevation, elevated, elevator

ELF elective low forceps; extremely low frequency

ELH egg-laying hormone

ELI exercise lability index

ELIA enzyme-linked immunoassay

ELICT enzyme-linked immunocytochemical technique

ELIEDA enzyme-linked immunoelectron diffusion assay

ELISA enzyme-linked immunosorbent assay

elix elixir

ELM external limiting membrane; extravascular lung mass

ELN electronic noise

ELOP estimated length of program

ELP elastase-like protein; endogenous limbic potential

ELS Eaton-Lambert syndrome; electron loss spectroscopy; extracorporeal life support; extralobar sequestration

ELSO Extracorporeal Life Support Organization

ELSS emergency life support system

ELT endless loop tachycardia; euglobulin lysis time

ELV erythroid leukemia virus

elx elixir

EM early memory; ejection murmur; electromagnetic; electron micrograph; electron microscopy, electron microscope; electrophoretic mobility; Embden-Meyerhof [pathway]; emergency medicine; emmetropia; emotional disorder, emotionally disturbed; ergonovine maleate; erythema migrans; erythema multiforme; erythrocyte mass; erythromycin; esophageal manometry; esophageal motility; extracellular matrix

E/M electron microscope, electron microscopy

E&M endocrine and metabolic

Em emmetropia

E$_m$ mid-point redox potential

EMA electronic microanalyzer; emergency assistance, emergency assistant; epithelial membrane antigen

EMAP evoked muscle action potential

EMB embryology; endomyocardial biopsy; engineering in medicine and biology; eosin-methylene blue; ethambutol; explosive mental behavior

emb embolism; embryo; embryology

EMBASE Excerpta Medica Database

EMBL European Molecular Biology Laboratory

embryol embryology

EMC electron microscopy; emergency medical care; emergency medical coordinator; encephalomyocarditis; essential mixed cryoglobulinemia

EMC&R emergency medical care and rescue

EMCRO Experimental Medical Care Review Organization

EMCV encephalomyocarditis virus

EMD Emery-Dreifuss muscular dystrophy; esophageal mobility disorder

EMEM Eagle's minimal essential medium

EMER electromagnetic molecular electron resonance

emer emergency

EMF electromagnetic flowmeter; electromotive force; Emergency Medicine Foundation; endomyocardial fibrosis; erythrocyte maturation factor; evaporated milk formula

emf electromotive force

EMG electromyogram, electromyography; eye movement gauge; exomphalos-macroglossia-gigantism [syndrome]

EMGN extramembranous glomerulonephritis

EMI electromagnetic interference; emergency medical information

EMIC emergency maternal and infant care

EMIC BACK Environmental Mutagen Information Center Backfile

EMIT enzyme multiplication immunoassay technique

EMJH Ellinghausen-McCullough-Johnson-Harris [medium]

EML erythema nodosum leprosum

EMM erythema multiforme major

EMMA eye movement measuring apparatus

EMO Epstein-Macintosh-Oxford [inhaler]; exophthalmos, myxedema circumscriptum praetibiale, and osteoarthropathia hypertrophicans [syndrome]

emot emotion, emotional

EMP electric membrane property; electromagnetic pulse; Embden-Meyerhof pathway; external membrane potential or protein; extramedullary plasmacytoma

emp as directed [Lat. *ex modo prescripto*]; plaster [Lat. *emplastrum*]

emp vesic blistering plaster [Lat. *emplastrum vesicatorium*]

EMPS exertional muscle pain syndrome

EMR educable mentally retarded; electromagnetic radiation; emergency mechanical restraint; essential metabolism ratio; eye movement record

EMRA Emergency Medicine Residents Association

EMRC European Medical Research Council

EMS early morning specimen; early morning stiffness; electrical muscle stimulation; Electronic Medical Service; emergency medical services; endometriosis; eosinophilia myalagia syndrome; ethyl methane-sulfonate

EMT emergency medical tag; emergency medical team; emergency medical technician; emergency medical treatment

EMTA endomethylene tetrahydrophthalic acid

EMT-A emergency medical technician-ambulance

EMT-I emergency medical technician-intermediate

EMT-M or **EMT-MAST** emergency medical technician–military antishock trousers

EMT-P emergency medical technician-paramedic

EMU early morning urine

emu electromagnetic unit

emul emulsion

EMV eye, motor, voice [Glasgow coma scale]

EMVC early mitral valve closure

EN endoscopy; enrolled nurse; enteral nutrition; epidemic nephritis; erythema nodosum

En, en enema

ENA extractable nuclear antigen

ENC environmental control

END early neonatal death; endocrinology; endorphin

end endoreduplication

Endo endocardial, endocardium; endocrine, endocrinology; endodontics; endotracheal

ENDOR electron nuclear double resonance

ENE ethylnorepinephrine

ENeG electroneurography

enem enema

ENG electronystagmogram, electronystagmography

Eng English

ENI elective neck irradiation

ENK enkephalin

ENL erythema nodosum leproticum

Eno enolase

ENOG electroneurography

ENP ethyl-p-nitrophenylthiobenzene phosphate; extractable nucleoprotein

ENR eosinophilic nonallergic rhinitis; extrathyroid neck radioactivity

ENS enteral nutritional support; ethylnorsuprarenin

ENT ear, nose, and throat; enzootic nasal tumor; extranodular tissue

ent enterotoxin

ent A enterotoxin A

Entom entomology

ENU N-ethyl-N-nitrosourea

env, environ environment, environmental

enz enzyme, enzymatic

EO eosinophil; ethylene oxide; eyes open

E_o skin dose

EOA effective orifice area; erosive osteoarthritis; esophageal obturator airway; examination, opinion, and advice

EOB emergency observation bed

EOCA early onset cerebellar ataxia

EOD entry on duty; every other day

EOF end of file

E of M error of measurement

EOG electro-oculogram, electro-oculography; electro-olfactogram, electro-olfactography

EOGBS early onset group B streptococcal [infection]

EOJ extrahepatic obstructive jaundice

EOL end of life

EOM end of message; equal ocular movement; external otitis media; extraocular movement; extraocular muscle

EOMA emergency oxygen mask assembly

EOMI extraocular muscles intact

EOM NL extraocular eye movements normal

EOP efficiency of plating; emergency outpatient

EOR exclusive operating room

EOS end of study; eosinophil; European Orthodontic Society

eos, eosin eosinophil

Eosm effective osmolarity

EOT effective oxygen transport

EOU epidemic observation unit

EP ectopic pregnancy; edible portion; electrophoresis; electrophysiologic; electroprecipitin; emergency physician; emergency procedure; endogenous pyrogen; endoperoxide; endorphin; end point; enteropeptidase; environmental protection; enzyme product; eosinophilic pneumonia; epicardial electrogram; epithelium, epithelial; epoxide; erythrocyte protoporphyrin; erythrophagocytosis; erythropoietic porphyria; erythropoietin; esophageal pressure; evoked potential; extreme pressure

EPA eicosapentaenoic acid; empiric phrase association; Environmental Protection Agency; erect posterior-anterior; erythroid potentiating activity; extrinsic plasminogen activator

EPAP expiratory positive airway pressure

EPAQ Extended Personal Attitudes Questionnaire

EPA/RCRA Environmental Protection Agency Resource Conservation and Recovery Act

EPB extensor pollicis brevis

EPC end-plate current; epilepsia partialis continua; external pneumatic compression

EPCA external pressure circulatory assistance

EPCG endoscopic pancreatocholangiography

EPDML epidemiology, epidemiologic

EPE erythropoietin-producing enzyme

EPEC enteropathogenic *Escherichia coli*

EPEG etoposide

EPF early pregnancy factor; endocarditis parietalis fibroplastica; endothelial proliferating factor; estrogenic positive feedback; exophthalmos-producing factor

EPG eggs per gram [count]; electropneumography, electropneumogram; ethanolamine phosphoglyceride

EPH edema-proteinuria-hypertension; extensor proprius hallucis

EPI Emotion Profile Index; epilepsy; epinephrine; epithelium, epithelial; evoked potential index; Expanded Programme of Immunization (WHO); extrapyramidal involvement

epid epidemic

epil epilepsy, epileptic

epineph epinephrine

epis episiotomy

epith epithelium

EPL effective patient's life; essential phospholipid; extensor pollicis longus; extracorporeal piezoelectric lithotriptor

EPM electron probe microanalysis; electrophoretic mobility; energy-protein malnutrition

EPN O-ethyl O-p-nitrophenylphosphonothionate

EPO erythropoiesis; erythropoietin; evening primrose-oil; expiratory port occlusion

EPP end-plate potential; equal pressure point; erythropoietic protoporphyria

EPPB end positive-pressure breathing

EPPS Edwards Personal Preference Schedule

EPQ Eysenck Personality Questionnaire
EPR early progressive resistance; electron paramagnetic resonance; electrophrenic respiration; emergency physical restraint; estradiol production rate; extraparenchymal resistance
EPROM erasable programmable read-only memory
EPS elastosis perforans serpiginosa; electrophysiologic study; enzyme pancreatic secretion; exophthalmos-producing substance; extracellular polysaccharide; extrapyramidal symptom, extrapyramidal syndrome
ep's epithelial cells
EPSDT early periodic screening, diagnosis, and treatment
EPSE extrapyramidal side effects
EPSEM equal probability of selection method
ε Greek letter *epsilon*; heavy chain of IgE; permittivity; specific absorptivity
EPSP excitatory postsynaptic potential
EPSS E-point septal separation
EPT early pregnancy test
EPTE existed prior to enlistment
EPTFE expanded polytetrafluoroethylene
EPTS existed prior to service
EPV entomopoxvirus
EPXMA electron probe x-ray microanalyzer
EQ educational quotient; encephalization quotient; energy quotient; equal to
Eq, eq equation; equivalent
equip equipment
equiv equivalency, equivalent
ER efficiency ratio; epigastric region; ejection rate; electroresection; emergency room; endoplasmic reticulum; enhanced reactivation; enhancement ratio; environmental resistance; equine rhinopneumonia; equivalent roentgen [unit]; erythrocyte receptor; estradiol receptor; estrogen receptor; etretinate; evoked response; expiratory reserve; extended release; extended resistance; external resistance; external rotation

ER⁻ decreased estrogen receptor
ER⁺ increased estrogen receptor
Er erbium; erythrocyte
er endoplasmic reticulum
ERA electrical response activity; electroencephalic response audiometry; Electroshock Research Association; estrogen receptor assay; estradiol receptor assay; evoked response audiometry
ERBF effective renal blood flow
ERC endoscopic retrograde cholangiography; enteric cytopathic human orphan-rhino-coryza [virus]; erythropoietin-responsive cell
Erc erythrocyte
ERCP endoscopic retrograde cholangiopancreatography
ERD evoked response detector
ERDA Energy Research and Development Administration
ERE external rotation in extension
ERF Education and Research Foundation; external rotation in flexion; Eye Research Foundation
E-RFC E-rosette forming cell
ERFS electrophysiological ring finger splinting
ERG electron radiography; electroretinography, electroretinogram
ERHD exposure-related hypothermic death
ERI E-rosette inhibitor
ERIA electroradioimmunoassay
ERIC Educational Resource Information Clearinghouse
ERISA Employee Retirement Income Security Act
ERM electrochemical relaxation method; extended radical mastectomy
ERP early receptor potential; effective refractory period; elodoisin-related peptide; endoscopic retrograde pancreatography; enzyme-releasing peptide; equine rhinopneumonitis; estrogen receptor protein; event-related potential
ERPF effective renal plasma flow
ERPLV effective refractory period of left ventricle

ERS endoscopic retrograde sphincterectomy

ERSP event-related slow potential

ERT esophageal radionuclide transit; estrogen replacement therapy; external radiation therapy

ERU endorectal ultrasound

ERV equine rhinopneumonitis virus; expiratory reserve volume

ERY erysipelas

Ery *Erysipelothrix*

ES ejection sound; electrical stimulus, electrical stimulation; electroshock; emergency service; emission spectrometry; endometritis-salpingitis; endoscopic sphincterotomy; end-to-side; enzyme substrate; epileptic syndrome; esophageal, esophagus; esophageal scintigraphy; esterase; exfoliation syndrome; Expectation Score; experimental study; exterior surface; extrasystole

Es einsteinium; estrid

es soap enema [Lat.*enema saponis*]

ESA Electrolysis Society of America; esterase

ESB electrical stimulation of the brain

ESC electromechanical slope computer; endosystolic count; erythropoietin-sensitive stem cell

ESCA electron spectroscopy for chemical analysis

ESCC epidural spinal cord compression

Esch *Escherichia*

ESCN electrolyte and steroid cardiopathy with necrosis

ESD electronic summation device; electrostatic discharge; emission spectrometric device; end-systolic dimension; esterase-D; exoskeletal device

ESE electrostatic unit [Ger. *electrostatische Einheit*]

ESF electrosurgical filter; erythropoietic stimulating factor

ESFL end-systolic force-length relationship

ESG estrogen; exfoliation syndrome glaucoma

ESI enzyme substrate inhibitor; epidural steroid injection

ESIMV expiratory synchronized intermittent mandatory ventilation

ESL end-systolic length; extracorporeal shockwave lithotripsy

ESLF end-stage liver failure

ESM ejection systolic murmur; endoscopic specular microscope; ethosuximide

ESMIS Emergency Medical Services Management Information System

ESN educationally subnormal; estrogen-stimulated neurophysin

ESN(M) educationally subnormal-moderate

ESN(S) educationally subnormal-severe

ESO electrospinal orthosis

eso esophagoscopy; esophagus

ESP early systolic paradox; effective sensory projection; effective systolic pressure; endometritis-salpingitis-peritonitis; end-systolic pressure; eosinophil stimulation promoter; epidermal soluble protein; especially; evoked synaptic potential; extrasensory perception

ESPA electrical stimulation–produced analgesia

ESR Einstein stoke radius; electric skin resistance; electron spin resonance; erythrocyte sedimentation rate

ESRD end-stage renal disease

ESRF end-stage renal failure

ESS empty sella syndrome; endostreptosin; erythrocyte-sensitizing substance; euthyroid sick syndrome; excited skin syndrome

ess essential

EST electric shock threshold; electroshock therapy; endometrial sinus tumor; endoscopic sphincterectomy; esterase; exercise stress test

est ester; estimation, estimated

esth esthetics, esthetic

ESU electrosurgical unit; electrostatic unit

E-sub excitor substance

ESV end-systolic volume; esophageal valve

ESVI end-systolic volume index
ESVS epiurethral suprapubic vaginal suspension
ESWL extracorporeal shock wave lithotripsy
ESWS end-systolic wall stress
ET educational therapy; effective temperature; ejection time; endotoxin; endotracheal; endotracheal tube; end-tidal; endurance time; enterotoxin; epidermolytic toxin; epithelial tumor; esotropia; essential thrombocythemia; essential tremor; ethanol; etiocholanolone test; etiology; eustachian tube; exchange transfusion; exercise test; exercise treadmill; exfoliative toxin; expiration time
ET₃ erythrocyte triiodothyronine
ET₄ effective thyroxine [test]
Et ethyl; etiology
et and [Lat. *et*]
ETA electron transfer agent; endotracheal airways; ethionamide
η Greek letter *eta*; absolute viscosity
ETAB extrathoracic assisted breathing
et al and others [Lat. *et alii*]
ETC electron transport chain; estimated time of conception
ET$_c$ corrected ejection time
ETD eustachian tube dysfunction
ETEC enterotoxin of *Escherichia coli*, enterotoxic *Escherichia coli*
ETF electron-transferring flavoprotein; eustachian tube function
ETH elixir terpin hydrate; ethanol; ethmoid
eth ether
ETHC elixir terpin hydrate with codeine
ETIBACK Environmental Teratology Information Center Backfile
ETIO etiocholanolone
etiol etiology
ETK erythrocyte transketolase
ETKTM every test known to man
ETL expiratory threshold load
ETM erythromycin
EtNU ethyl nitrosourea
ETO estimated time of ovulation
Eto ethylene oxide

ETOH, EtOH ethyl alcohol
ETOX ethylene oxide
ETP electron transport particle; entire treatment period; ephedrine, theophylline, phenobarbital; eustachian tube pressure
ETR effective thyroxine ratio
ETS electrical transcranial stimulation
ETT endotracheal tube; epinephrine tolerance test; exercise tolerance test; extrathyroidal thyroxine
ETU emergency and trauma unit; emergency treatment unit
ETV extravascular thermal volume
EU Ehrlich unit; emergency unit; endotoxin unit; entropy unit; enzyme unit; esterase unit; etiology unknown
Eu europium; euryon
EUA examination under anesthesia
EUL expected upper limit
EUM external urethral meatus
EUP extrauterine pregnancy
EURONET European On-Line Network
EUROTOX European Committee on Chronic Toxicity Hazards
EUS endoscopic ultrasound; external urethral sphincter
Eust eustachian
EUV extreme ultraviolet laser
EV emergency vehicle; enterovirus; epidermodysplasia verruciformis; estradiol valerate; evoked potential [response]; excessive ventilation; expected value; extravascular
Ev, ev eversion
eV, ev electron volt
EVA ethyl violet azide; ethylene vinyl acetate
evac evacuate, evacuated, evacuation
eval evaluate, evaluated, evaluation
evap evaporation, evaporated
EVB esophageal variceal bleeding
EVC Ellis-van Creveld [syndrome]
EVCI expected value of clinical information
EVD external ventricular drainage; extravascular [lung] density
ever eversion, everted

EVF ethanol volume fraction
EVFMG exchange visitor foreign medical graduate
EVG electroventriculography
EVLW extravascular lung water
EVM electronic voltmeter; extravascular mass
EVP episcleral venous pressure; evoked visual potential
EVR evoked visual response
EVRS early ventricular repolarization syndrome
EVTV extravascular thermal volume
EW emergency ward
E-W Edinger-Westphal [nucleus]
EWB estrogen withdrawal bleeding
EWHO elbow-wrist-hand orthosis
EWL egg-white lysozyme; evaporation water loss
EX exfoliation; exsmoker
E(X) expected value of the random variable X
ex exacerbation; examination, examined, examiner; example; excision; exercise; exophthalmos; exposure; extraction
exac exacerbation
EXAFS extended x-ray absorption fine structure
exam examination, examine, examined
EXBF exercise hyperemia blood flow
exc excision
exch exchange
excr excretion
ExEF ejection fraction during exercise

EXELFS extended electron-loss line fine structure
exer exercise
exhib let it be given [Lat. *exhibeatur*]
EXO exonuclease; exophoria
exog exogenous
exoph exophthalmia
exos exostosis
exp expansion; expectorant; experiment, experimental; expiration, expired; exponential function; exposure
exp lap exploratory laparotomy
expect expectorant
exper experiment, experimental
ExPGN extracapillary proliferative glomerulonephritis
expir expiration, expiratory, expired
expl exploratory
exptl experimental
EXREM external radiation-emission man [dose]
EXS external support
EXT exercise testing
Ext extraction, extract
ext extension; extensive; extensor; exterior; external; extract; extreme, extremity
extrav extravasation
ext rot external rotation
extub extubation
EXU excretory urogram
exud exudate, exudation
EY egg yolk; epidemiological year
EYA egg yolk agar
Ez eczema

F

F bioavailability; a cell that donates F factor in bacterial conjugation; a conjugative plasmid in F⁺ bacterial cells; degree of fineness of abrasive particles; facies; factor; Fahrenheit; failure; false; family; farad; Faraday constant; fascia; fasting; fat; father; feces; fellow; female; fermentation; fertility; fetal; fiat; fibroblast; fibrous; field of vision; filament; *Filaria*; fine; finger; flexion; flow; fluorine; flux; focus; foil; fontanel; foramen; force; form, forma; formula; fornix; fossa; fraction, fractional; fracture; fragment; free; French [catheter]; frequency; frontal; frontal electrode placement in electroencephalography; function; fundus; *Fusiformis*; *Fusobacterium*; gilbert; Helmholz free energy; hydrocortisone [compound F]; inbreeding coefficient; left foot electrode in vectorcardiography; phenylalanine; variance ratio

F₁, F₂ etc. first, second, etc., filial generation

FI, FII, etc. factors I, II, etc.

F344 Fischer 344 [rat]

°F degree on the Fahrenheit scale

F' a hybrid F plasmid

F⁻ a bacterial cell lacking an F plasmid

F⁺ a bacterial cell having an F plasmid

f atomic orbital with angular momentum quantum number 3; farad; father; female; femto; fiber, fibrous; fingerbreadth; fission; flexion; fluid; focal; foot; form, forma; formula; fostered [experimental animal]; fraction; fracture; fragment; frequency; frontal; function; fundus; make [Lat. *fiat*]; numerical expression of the relative aperture of a camera lens

FA false aneurysm; Families Anonymous; Fanconi's anemia; far advanced; fatty acid; febrile antigen; femoral artery; fibrinolytic activity; fibroadenoma; fibrosing alveolitis; field ambulance; filterable agent; filtered air; first aid; fluorescent antibody; fluorescent assay; fluoroalanine; folic acid; follicular area; food allergy; forearm; fortified aqueous [solution]; free acid; Freund's adjuvant; Friedreich's ataxia; functional activity

F/A fetus active

fa fatty [rat]

FAA folic acid antagonist; formaldehyde, acetic acid, alcohol

FAB fast atom bombardment; formalin ammonium bromide; fragment, antigen-binding [of immunoglobulins]; French-American-British [carcinoma staging]; functional arm brace

Fab fragment, antigen-binding [of immunoglobulins]

F(ab')₂ fragment, antigen-binding [of immunoglobulins]

Fabc fragment, antigen and complement binding [of immunoglobulins]

FABER flexion in abduction and external rotation

FABF femoral artery blood flow

FABP fatty acid-binding protein; folate-binding protein

FAC familial adenomatosis coli; femoral arterial cannulation; ferric ammonium citrate; 5-fluorouracil, Adriamycin, and cyclophosphamide; foamy alveolar cast; fractional area changes; free available chlorine

Fac factor

fac facility; to make [Lat. *facere*]

FACA Fellow of the American College of Anesthetists; Fellow of the American College of Angiology; Fellow of the American College of Apothecaries

FACAI Fellow of the American College of Allergy and Immunology

Facb fragment, antigen, and complement binding

FACC Fellow of the American College of Cardiologists

FACCP Fellow of the American College of Chest Physicians

FACD Fellow of the American College of Dentists

FACEB Federation of American Societies for Experimental Biology

FACEP Fellow of the American College of Family Physicians

FACES unique facies, anorexia, cachexia, and eye and skin lesions [syndrome]

FACFS Fellow of the American College of Foot Surgeons

FACG Fellow of the American College of Gastroenterology

FACH forceps to after-coming head

FACHA Fellow of the American College of Health Administrators

FACMTA Federal Advisory Council on Medical Training Aids

FACNHA Foundation of American College of Nursing Home Administrators

FACO Fellow of the American College of Otolaryngology

FACOG Fellow of the American College of Obstetricians and Gynecologists

FACOSH Federal Advisory Committee on Occupational Safety and Health

FACP Fellow of the American College of Physicians

FACPM Fellow of the American College of Preventive Medicine

FACS Fellow of the American College of Surgeons; fluorescence-activated cell sorter

FACSM Fellow of the American College of Sports Medicine

FACT Flannagan Aptitude Classification Test

FACWA familial amyotrophic chorea with acanthocytosis

FAD familial Alzheimer's dementia; familial autonomic dysfunction; fetal activity-acceleration determination; flavin adenine dinucleotide

FADF fluorescent antibody dark field

FADH$_2$ reduced form of flavin adenine dinucleotide

FADIR flexion in adduction and internal rotation

FADN flavin adenine dinucleotide

FADS fetal akinesia deformation sequence

FAE fetal alcohol effect

FAF fatty acid free; fibroblast-activating factor

FAH Federation of American Hospitals

Fahr Fahrenheit

FAI first aid instruction; free androgen index; functional aerobic impairment

FAJ fused apophyseal joint

FALG fowl antimouse lymphocyte globulin

FALP fluoro-assisted lumbar puncture

FAM 5-fluorouracil, Adriamycin, and mitomycin C

Fam, fam family, familial

FAMA Fellow of the American Medical Association; fluorescent antibody to membrane antigen

FAME fatty acid methyl ester

fam hist family history

FAMMM familial atypical multiple mole–melanoma [syndrome]

FAN fuchsin, amido black, and naphthol yellow

FANA fluorescent antinuclear antibody

F and R force and rhythm [of pulse]

FANPT Freeman Anxiety Neurosis and Psychosomatic Test

FANY first aid nursing yeomanry

FAP familial adenomatous polyposis; familial amyloid polyneuropathy; fatty acid polyunsaturated; fatty acid poor; femoral artery pressure; fibrillating action potential; fixed action potential; frozen animal procedure

FAPA Fellow of the American Psychiatric Association; Fellow of the American Psychoanalytical Association

FAPHA Fellow of the American Public Health Association

FAR fractional albumin rate

far faradic

FARE Federation of Alcoholic Rehabilitation Establishments

FAS fatty acid synthetase; Federation of American Scientists; fetal alcohol syndrome

FASC free-standing ambulatory surgical center

fasc fasciculus, fascicular

FASEB Federation of American Societies for Experimental Biology

FASHP Federation of Associations of Schools of the Health Professions

FAST flow-assisted, short-term [balloon catheter]; fluorescent antibody staining technique; fluoro-allergosorbent test; Frenchay Aphasia Screening Test

FAT family attitudes test; fluorescent antibody technique; fluorescent antibody test

FAV feline ataxia virus; floppy aortic valve; fowl adenovirus

FAX, fax facsimile

FAZ Fanconi-Albertini-Zellweger [syndrome]; foveal avascular zone; fragmented atrial activity zone

FB fasting blood [sugar]; feedback; fiberoptic bronchoscopy; fingerbreadth; foreign body; *Fusobacterium*

FBA fecal bile acid

FBCOD foreign body of the cornea, oculus dexter (right eye)

FBCOS foreign body of the cornea, oculus sinister (left eye)

FBCP familial benign chronic pemphigus

FBD functional bowel disorder

FbDP fibrin degradation products

FBE full blood examination

FBEC fetal bovine endothelial cell

FBF forearm blood flow

FBG fasting blood glucose; fibrinogen

fbg fibrinogen

FBHH familial benign hypocalciuric hypercalcemia

FBI flossing, brushing, and irrigation

FBL follicular basal lamina

FBM fetal breathing movements

FBN Federal Bureau of Narcotics

FBP femoral blood pressure; fibrin breakdown product

FBPsS Fellow of the British Psychological Society

FBS fasting blood sugar; feedback system; fetal bovine serum

FBSS failed back surgery syndrome

FC fasciculus cuneatus; fast component [of a neuron]; febrile convulsions; feline conjunctivitis; ferric citrate; fibrocyte; finger clubbing; finger counting; fluorocarbon; fluorocytosine; Foley catheter; foster care; fowl cholera; free cholesterol; frontal cortex; functional castration

5-FC 5-fluorocytosine

Fc centroid frequency; fragment, crystallizable [of immunoglobulin]

Fc' a fragment of an immunoglobulin molecule produced by papain digestion

fc foot candles

F + C flare + cells

FCA ferritin-conjugated antibodies; Freund's complete adjuvant

FCAP Fellow of the College of American Pathologists

F cath Foley catheter

FCC follicular center cells

fcc face-centered-cubic

f/cc fibers per cubic centimeter of air

FCCL follicular center cell lymphoma

FCD feces collection device; fibrocystic disease; fibrocystic dysplasia; focal cytoplasmic degradation

FCE fibrocartilaginous embolism

FCF fetal cardiac frequency; fibroblast chemotactic factor

FCFC fibroblast colony-forming cell

FCHL familial combined hyperlipidemia

FChS Fellow of the Society of Chiropodists

FCI fixed-cell immunofluorescence; food chemical intolerance

FCIM Federated Council for Internal Medicine

FCL fibroblast cell line

fcly face lying

FCM flow cytometry

FCMC family centered maternity care

FCMD Fukuyama-type congenital muscular dystrophy

FCMS Fellow of the College of Medicine and Surgery; Foix-Chavany-Marie syndrome

FCMW Foundation for Child Mental Welfare

FCO Fellow of the College of Osteopathy

FCP final common pathway; Functional Communication Profile

FCPS Fellow of the College of Physicians and Surgeons

FCR flexor carpi radialis; fractional catabolic rate

FcR Fc receptor

FCRA fecal collection receptacle assembly; Fellow of the College of Radiologists of Australasia

FCRC Frederick Cancer Research Center

FCS fecal containment system; feedback control system; fetal calf serum; foot compartment syndrome

FCSP Fellow of the Chartered Society of Physiotherapy

FCST Fellow of the College of Speech Therapists

FCT food composition table

FCU flexor carpi ulnaris

FCx frontal cortex

FD familial dysautonomia; family doctor; fan douche; fatal dose; fetal danger; fibrin derivative; focal distance; Folin-Denis [assay]; follicular diameter; foot drop; forceps delivery; freeze drying

Fd the amino-terminal portion of the heavy chain of an immunoglobulin molecule; ferredoxin

fd fundus

FD$_{50}$ median fatal dose

FDA fluorescein diacetate; Food and Drug Administration; right frontoanterior [position of the fetus]

FDBL fecal daily blood loss

FDC follicular dendritic cell

FD&C Food, Drug and Cosmetic Act; food, drugs, and cosmetics

FDCPA Food, Drug, and Consumer Product Agency

FDD Food and Drugs Directorate

FDDC ferric dimethyldithiocarbonate

FDDS Family Drawing Depression Scale

FDE female day-equivalent; final drug evaluation

FDF fast death factor

FDFQ Food/Drink Frequency Questionnaire

FDG fluorodeoxyglucose

fdg feeding

FDGF fibroblast-derived growth factor

FDH familial dysalbuminemic hyperthyroxinemia; focal dermal hypoplasia; formaldehyde dehydrogenase

FDI International Dental Federation [Fédération Dentaire Internationale]

FDIU fetal death in utero

FDL flexor digitorum longus

FDLMP first day of last menstrual period

FDLV fer de lance virus

FDM fetus of diabetic mother; fibrous dysplasia of the mandible

FDNB fluorodinitrobenzene

FDO Fleet Dental Officer

FDP fibrin degradation product; fibrinogen degradation product; flexor digitorum profundus; frontodextra posterior [position of fetus]; fructose-1,6-diphosphate

FDPase fructose-1,6-diphosphatase

FDQB flexor digiti quinti brevis

FDR fractional disappearance rate

FDS Fellow in Dental Surgery; fiber duodenoscope; flexor digitorum superficialis

FDSRCSEng Fellow in Dental Surgery of the Royal College of Surgeons of England

FDT frontodextra transversa [position of fetus]

FDV Friend disease virus

FDZ fetal danger zone

FE fatty ester; fecal emesis; fetal erythroblastosis; fetal erythrocyte; fluid extract; fluorescent erythrocyte; forced expiration; formaldehyde-ethanol

Fe female; ferret; iron [Lat. *ferrum*]
fe female
feb fever [Lat. *febris*]
feb dur while the fever lasts [Lat. *febre durante*]
FEBP fetal estrogen-binding protein
FEBS Federation of European Biochemical Societies
FEC forced expiratory capacity; free erythrocyte coproporphyrin; Friend erythroleukemia cell
FECG fetal electrocardiogram
F_{ECO_2} fractional concentration of carbon dioxide in expired gas
FECP free erythrocyte coproporphyrin
FECT fibroelastic connective tissue
FECV feline enteric coronavirus
FECVC functional extracellular fluid volume
FeD iron deficiency
Fed federal
FEDRIP Federal Research in Progress [database]
FEE forced equilibrating expiration
FEEG fetal electroencephalography
FEF forced expiratory flow
FEF$_{50}$ forced expiratory flow at 50% of forced vital capacity
FEF$_{50}$/FIF$_{50}$ ratio of expiratory flow to inspiratory flow at 50% of forced vital capacity
FEFV forced expiratory flow volume
FEGO International Federation of Gynecology and Obstetrics
FEHBP Federal Employee Health Benefits Program
FEKG fetal electrocardiogram
FEL familial erythrophagocytic lymphohistiocytosis
FELC Friend erythroleukemia
FeLV feline leukemia virus
FEM, fem female; femur, femoral
fem intern at inner side of the thighs [Lat. *femoribus internus*]
FENa, FE$_{Na}$ fractional excretion of sodium
FE$_{O_2}$, F$_{EO_2}$ fractional concentration of oxygen in expired gas

FEP fluorinated ethylene-propylene; free erythrocyte protoporphyrin
FEPB functional electronic peroneal brace
FEPP free erythrocyte protoporphyrin
FER flexion, extension, rotation; fractional esterification rate
fert fertility, fertilized
ferv boiling [Lat. *fervens*]
FES fat embolism syndrome; flame emission spectroscopy; forced expiratory spirogram; functional electrical stimulation
Fe/S iron/sulfur [protein]
FeSV feline sarcoma virus
FET field-effect transistor; forced expiratory time
FETE Far Eastern tick-borne encephalitis
FETs forced expiratory time in seconds
FEUO for external use only
FEV familial exudative vitreoretinopathy; forced expiratory volume
fev fever
FEV1, FEV$_1$ forced expiratory volume in one second
FEVB frequency ectopic ventricular beat
FEVR familial exudative vitreoretinopathy
FF degree of fineness of abrasive particles; fat-free; father factor; fecal frequency; fertility factor; field of Forel; filtration fraction; fine fiber; finger flexion; finger-to-finger; fixation fluid; flat feet; flip-flop; fluorescent focus; follicular fluid; force fluids; forearm flow; forward flexion; foster father; free fraction; fresh frozen; fundus firm
ff$^+$ fertility inhibition positive
ff$^-$ fertility inhibition negative
FFA Fellow of the Faculty of Anaesthetists; free fatty acid
FFAP free fatty acid phase
FFARCS Fellow of the Faculty of Anaesthetists of the Royal College of Surgeons
FFB flexible fiberoptic bronchoscopy

FFC fixed flexion contracture; fluorescence flow cytometry; free from chlorine

FFCM Fellow of the Faculty of Community Medicine

FFD Fellow in the Faculty of Dentistry; focus-film distance

FFDCA Federal Food, Drug, and Cosmetic Act

FFDSRCS Fellow of the Faculty of Dental Surgery of the Royal College of Surgeons

FFDW fat-free dry weight

FFE fecal fat excretion

FFF degree of fineness of abrasive particles; field-flow fractionation; flicker fusion frequency

FFG free fat graft

FFHom Fellow of the Faculty of Homeopathy

FFI free from infection; fundamental frequency indicator

FFIT fluorescent focus inhibition test

FFM fat-free mass

FFOM Fellow of the Faculty of Occupational Medicine

FFP fresh frozen plasma

FFR Fellow of the Faculty of Radiologists

FFROM full and free range of motion

FFS fat-free solids; fee for services

FFT flicker fusion test or threshold

FFU femur-fibula-ulna [syndrome]; focal forming unit

FFW fat-free weight

FFWC fractional free water clearance

FFWW fat-free wet weight

FG fasciculus gracilis; fast-glycolytic [fiber]; Feeley-Gorman [agar]; fibrinogen; Flemish giant [rabbit]

fg femtogram

FGC fibrinogen gel chromatography

FGD fatal granulomatous disease

FgDP fibrinogen degradation products

FGDS fibrogastroduodenoscopy

FGF father's grandfather; fibroblast growth factor; fresh gas flow

FGG focal global glomerulosclerosis; fowl gamma-globulin

FGL fasting gastrin level

FGM father's grandmother

FGN fibrinogen; focal glomerulonephritis

FGP fundic gland polyp

FGS fibrogastroscopy; focal glomerular sclerosis

FGT fluorescent gonorrhea test

FH facial hemihyperplasia; familial hypercholesterolemia; family history; fasting hyperbilirubinemia; femoral hypoplasia; fetal head; fetal heart; fibromuscular hyperplasia; follicular hyperplasia; Frankfort horizontal [plane]

FH+ family history positive

FH− family history negative

FH₄ tetrahydrofolic acid

fh fostered by hand [experimental animal]; let a draught be made [Lat. *fiat haustus*]

FHA familial hypoplastic anemia; Fellow of the Institute of Hospital Administrators; filamentous hemagglutinin

FH/BC frontal horn/bicaudate [ratio]

FHC familial hypercholesterolemia; family health center; Ficoll-Hypaque centrifugation; Fuchs' heterochromic cyclitis

FHD familial histiocytic dermatoarthritis; family history of diabetes

FHF fetal heart frequency; fulminant hepatic failure

fHg free hemoglobin

FHH familial hypocalciuric hypercalcemia; fetal heart heard

FHI Fuchs' heterochromic iridocyclitis

FHIP family health insurance plan

FHL flexor hallucis longus; functional hearing loss

FHM fathead minnow [cells]

FHN family history negative

FHNH fetal heart not heard

FHP family history positive

FHR familial hypophosphatemic rickets; fetal heart rate

FHRNST fetal heart rate nonstress test

FHS fetal heart sound; fetal hydantoin syndrome

FHT fetal heart; fetal heart tone
FHTG familial hypertriglyceridemia
FH-UFS femoral hypoplasia-unusual facies syndrome
FHV falcon herpesvirus
FHVP free hepatic vein pressure
FHx family history
FI fasciculus intrafascicularis; fever caused by infection; fibrinogen; fixed interval; flame ionization; follicular involution; food intolerance; forced inspiration; frontoiliac
FIA fluorescent immunoassay; focal immunoassay; Freund's incomplete adjuvant
FIAC 2'-fluoro-5-iodo-aracytosine
FIB Fellow of the Institute of Biology; fibrin; fibrinogen; fibrositis; fibula
fib fiber; fibrillation; fibrin; fibrinogen; fibula
FIC Fogarty International Center; fractional inhibitory concentration
FICA Federal Insurance Contributions Act
FICD Fellow of the Institute of Canadian Dentists; Fellow of the International College of Dentists
FiCO₂, FI_CO₂ fractional concentration of carbon dioxide in inspired gas
FICS Fellow of the International College of Surgeons
FID flame ionization detector; free induction decay; fungal immunodiffusion
FIF feedback inhibition factor; fibroblast interferon; forced inspiratory flow; formaldehyde-induced fluorescence
FIFO first in, first out
FIFR fasting intestinal flow rate
FIGD familial idiopathic gonadotropin deficiency
FIGLU formiminoglutamic acid
FIGO International Federation of Gynecology and Obstetrics
FIH familial isolated hypoparathyroidism; fat-induced hyperglycemia
fil filament; filial
filt filter, filtration

FIM field ion microscopy
FIMLT Fellow of the Institute of Medical Laboratory Technology
FIN fine intestinal needle
FINCC familial idiopathic nonarteriosclerotic cerebral calcification
FI_O₂ forced inspiratory oxygen; fractional concentration of oxygen in inspired gas
FiO₂ fractional concentration of oxygen in inspired gas
FIP feline infectious peritonitis
FIPV feline infectious peritonitis virus
FIQ full-scale intelligence quotient
FIR far infrared; fold increase in resistance
FIRDA frontal, intermittent delta activity
FIS forced inspiratory spirogram
fist fistula
FIT fluorescein isothiocyanate; fusion inferred threshold
FITC fluorescein isothiocyanate
FIUO for internal use only
FIV feline immunodeficiency; forced inspiratory volume
FIV₁ forced inspiratory volume in one second
FIVC forced inspiratory vital capacity
FJN familial juvenile nephrophthisis
FJRM full joint range of movement
FJS finger joint size
FK feline kidney
FL fatty liver; feline leukemia; fibers of Luschka; fibroblast-like; filtration leukapheresis; focal length; Friend leukemia; frontal lobe; full liquid [diet]; functional length
FL-2 feline lung [cells]
Fl fluid; fluorescence
fl femtoliter; filtered load; flexion, flexible; fluorescent; flow; fluid; flutter; foot lambert
FLA fluorescent-labeled antibody; left frontoanterior [position of the fetus] [Lat. *fronto-laeva anterior*]
Fla let it be done according to rule [Lat. *fiat lege artis*]

flac flaccidity, flaccid
flav yellow [Lat. *flavus*]
FLC fatty liver cell; fetal liver cell; Friend leukemia cell
FLD fibrotic lung disease
fld fluid
fl dr fluid dram
FLEX Federation Licensing Examination
flex flexor, flexion
FLK funny looking kid
FLKS fatty liver and kidney syndrome
FLM fasciculus longitudinalis medialis
floc flocculation
fl oz fluid ounce
FLP left frontoposterior [position of the fetus] [Lat. *fronto-laeva posterior*]
FLR funny looking rash
FLS fatty liver syndrome; Fellow of the Linnean Society; fibrous long-spacing [collagen]; flow-limiting segment
FLSP fluorescein-labeled serum protein
FLT left frontotransverse [position of the fetus] [Lat. *fronto-laeva transversa*]
FLU flunitrazepam; fluphenazine
flu influenza
fluor fluorescence; fluorescent; fluorometry; fluoroscopy
fluoro fluoroscope, fluoroscopy
FLV feline leukemia virus; Friend leukemia virus
FM face mask; facilities management; family medicine; feedback mechanism; fetal movement; fibromuscular; filtered mass; flavin mononucleotide; flowmeter; foramen magnum; forensic medicine; foster mother; frequency modulation; functional movement; make a mixture [Lat. *fiat mistura*]
Fm fermium
f-M free metanephrine
fm femtometer
FMA Frankfort mandibular plane angle
FMAT fetal movement acceleration test
FMC family medicine center; flight medicine clinic; focal macular choroidopathy
FMD family medical doctor; fibromus-

cular dysplasia; foot and mouth disease; frontometaphyseal dysplasia
FMDV foot and mouth disease virus
FME full mouth extraction
Fmed median frequency
FMEL Friend murine erythroleukemia
FMEN familial multiple endocrine neoplasia
F-met, fMet formyl methionine
FMF familial Mediterranean fever; fetal movement felt; flow microfluorometry; forced midexpiratory flow
FMG five-mesh gauze; foreign medical graduate
FMGEMS Foreign Medical Graduate Examination in Medical Sciences
FMH family medical history; fat-mobilizing hormone; feto-maternal hemorrhage; fibromuscular hyperplasia
FMI Foods and Moods Inventory
FML flail mitral leaflet; fluorometholone
FMLP, f-MLP N-formyl-methionyl-leucyl-phenylalanine
FMN first malignant neoplasm; flavin mononucleotide; frontomaxillonasal [suture]
FMNH, FMNH $_2$ reduced form of flavin mononucleotide
FMO Fleet Medical Officer; Flight Medical Officer
fmol femtomole
FMP first menstrual period; fructose monophosphate
FMR Friend-Moloney-Rauscher [antigen]
FMS fat-mobilizing substance; Fellow of the Medical Society; fibromyalgia syndrome; full mouth series
FMU first morning urine
F-MuLV Friend murine leukemia virus
FMX full mouth x-ray
FN false negative; fibronectin; fluoride number
F-N finger to nose
FNA fine-needle aspiration
FNAB fine-needle aspiration biopsy
FNAC fine-needle aspiration cytology
FNC fatty nutritional cirrhosis

FNCJ fine needle catheter jejunostomy

FND febrile neutrophilic dermatosis; frontonasal dysplasia

f-NE free norepinephrine

Fneg false negative

FNF false-negative fraction; femoral neck fracture

FNH focal nodular hyperplasia

f-NM free normetanephrine

FNP family nurse practitioner

FNS functional neuromuscular stimulation

FNT false neurochemical transmitter

FO fiberoptic; fish oil; foramen ovale; forced oscillation; fronto-occipital

Fo fomentation, fomenting

FOA Federation of Orthodontic Associations

FOAVF failure of all vital forces

FOB fecal occult blood; feet out of bed; fiberoptic bronchoscopy; foot of bed; functional observational battery

FOBT fecal occult blood test

FOC fronto-occipital circumference

FOCAL formula calculation

FOD free of disease

FOG fast oxidative glycolytic [fiber]

fol leaf [Lat. *folium*]

FOMi 5-fluorouracil, vincristine, and mitomycin C

FOOB fell out of bed

FOOSH fell onto [his or her] outstretched hand

FOP fibrodysplasia ossificans progressiva; forensic pathology

FOPR full outpatient rate

For forensic

for foreign; formula

form formula

fort strong [Lat. *fortis*]

FORTRAN formula translation

FOS fiberoptic sigmoidoscopy; fractional osteoid surface

FOV field of view

FP false positive; family physician; family planning; family practice; family practitioner; Fanconi's pancytopenia; femoropopliteal; fibrinopeptide; filling pressure; filter paper; fixation protein; flash point; flavin phosphate; flavoprotein; flexor profundus; fluid pressure; fluorescence polarization; food poisoning; forearm pronated; freezing point; frontoparietal; frozen plasma; full period; fusion point

F-6-P fructose-6-phosphate

Fp frontal polar electrode placement in electroencephalography

fp flexor pollicis; foot-pound; forearm pronated; freezing point; let a potion be made [Lat. *fiat potio*]

FPA Family Planning Association; fibrinopeptide A; filter paper activity; fluorophenylalanine

FPB femoral popliteal bypass; fibrinopeptide B; flexor pollicis brevis

FPC familial polyposis coli; family planning clinic; fish protein concentrate

FpCA 1-fluoromethyl-2-p-chlorophenyl-ethylamine

FPD feto-pelvic disproportion; flame photometric detector

FPE fatal pulmonary embolism

FPF fibroblast pneumocyte factor

FPG fasting plasma glucose; fluorescence plus Giemsa; focal proliferative glomerulonephritis

FPGS folylpolyglutamate synthetase

FPH$_2$ reduced form of flavin phosphate

FPHE formaldehyde-treated pyruvaldehyde-stabilized human erythrocytes

FPI femoral pulsatility index; formula protein intolerance; Freiburg Personality Identification Questionnaire

f pil let pills be made [Lat. *fiat pilulae*]

FPK fructose phosphokinase

FPL fasting plasma lipids; flexor pollicis longus

FPM filter paper microscopic [test]; full passive movements

fpm feet per minute

FPN ferric chloride, perchloric acid, and nitric acid [solution]

FPO Federation of Prosthodontic Organizations; freezing point osmometer

FPP free portal pressure

FPPH familial primary pulmonary hypertension

FPR false-positive rate; finger peripheral resistance; fluorescence photobleaching recovery; fractional proximal resorption

FPRA first pass radionuclide angiogram

FPS Fellow of the Pathological Society; Fellow of the Pharmaceutical Society; fetal PCB (polychlorinated biphenyl) syndrome; footpad swelling

fps feet per second; frames per second

FPV fowl plague virus

FPVB femoral popliteal vein bypass

FR failure rate; fasciculus retroflexus; febrile reaction; feedback regulation; Fischer-Race [notation]; fixed ratio; flocculation reaction; flow rate; fluid restriction; fluid retention; free radical; frequency of respiration; frequent relapses

F&R force and rhythm [pulse]

Fr fracture; francium; franklin [unit charge]; French

Fr1 first fraction

FRA fibrinogen-related antigen; fluorescent rabies antibody

fra fragile [site]

FRAC Food Research and Action Center

frac fracture

fract fracture

fract dos in divided doses [Lat. *fracta dosi*]

FRAP fluorescence recovery after photobleaching

FRAT free radical assay technique

FRAX fragile [chromosome] X

fra(X) fragile X chromosome, fragile X syndrome

FRAX-MR fragile X-mental retardation [syndrome]

Fr BB fracture of both bones

FRC Federal Radiation Council; frozen red cells; functional reserve capacity; functional residual capacity

FRCD Fellow of the Royal College of Dentists; fixed ratio combination drug

FRCGP Fellow of the Royal College of General Practitioners

FRCOG Fellow of the Royal College of Obstetricians and Gynaecologists

FRCP Fellow of the Royal College of Physicians

FRCPA Fellow of the Royal College of Pathologists of Australia

FRCPath Fellow of the Royal College of Pathologists

FRCP(C) Fellow of the Royal College of Physicians of Canada

FRCPE Fellow of the Royal College of Physicians of Edinburgh

FRCPI Fellow of the Royal College of Physicians of Ireland

FRCPsych Fellow of the Royal College of Psychiatrists

FRCS Fellow of the Royal College of Surgeons

FRCS(C) Fellow of the Royal College of Surgeons of Canada

FRCSEd Fellow of the Royal College of Surgeons of Edinburgh

FRCSEng Fellow of the Royal College of Surgeons of England

FRCSI Fellow of the Royal College of Surgeons of Ireland

FRCVS Fellow of the Royal College of Veterinary Surgeons

FRE Fischer rat embryo

FREIR Federal Research on Biological and Health Effects of Ionizing Radiation

frem fremitus

freq frequency

FRES Fellow of the Royal Entomological Society

FRF Fertility Research Foundation; follicle-stimulating hormone-releasing factor

FRFC functional renal failure of cirrhosis

FRH follicle-stimulating hormone-releasing hormone

FRh fetal rhesus monkey kidney [cell]

FRHS fast-repeating high sequence

frict friction

frig cold [Lat. *frigidus*]

FRIPHH Fellow of the Royal Institute of Public Health and Hygiene

FRJM full range joint movement

FRMedSoc Fellow of the Royal Medical Society

FRMS Fellow of the Royal Microscopical Society

FROM full range of movements

FRP functional refractory period

FRS Fellow of the Royal Society; ferredoxin-reducing substance; first rank symptom; furosemide

FRSH Fellow of the Royal Society of Health

FRT Family Relations Test; full recovery time

Fru fructose

frust in small pieces [Lat. *frustillatim*]

Frx fracture

FS factor of safety; Fanconi syndrome; Felty syndrome; fibromyalgia syndrome; field stimulation; Fisher syndrome; food service; forearm supination; fracture site; fragile site; Friesinger score; frozen section; full scale [IQ]; full soft [diet]; full strength; function study; human foreskin [cells]; simple fracture

F/S female, spayed [animal]

fsa let it be made skillfully [Lat. *fiat secundum artem*]

fsar let it be made according to the rules [Lat. *fiat secundum artem reglas*]

FSB fetal scalp blood

FSBP finger systolic blood pressure

FSBT Fowler single breath test

FSC Food Standards Committee

FSD focus-skin distance

FSE filtered smoke exposure

FSF fibrin stabilizing factor

FSG fasting serum glucose; focal segmental sclerosis

FSGHS focal segmental glomerular hyalinosis and sclerosis

FSGN focal sclerosing glomerulonephritis

FSGS focal segmental glomerulosclerosis

FSH fascioscapulohumeral; focal and segmental hyalinosis; follicle-stimulating hormone

FSHB follicle-stimulating hormone, beta chain

FSHD facioscapulohumeral dystrophy

FSH/LR-RH follicle-stimulating hormone and luteinizing hormone releasing hormone

FSH-RF follicle-stimulating hormone-releasing factor

FSH-RH follicle-stimulating hormone-releasing hormone

FSI foam stability index; Food Sanitation Institute; function status index

FSIQ full-scale intelligence quotient

FSL fasting serum level

FSMB Federation of State Medical Boards

FSP familial spastic paraplegia; fibrin split products; fibrinogen split products; fine suspended particles

F-SP special form [Lat. *forma specialis*]

FSQ Functional Status Questionnaire

FSR Fellow of the Society of Radiographers; film screen radiography; fragmented sarcoplasmic reticulum; fusiform skin revision

FSS focal segmental sclerosis; Freeman-Sheldon syndrome; French steel sound

FST foam stability test

FSU family service unit; functional spine unit

FSV feline fibrosarcoma virus

FSW field service worker

FT false transmitter; family therapy; fast twitch; fibrous tissue; fingertip; follow through; free testosterone; free thyroxine; full term; function test

FT$_3$ free triiodothyronine

FT$_4$ free thyroxine

Ft ferritin

fT free testosterone

ft foot, feet; let there be made [Lat. *fiat* or *fiant*]

FTA fluorescent titer antibody; fluorescent treponemal antibody

FTA-ABS, FTA-Abs fluorescent treponemal antibody, absorbed [test]

FTAG, F-TAG fast-binding target-attaching globulin

FTAT fluorescent treponemal antibody test

FTBD fit to be detained; full-term born dead

FTBE focal tick-borne encephalitis

FTBS Family Therapist Behavioral Scale

FTC Federal Trade Commission; frequency threshold curve

ftc foot candle

ft cataplasm let a poultice be made [Lat. *fiat cataplasma*]

ft cerat let a cerate be made [Lat. *fiat ceratum*]

ft collyr let an eyewash be made [Lat. *fiat collyrium*]

FTD femoral total density

FTE full-time equivalent

ft emuls let an emulsion be made [Lat. *fiat emulsio*]

ft enem let an enema be made [Lat. *fiat enema*]

FTF finger to finger

FTG full-thickness graft

ft garg let a gargle be made [Lat. *fiat gargarisma*]

FTH ferritin heavy chain

FTI free thyroxine index

FT₃I free triiodothyronine index

ft infus let an injection be made [Lat. *fiat infusum*]

FTIR functional terminal innervation ratio

FTKA failed to keep appointment

FTL ferritin light chain

ftL foot lambert

FTLB full-term live birth

ft lb foot pound

ft linim let a liniment be made [Lat. *fiat linimentum*]

FTLV feline T-lymphotropic lentivirus

FTM fluid thioglycolate medium; fractional test meal

ft mas let a mass be made [Lat. *fiat massa*]

ft mas div in pil let a mass be made and divided into pills [Lat. *fiat massa dividenda in pilulae*]

ft mist let a mixture be made [Lat. *fiat mistura*]

FTN finger to nose

FTNB full-term newborn

FTND full-term normal delivery

FTO fructose-terminated oligosaccharide

ft pil let pills be made [Lat. *fiat pilulae*]

ft pulv let a powder be made [Lat. *fiat pulvis*]

FTR fractional tubular reabsorption

FTS family tracking system; feminizing testis syndrome; fetal tobacco syndrome; fissured tongue syndrome; flexortenosynovitis; thymulin [Fr. *facteur thymique sérique*]

FTSG full thickness skin graft

ft solut let a solution be made [Lat. *fiat solutio*]

ft suppos let a suppository be made [Lat. *fiat suppositorium*]

FTT failure to thrive; fat tolerance test

FTU fluorescence thiourea

ft ung let an ointment be made [Lat. *fiat unguentum*]

FU fecal urobilinogen; fetal urobilinogen; fluorouracil; follow-up; fractional urinalysis; fundus

Fu Finsen unit

F/U follow-up, fundus of umbilicus

F&U flanks and upper quadrants

5-FU 5-fluorouracil

FUB functional uterine bleeding

Fuc fucose

FUDR, FUdR fluorodeoxyuridine

FUFA free volatile fatty acid

FUM 5-fluorouracil and methotrexate; fumarate; fumigation

FUMP fluorouridine monophosphate

FUN follow-up note

funct function, functional

FUO fever of unknown origin

FUOV follow-up office visit

FUR fluorouracil riboside; fluorouridine

FUS feline urologic syndrome; first-use syndrome

FUT fibrinogen uptake test

FUTP fluoridine triphosphate

FV femoral vein; fluid volume; Friend virus

FVA Friend virus anemia

FVC false vocal cord; forced vital capacity

FVE forced volume expiration

FVIC forced inspiratory vital capacity

FVL femoral vein ligation; flow volume loop; force, velocity, length

FVOP finger venous opening pressure

FVP Friend virus polycythemia

FVR feline viral rhinotracheitis; forearm vascular resistance

FVS fetal valproate syndrome

FW Felix-Weil [reaction]; Folin-Wu [reaction]; fragment wound

Fw F wave

fw fresh water

FWA Family Welfare Association

FWB full weight bearing

FWHM full width at half maximum

FWPCA Federal Water Pollution Control Administration

FWR Felix-Weil reaction; Folin-Wu reaction

FX fluoroscopy; fornix; fracture frozen section

Fx fracture

fx fracture; friction

Fx-dis fracture-dislocation

FXN function

FXS fragile X syndrome

FY fiscal year

FYI for your information

FZ focal zone; furazolidone

Fz frontal midline placement of electrodes in electroencephalography

FZS Fellow of the Zoological Society

G acceleration [force]; conductance; free energy; gallop; ganglion; gap; gas; gastrin; gauge; gauss; geometric efficiency; giga; gingiva; gingival; glabella; globular; globulin; glucose; glycine; glycogen; goat; gold inlay; gonidial; good; goose; grade; Grafenberg spot; gram; gravida; gravitation constant; Greek; green; guanidine; guanine; guanosine; gynecology; unit of force of acceleration

G₀ quiescent phase of cells leaving the mitotic cycle

G₁ presynthetic gap [phase of cells prior to DNA synthesis]

G₂ postsynthetic gap [phase of cells following DNA synthesis]

GI primigravida

GII secundigravida

GIII tertigravida

G° standard free energy

g force [pull of gravity]; gap; gender; grain; gram; gravity; group; ratio of magnetic moment of a particle to the Bohr magneton; standard acceleration due to gravity, $9.80665 \ m/s^2$

g relative centrifugal force

γ see *gamma*

GA Gamblers Anonymous; gastric analysis; gastric antrum; general anesthesia; general appearance; gentisic acid; gestational age; gingivoaxial; glucoamylase; glucose; glucose/acetone; glucuronic acid; Golgi apparatus; gramicidin A; granulocyte adherence; granuloma annulare; guessed average; gut-associated; gyrate atrophy

G/A globulin/albumin [ratio]

Ga gallium; granulocyte agglutination

ga gauge

GAA gossypol acetic acid

GAAS Goldberg Anorectic Attitude Scale

GABA, gaba gamma-aminobutyric acid

GABAT, GABA-T gamma-aminobutyric acid transaminase

GABHS group A beta-hemolytic streptococcus

GABOA gamma-amino-beta-hydroxybutyric acid

GAD glutamic acid decarboxylase

GADH gastric alcohol dehydrogenase

GADS gonococcal arthritis/dermatitis syndrome

GAG glycosaminoglycan; group-specific antigen gene

GAHS galactorrhea-amenorrhea hyperprolactinemia syndrome

GAIPAS General Audit Inpatient Psychiatric Assessment Scale

GAL galactosyl; glucuronic acid lactone

Gal galactose

gal galactose; gallon

GalC galactocerebroside

GalN galactosamine

GALT galactose-1-p-uridyltransferase; gut-associated lymphoid tissue

GALV gibbon ape leukemia virus

Galv, galv galvanic

γ Greek letter *gamma*; a carbon separated from the carboxyl group by two other carbon atoms; a constituent of the gamma protein plasma fraction; heavy chain of immunogammaglobulin; a monomer in fetal hemoglobin; photon

γG immunoglobulin G

GAN giant axon neuropathy

G and D growth and development

gang, gangl ganglion, ganglionic

GANS granulomatous angiitis of the nervous system

GAP D-glyceraldehyde-3-phosphate; guanosine triphosphatase activating protein

GAPD glyceraldehyde-3-phosphate dehydrogenase

GAPDH reduced glyceraldehyde-phosphate dehydrogenase

GAPO growth retardation, alopecia,

pseudo-anodontia, and optic atrophy [syndrome]

Garg, garg gargle

GARS glycine amide phosphoribosyl synthetase

GAS galactorrhea-amenorrhea syndrome; gastric acid secretion; gastroenterology; general adaptation syndrome; generalized arteriosclerosis

GASA growth-adjusted sonographic age

gastroc gastrocnemius [muscle]

GAT gelatin agglutination test; Gerontological Apperception Test; group adjustment therapy

GB gallbladder; glial bundle; goof balls; Guillain-Barré [syndrome]

Gb gilbert

GBA ganglionic blocking agent; gingivobuccoaxial

GBD gallbladder disease; gender behavior disorder; glass blower's disease; granulomatous bowel disease

GBG glycine-rich beta-glycoprotein; gonadal steroid-binding globulin

GBH gamma-benzene hexachloride; graphite benzalkonium-heparin

GBHA glyoxal-bis-(2-hydroxyanil)

GBI globulin-binding insulin

GBIA Guthrie bacterial inhibition assay

GBL glomerular basal lamina

GBM glomerular basement membrane

GBP galactose-binding protein; gastric bypass; gated blood pool

GBS gallbladder series; gastric bypass surgery; group B *Streptococcus*; Guillain-Barré syndrome; glycerine-buffered saline [solution]

GBSS Gey's balanced saline solution; Guillain-Barré-Strohl syndrome

GC ganglion cell; gas chromatography; general circulation; general closure; general condition; geriatric care; germinal center; glucocorticoid; goblet cell; Golgi cell; gonococcus; gonorrhea; granular casts; granulomatous colitis; granulosa cell; group-specific component; guanine cytosine; guanylcyclase

Gc gigacycle; gonococcus; group-specific component

GCA gastric cancer area; giant cell arteritis

g-cal gram calorie

GCB gonococcal base

GCBM glomerular capillary basement membrane

GCF growth-rate-controlling factor

GCFT gonococcal/gonorrhea complement fixation test

GCI General Cognitive Index

GCIIS glucose controlled insulin infusion system

GCLO gastric *Campylobacter*-like organism

g-cm gram-centimeter

GC-MS gas chromatography-mass spectrometry

GCN giant cerebral neuron

g-coef generalizability coefficient

GCR glucocorticoid receptor; Group Conformity Rating

GCRS gynecological chylous reflux syndrome

GCS general clinical services; Gianotti-Crosti syndrome; Glasgow Coma Scale; glucocorticosteroid; glutamylcysteine synthetase

GCSA Gross cell surface antigen

G-CSF granulocyte colony-stimulating factor

GCT general care and treatment; giant cell thyroiditis; giant cell tumor

GC(T)A giant cell (temporal) arteritis

GCU gonococcal urethritis

GCV great cardiac vein

GCVF great cardiac vein flow

GCW glomerular capillary wall

GCWM General Conference on Weights and Measures

GCY gastroscopy

GD gastroduodenal; general diagnostics; general dispensary; gestational day; Gianotti's disease; gonadal dysgenesis; Graves' disease; growth and development

Gd gadolinium

G&D growth and development

GDA germine diacetate

GDB gas density balance; guide dogs for the blind

GDC giant dopamine-containing cell; General Dental Council

Gd-DTPA gadolinium-diethylene-triamine-pentaacetic acid

GDF gel diffusion precipitin

GDH glucose dehydrogenase; glutamate dehydrogenase; glycerophosphate dehydrogenase; glycol dehydrogenase; gonadotropin hormone; growth and differentiation hormone

GDID genetically determined immunodeficiency disease

g/dl grams per deciliter

GDM gestational diabetes mellitus

GDMO General Duties Medical Officer

GDP gel diffusion precipitin; guanosine diphosphate

GDS Global Deterioration Scale; Gordon Diagnostic System [for attention disorders]; gradual dosage schedule

GDW glass-distilled water

GDXY XY gonadal dysgenesis

GE gastric emptying; gastroemotional; gastroenteritis; gastroenterology; gastroenterostomy; gastroesophageal; gastrointestinal endoscopy; gel electrophoresis; generalized epilepsy; generator of excitation; gentamicin; glandular epithelium

Ge germanium

G/E granulocyte/erythroid [ratio]

GEC galactose elimination capacity; glomerular epithelial cell

GECC Government Employees' Clinic Centre

GEF gastroesophageal fundoplication; glossoepiglottic fold; gonadotropin enhancing factor

GEH glycerol ester hydrolase

gel gelatin

gel quav in any kind of jelly [Lat. *gelatina quavis*]

GEN gender; generation

Gen genetics, genetic; genus

gen general; genital

genet genetic, genetics

GENETOX Genetic Toxicology [data base]

gen et sp nov new genus and species [Lat. *genus et species nova*]

genit genitalia, genital

gen nov new genus [Lat. *genus novum*]

GENOVA generalized analysis of variance

GENPS genital neoplasm-papilloma syndrome

GENT gentamicin

GEP gastroenteropancreatic

GEPG gastroesophageal pressure gradient

GER gastroesophageal reflux; geriatrics; granular endoplasmic reticulum

Ger geriatric(s); German

GERD gastroesophageal reflux disease

geriat geriatrics, geriatric

GERL Golgi-associated endoplasmic reticulum lysosome

Geront gerontology, gerontologist, gerontologic

GES glucose-electrolyte solution

GEST gestation

GET gastric emptying time; general endotracheal [anesthesia]; graded treadmill exercise test

Gev giga electron volt

GEWS Gianturco expandable wire stent

GEX gas exchange

GF gastric fistula; gastric fluid; germ-free; glass factor; glomerular filtration; gluten-free; grandfather; growth factor; growth failure

gf gram-force

GFA glial fibrillary acidic [protein]

GFAP glial fibrillary acidic protein

GFD gluten-free diet

GFFS glycogen and fat-free solid

GFH glucose-free Hanks [solution]

GFI glucagon-free insulin; ground-fault interrupter

GFL giant follicular lymphoma

GFP gamma-fetoprotein; gel-filtered platelet; glomerular filtered phosphate

GFR glomerular filtration rate
GFS global focal sclerosis; guafenesin
GG gamma globulin; genioglossus; glycylglycine
GGA general gonadotropic activity
GGCS gamma-glutamyl cysteine synthetase
GGE generalized glandular enlargement; gradient gel electrophoresis
GGFC gamma-globulin-free calf [serum]
GGG gamboge [Lat. *gummi guttae gambiae*]; glycine-rich gamma-glycoprotein
GGM glucose-galactose malabsorption
GG or S glands, goiter, or stiffness [of neck]
GGPNA gamma-glutamyl-p-nitroanilide
GGT gamma-glutamyl transferase; gamma-glutamyl transpeptidase
GGTP gamma-glutamyl transpeptidase
GGVB gelatin, glucose, and veronal buffer
GH general health; general hospital; genetic hypertension; genetically hypertensive [rat]; geniohyoid; growth hormone
GHA Group Health Association
GHAA Group Health Association of America
GHB gamma hydroxybutyrate
GHb glycated hemoglobin
GHBA gamma-hydroxybutyric acid
GHD growth hormone deficiency
GHPQ General Health Perception Questionnaire
GHQ General Health Questionnaire
GHR granulomatous hypersensitivity reaction
GHRF growth hormone-releasing factor
GH-RH growth hormone-releasing hormone
GH-RIF growth hormone-release inhibiting factor
GH-RIH growth hormone release-inhibiting hormone
GHV goose hepatitis virus
GHz gigahertz
GI gastrointestinal; gelatin infusion

[medium]; gingival index; globin insulin; glomerular index; glucose intolerance; granuloma inguinale; growth inhibition
gi gill
GIA gastrointestinal anastomosis
GIB gastrointestinal bleeding
GIBF gastrointestinal bacterial flora
GICA gastrointestinal cancer
GID gender identity disorder
GIF growth hormone-inhibiting factor
GIFT gamete intrafallopian transfer; granulocyte immunofluorescence test
GIGO garbage in, garbage out
GIH gastrointestinal hemorrhage; growth-inhibiting hormone
GII gastrointestinal infection
GIK glucose-insulin-potassium [solution]
GIM gonadotropin-inhibiting material
Ging, ging gingiva, gingival
g-ion gram-ion
GIP gastric inhibitory peptide or polypeptide; giant cell interstitial pneumonia; glucose-dependent insulinotropic peptide; gonorrheal invasive peritonitis
GIR global improvement rating
GIS gas in stomach; gastrointestinal series
GIT gastrointestinal tract
GITS gastrointestinal therapeutic system
GITT gastrointestinal transit time; glucose insulin tolerance test
GJ gap junction; gastric juice; gastrojejunostomy
GJA-S gastric juice aspiration syndrome
GK galactokinase; glomerulocystic kidney; glycerol kinase
GKD glycerol kinase deficiency
GL gland; glomerular layer; glycolipid; glycosphingolipid; glycyrrhizin; greatest length; gustatory lacrimation
Gl beryllium [Lat. *glucinium*]; glabella
gl gill; gland, glandular
g/l grams per liter
GLA galactosidase A; gamma-linolenic acid; gingivolinguoaxial
glac glacial

GLAD gold-labelled antigen detection
gland glandular
GLC gas-liquid chromatography
Glc glucose
glc glaucoma
GlcA gluconic acid
GLC-MS gas-liquid chromatography–mass spectrometry
GlcN glucosamine
GlcUA D-glucuronic acid
GLD globoid leukodystrophy; glutamate dehydrogenase
GLDH glutamic dehydrogenase
GLH germinal layer hemorrhage; giant lymph node hyperplasia
GLI glicentin; glucagon-like immunoreactivity
GLIM generalized linear interactive model
GLM general linear model
Gln glucagon; glutamine
GLNH giant lymph node hyperplasia
GLO glyoxylase
GLO1 glyoxylase 1
glob globular; globulin
GLP glucose-L-phosphate; glycolipoprotein; good laboratory practice; group living program
GLR graphic level recorder
GLS generalized lymphadenopathy syndrome
GLTN glomerulotubulonephritis
GLTT glucose-lactate tolerance test
GLU glucose; glucuronidase; glutamic acid, glutamine
Glu glucuronidase; glutamic acid, glutamine
glu glucose; glutamate
GLU-5 five-hour glucose tolerance test
GLUC glucosidase
gluc glucose
GLUD glutamate dehydrogenase
GLV Gross leukemia virus
GLY, gly glycine
glyc glyceride
GM gastric mucosa; Geiger-Müller [counter]; general medicine; genetic manipulation; geometric mean; giant melanosome; gram; grand mal [epilepsy]; grandmother; grand multiparity; granulocyte-macrophage; growth medium
GM⁺ gram-positive
GM⁻ gram-negative
G-M Geiger-Müller [counter]
Gm an allotype marker on the heavy chains of immunoglobins
gm gram
g-m gram-meter
GMA glyceral methacrylate
GMB gastric mucosal barrier; granulomembranous body
GMBF gastric mucosa blood flow
GMC general medical clinic; general medical council; grivet monkey cell
gm cal gram calorie
gm/cc grams per cubic centimeter
GMCD grand mal convulsive disorder
GM-CFU granulocyte-macrophage colony forming unit
GM-CSF granulocyte-macrophage colony-stimulating factor
GMD geometric mean diameter; glycopeptide moiety modified derivative
GME graduate medical education
GMENAC Graduate Medical Education National Advisory Committee
GMH germinal matrix hemorrhage
GMK green monkey kidney [cells]
GML gut mucosa lymphocyte
g/ml grams per milliliter
gm/l grams per liter
gm-m gram-meter
g-mol gram-molecule
GMP glucose monophosphate; guanosine monophosphate
3':5'-GMP guanosine 3':5'-cyclic phosphate
GMR gallops, murmurs, rubs
GMS General Medical Service; Gilbert-Meulengracht syndrome; Gomori methenamine silver [stain]; glyceryl monostearate
GM&S general medicine and surgery
GMSC General Medical Services Committee

GMT geometric mean titer; gingival margin trimmer
GMV gram molecular volume
GMW gram molecular weight
GN gaze nystagmus; glomerulonephritis; glucose nitrogen [ratio]; gnotobiote; graduate nurse; gram-negative
G/N glucose/nitrogen ratio
Gn gnathion; gonadotropin
GNA general nursing assistance
GNB ganglioneuroblastoma; gram-negative bacillus
GNBM gram-negative bacillary meningitis
GNC general nursing care; General Nursing Council
GND Gram-negative diplococci
GNID gram-negative intracellular diplococci
GNP gerontologic nurse practitioner
GNR gram-negative rods
GnRF gonadotropin-releasing factor
GnRH gonadotropin-releasing hormone
G/NS glucose in normal saline [solution]
GNTP Graduate Nurse Transition Program
GO gastro-[o]esophageal; gonorrhea; glucose oxidase
G&O gas and oxygen
Go gonion
GOAT Galveston Orientation and Amnesia Test
GOBAB gamma-hydroxy-beta-aminobutyric acid
GOE gas, oxygen, and ether
GOG Gynecologic Oncology Group
GOH geroderma osteodysplastica hereditaria
GΩ gigohm [one billion ohms]
GON gonococcal ophthalmia neonatorum
GOND glaucomatous optic nerve damage
GOQ glucose oxidation quotient
GOR gastroesophageal reflux; general operating room
GOT aspartate aminotransferase; glucose oxidase test; glutamate oxaloacetate transaminase; goal of treatment
GOTM glutamic-oxaloacetic transaminase, mitochondrial
GP gangliocytic paraganglioma; gastroplasty; general paralysis, general paresis; general practice, general practitioner; genetic prediabetes; geometric progression; globus pallidus; glucose phosphate; glutathione peroxidase; glycerophosphate; glycopeptide; glycoprotein; Goodpasture syndrome; gram-positive; guinea pig; gutta percha
G/P gravida/para
G-1-P glucose-1-phosphate
G3P, G-3-P glyceraldehyde-3-phosphate; glycerol-3-phosphate
G6P, G-6-P glucose-6-phosphate
gp gene product; glycoprotein; group
GPA Goodpasture antigen; grade point average; Group Practice Association; guinea pig albumin
GPAIS guinea pig anti-insulin serum
G6Pase, G-6-Pase glucose-6-phosphatase
GPB glossopharyngeal breathing
GPC gastric parietal cell; gel permeation chromatography; giant papillary conjunctivitis; granular progenitor cell; guinea pig complement
GPD glucose-6-phosphate dehydrogenase
G6PD, G-6-PD glucose-6-phosphate dehydrogenase
G-6-PDA glucose-6-phosphate dehydrogenase enzyme variant A
G6PDH, G-6-PDH glucose-6-phosphate dehydrogenase reduced
GPE guinea pig embryo
GPEP General Professional Education of the Physician
GPF glomerular plasma flow; granulocytosis-promoting factor
GPGG guinea pig gamma-globulin
GPh Graduate in Pharmacy
GPHN giant pigmented hairy nevus
GPHV guinea pig herpes virus
GPI general paralysis of the insane; glu-

cose phosphate isomerase; glycoprotein I; guinea pig ileum

GpIb glycoprotein Ib

GPIMH guinea pig intestinal mucosal homogenate

GPIPID guinea pig intraperitoneal infectious dose

GPK guinea pig kidney [antigen]

GPKA guinea pig kidney absorption [test]

GPLV guinea pig leukemia virus

Gply gingivoplasty

GPM general preventive medicine; giant pigmented melanosome

GPMAL gravida, para, multiple births, abortions, and live births

GPN graduate practical nurse

GPPQ General Purpose Psychiatric Questionnaire

GPRBC guinea pig red blood cell

GPS Goodpasture's syndrome; gray platelet syndrome; guinea pig serum; guinea pig spleen

GPT glutamate-pyruvate transaminase; glutamic-pyruvic transaminase

GpTh group therapy

GPU guinea pig unit

GPUT galactose phosphate uridyl transferase

GPx glutathione peroxidase

GQAP general question-asking program

GR gamma-rays; gastric resection; general research; generalized rash; glucocorticoid receptor; glutathione reductase

gr grade; graft; grain; gram; gravity; gray; gross

gr⁻ gram-negative

gr⁺ gram-positive

GRA gated radionuclide angiography; glucocorticoid-remedial aldosteronism; gonadotropin-releasing agent

GRABS group A beta-hemolytic streptococcal pharyngitis

Grad by degrees [Lat. *gradatim*]

grad gradient; gradually; graduate

GRAE generally regarded as effective

gran granule, granulated

GRAS generally recognized as safe

GRASS gradient recalled acquisition in the steady state

grav gravid

grav I pregnancy one; primigravida

GRD gastroesophageal reflux disease; gender role definition

grd ground

GRE gradient-recalled echo; Graduate Record Examination

GRF gastrin-releasing factor; genetically related macrophage factor; gonadotropin-releasing factor; growth hormone-releasing factor

GRG glycine-rich glycoprotein

GRH growth hormone-releasing hormone

GRID gay-related immunodeficiency [syndrome]

GRIF growth hormone release-inhibiting factor

GRN granules

GrN gram-negative

Grn green

GRP gastrin-releasing peptide; glucose-regulated protein

GrP gram-positive

Gr₁P₀AB₁ one pregnancy, no births, one abortion

GRPS glucose-Ringer-phosphate solution

GRS Golabi-Rosen syndrome

GRW giant ragweed [test]

gr wt gross weight

GS gallstone; Gardner syndrome; gastric shield; general surgery; Gilbert syndrome; glomerular sclerosis; glutamine synthetase; goat serum; Goldenhar syndrome; Goodpasture's syndrome; graft survival; granulocytic sarcoma; grip strength; group section; group-specific

G6S glucosamine-6-sulfatase

gs group specific

G/S glucose and saline

g/s gallons per second

GSA general somatic afferent; group-specific antigen; Gross virus antigen; guanidinosuccinic acid

GSBG gonadal steroid-binding globulin

GSC gas-solid chromatography; gravity settling culture

GSCN giant serotonin-containing neuron

GSD genetically significant dose; Gerstmann-Sträussler disease; glutathione synthetase deficiency; glycogen storage disease

GSE general somatic efferent; gluten-sensitive enteropathy

GSF galactosemic fibroblast; genital skin fibroblast

GSH glomerulus-stimulating hormone; golden Syrian hamster; reduced glutathione

GSN giant serotonin-containing neuron

GSoA Gerontological Society of America

GSP galvanic skin potential

GSR galvanic skin response; generalized Shwartzman reaction; glutathione reductase

GSS gamete-shedding substance; General Social Survey; Gerstmann-Sträussler-Scheinker [disease]

GSSG oxidized glutathione

GSSR generalized Sanarelli-Shwartzman reaction

GST glutathione-S-transferase; gold salt therapy; gold sodium thiomalate; graphic stress telethermometry; group striction

GSW gunshot wound

GSWA gunshot wound, abdominal

GT gait training; gastrostomy; generation time; genetic therapy; gingiva treatment; Glanzmann's thrombasthenia; glucose therapy; glucose tolerance; glucose transport; glucuronyl transferase; glutamyl transpeptidase; glycityrosine; granulation tissue; great toe; greater trochanter; group tensions; group therapy

GT1-GT10 glycogen storage disease, types 1 to 10

gt drop [Lat. *gutta*]

g/t granulation time; granulation tissue

G&T gowns and towels

GTA gene transfer agent; Glanzmann's thrombasthenia; glycerol teichoic acid

GTB gastrointestinal tract bleeding

GTD gestational trophoblastic disease

GTF glucose tolerance factor; glucosyltransferase

GTH gonadotropic hormone

GTHR generalized thyroid hormone resistance

GTM generalized tendomyopathy

GTN gestational trophoblastic neoplasia; glomerulotubulonephritis; glyceryl trinitrate

GTO Golgi tendon organ

GTP glutamyl transpeptidase; guanosine triphosphate

GTR galvanic tetanus ratio; granulocyte turnover rate

GTS Gilles de la Tourette syndrome; glucose transport system

GTT gelatin-tellurite-taurocholate [agar]; glucose tolerance test

gtt drops [Lat. *guttae*]

GU gastric ulcer; genitourinary; glucose uptake; glycogenic unit; gonococcal urethritis; gravitational ulcer; guanethidine

GUA group of units of analysis

Gua guanine

GULHEMP general physique, upper extremity, lower extremity, hearing, eyesight, mentality, and personality

Guo guanosine

GUS genitourinary sphincter; genitourinary system

gutt to the throat [Lat. *gutturi*]

guttat drop by drop [Lat. *guttatim*]

gutt quibusd with a few drops [Lat. *guttis quibusdam*]

GV gastric volume; gentian violet; germinal vesicle; granulosis virus; griseoviridan; Gross virus

GVA general visceral afferent [nerve]

GVB gelatin-Veronal buffer

GVBD germinal vesicle breakdown

GVE general visceral efferent [nerve]

GVF good visual fields

GVG gamma-vinyl-gamma-aminobutyric acid

GVH, GvH graft-versus-host

GVHD, GvHD graft-versus-host disease

GVHR, GvHR graft-versus-host reaction

GVTY gingivectomy

GW germ warfare; gigawatt; glycerin in water; gradual withdrawal; group work

G/W glucose in water

GWE glycerol and water enema

GWG generalized Wegener's granulomatosis

GX glycinexylidide

GXT graded exercise test

Gy gray

GYN, Gyn, gyn gynecologic, gynecologist, gynecology

GZ Guilford-Zimmerman [test]

H

H bacterial antigen in serologic classification of bacteria [Ger. *Hauch,* film]; deflection in the His bundle in electrogram [spike]; draft [Lat. *haustus*]; electrically induced spinal reflex; enthalpy; fucosal transferase-producing gene; heart; heavy; height; hemagglutination; hemisphere; hemolysis; *Hemophilus;* henry; heparin; heroin; high; histidine; *Histoplasma;* histoplasmosis; Holzknecht unit; homosexual; horizontal; hormone; horse; hospital; Hounsfield unit; hour; human; hydrogen; hydrolysis; hygiene; hyoscine; hypermetropia; hyperopia; hypodermic; hypothalamus; magnetic field strength; magnetization; mustard gas; oersted; the region of a sarcomere containing only myosin filaments [Ger. *heller,* lighter] [band]

H^+ hydrogen ion

$[H^+]$ hydrogen ion concentration

H_0 null hypothesis

H1, ^{1}H, H^1 protium

H_1 alternative hypothesis

H2, ^{2}H, H^2 deuterium

H$_2$ blockers histamine blockers

H3, ^{3}H, H^3 tritium

h hand-rearing [of experimental animals]; heat transfer coefficient; hecto; height; henry; hour [Lat. *hora*]; human; hundred; negatively staining region of a chromosome; Planck's constant; secondary constriction; specific enthalpy

HA H antigen; Hakim-Adams [syndrome]; halothane anesthesia; Hartley [guinea pig]; headache; hearing aid; height age; hemadsorption; hemagglutinating antibody; hemagglutination; hemagglutinin; hemolytic anemia; hemophiliac with adenopathy; hepatic adenoma; hepatic artery; hepatitis A; hepatitis-associated; heterophil antibody; Heyden antibiotic; high anxiety; hippuric acid; histamine; histocompatibility antigen; Horton's arteritis; hospital administration; hospital admission; hospital apprentice; Hounsfield unit; human albumin; hyaluronic acid; hydroxyapatite; hyperalimentation; hyperandrogenism; hypersensitivity alveolitis; hypothalamic amenorrhea

H/A head to abdomen

HA2 hemadsorption virus 2

Ha absolution hypermetropia; hafnium; hamster; Hartmann number

ha hectare

HAA hearing aid amplifier; hemolytic anemia antigen; hepatitis-associated antigen; hospital activity analysis

HA Ag hepatitis A antigen

HABA 2(4'-hydroxyazobenzene) benzoic acid

HABF hepatic artery blood flow

HAChT high affinity choline transport

HACR hereditary adenomatosis of the colon and rectum

hACSP human adenylate cyclase-stimulating protein

HACS hyperactive child syndrome

HAD hemadsorption; hospital administration, hospital administrator

HAd hemadsorption; hospital administrator

HADH hydroxyacyl CoA dehydrogenase

HAd-I hemadsorption-inhibition

HAE health appraisal examination; hearing aid evaluation; hepatic artery embolism; hereditary angioneurotic edema

HaF Hageman factor

HAFP human alpha-fetoprotein

HAG heat-aggregated globulin

HAGG hyperimmune antivariola gammaglobulin

HAGH hydroxyacyl-glutathione hydrolase

HAHTG horse antihuman thymus globulin

HAI hemagglutination inhibition; hepatic arterial infusion

H&A Ins health and accident insurance

HAIR-AN hyperandrogenism, insulin resistance, and acanthosis nigricans [syndrome]

HaK hamster kidney

HAL hepatic artery ligation; hypoplastic acute leukemia

hal halogen; halothane

HALC high affinity-low capacity

halluc hallucinations

HALP hyperalphalipoproteinemia

HaLV hamster leukemia virus

HAM hearing aid microphone; helical axis in motion; human alveolar macrophage; hypoparathyroidism, Addison's disease, and mucocutaneous candidiasis [syndrome]

HAm human amnion

HAMA Hamilton anxiety [scale]; human anti-murine antibody

HAMD Hamilton depression [scale]

Ha-MSV Harvey murine sarcoma virus

HAN heroin-associated nephropathy; hyperplastic alveolar nodule

HANA hemagglutinin neuraminidase

H and E hematoxylin and eosin [stain]

Handicp handicapped

HANE hereditary angioneurotic edema

HANES Health and Nutrition Examination Survey

hANF human atrial natriuretic factor

h-ANP human atrial natriuretic polypeptide

HAP Handicapped Aid Program; heredopathia atactica polyneuritiformis; high-altitude peristalsis; histamine acid phosphate; humoral antibody production; hydrolyzed animal protein; hydroxyapatite

HAPA hemagglutinating anti-penicillin antibody

HAPC high-amplitude peristaltic contraction; hospital-acquired penetration contact

HAPE high-altitude pulmonary edema

HAPPHY Heart Attack Primary Prevention in Hypertension

HAPS hepatic arterial perfusion scintigraphy

HAR high-altitude retinopathy

HAREM heparin assay rapid easy method

HARH high-altitude retinal hemorrhage

HARM heparin assay rapid method

HARS histidyl-RNA synthetase

HART Heparin-Aspirin Reinfarction Trial

HAS Hamilton Anxiety Scale; health advisory service; highest asymptomatic [dose]; hospital administrative service; hospital advisory service; human albumin solution; hyperalimentation solution; hypertensive arteriosclerotic

HASCVD hypertensive arteriosclerotic cardiovascular disease

HASHD hypertensive arteriosclerotic heart disease

HASP Hospital Admissions and Surveillance Program

HAT Halsted Aphasia Test; head, arm, trunk; heparin-associated thrombocytopenia; heterophil antibody titer; hospital arrival time; hypoxanthine, aminopterin, and thymidine; hypoxanthine, azaserine, and thymidine

HATG horse antihuman thymocyte globulin

HATH Heterosexual Attitudes Toward Homosexuality [scale]

HATT heparin-associated thrombocytopenia and thrombosis

HATTS hemagglutination treponemal test for syphilis

HAU hemagglutinating unit

haust a draft [Lat. *haustus*]

HAV hemadsorption virus; hepatitis A virus

HAWIC Hamburg-Wechsler Intelligence Test for Children

HAZ MAT hazardous material

HB health board; heart block; heel to buttock; held back; hemoglobin; hepatitis B; His bundle; hold breakfast; housebound; hybridoma bank; hyoid body

Hb hemoglobin

HbA hemoglobin A, adult hemoglobin

HBA₁ glycosylated hemoglobin

HBAb hepatitis B antibody

HBABA hydroxybenzeneazobenzoic acid

HBAg hepatitis B antigen

HBB hemoglobin beta-chain; hospital blood bank; hydroxybenzyl benzimidazole

HbBC hemoglobin binding capacity

HBBW hold breakfast blood work

HB$_c$, HBC, HBc hepatitis B core [antigen]

HbC hemoglobin C

HB$_c$Ag, HBcAg, HBCAG hepatitis B core antigen

HBCG heat-aggregated Calmette-Guérin bacillus

HbCO carboxyhemoglobin

Hb CS hemoglobin Constant Spring

HBD has been drinking; hydroxybutyric dehydrogenase; hypophosphatemic bone disease

HbD hemoglobin D

HBDH hydroxybutyrate dehydrogenase

HBDT human basophil degranulation test

HBE His bundle electrogram

HbE hemoglobin E

HB$_e$Ag, HBeAg, HBEAG hepatitis B early [antigen]

HBF hand blood flow; hemispheric blood flow; hemoglobinuric bilious fever; hepatic blood flow; hypothalamic blood flow

HbF fetal hemoglobin, hemoglobin F

Hbg hemoglobin

HBGM home blood glucose monitoring

HBGR hemoglobin-gamma regulator

HbH hemoglobin H

Hb-Hp hemoglobin-haptoglobin [complex]

HBI high serum-bound iron

HBIG, HBIg hepatitis B immunoglobulin

HBL hepatoblastoma

HBLA human B-cell lymphocyte antigen

HBLV human B-cell lymphotropic virus

HBM Health Belief Model; hypertonic buffered medium

HbM hemoglobin Milwaukee

HbMet methemoglobin

HBO hyperbaric oxygenation, hyperbaric oxygen

HbO oxyhemoglobin

HbO₂ oxyhemoglobin

HBOT hyperbaric oxygen therapy

HBP hepatic binding protein; high blood pressure

HbP primitive hemoglobin

HBr hydrobromic acid

HBS hepatitis B surface [antigen]; hyperkinetic behavior syndrome

HB$_s$ hepatitis B surface [antigen]

HbS hemoglobin S, sickle-cell hemoglobin

HBSAg IgG antibody to HBsAg

HB$_s$Ag, HBsAg, HBSAG hepatitis B surface antigen

HBsAg/adr hepatitis B surface antigen manifesting group-specific determinant *a* and subtype-specific determinants *d* and *r*

HBSC hematopoietic blood stem cell

HBSS Hank's balanced salt solution

HbSS hemoglobin SS

HBT human brain thromboplastin; human breast tumor

HBV hepatitis B vaccine; hepatitis B virus

HBV-MN membranous nephropathy associated with hepatitis B virus

HBW high birth weight

HbZ hemoglobin Z, hemoglobin Zürich

HC hair cell; hairy cell; handicapped; head circumference; head compression; healthy control; heat conservation; heavy chain; hemoglobin concentration; hemorrhagic colitis; heparin cofactor; hepatic catalase; hepatocellular; hereditary coproporphyria; hippocampus; histamine challenge; histochemistry; home care; Hospital Corps; house call; Huntington's chorea; hyaline casts; hydraulic concussion; hydrocarbon; hydrocortisone; hydroxycorticoid; hyoid cornu;

hypercholesterolemia; hypertrophic cardiomyopathy

H&C hot and cold

Hc hydrocolloid

HCA heart cell aggregate; hepatocellular adenoma; home care aide; Hospital Corporation of America; hydrocortisone acetate

HCAP handicapped

HCB hexachlorobenzene

HCC hepatitis contagiosa canis; hepatocellular carcinoma; history of chief complaint; hydroxycholecalciferol

25-HCC 25-hydroxycholecalciferol

HCD health care delivery; heavy-chain disease; high-calorie diet; high-carbohydrate diet; homologous canine distemper

HCE hypoglossal carotid entrapment

HCF hereditary capillary fragility; highest common factor; hypocaloric carbohydrate feeding

HCFA Health Care Financing Administration

hCFSH human chorionic follicle-stimulating hormone

HCG, hCG human chorionic gonadotropin

HCH hexachlorocyclohexane; hemochromatosis

HCHWA hereditary cerebral hemorrhage with amyloidosis

HcImp hydrocolloid impression

HCIS Health Care Information System

HCL hairy-cell leukemia; human cultured lymphoblasts

HCLF high carbohydrate, low fiber [diet]

HCM health care management; hypertrophic cardiomyopathy

HCMM hereditary cutaneous malignant melanoma

HCMV human cytomegalovirus

HCN hereditary chronic nephritis

HCO₃⁻ bicarbonate

HCP handicapped; hepatocatalase peroxidase; hereditary coproporphyria; hexachlorophene; high cell passage

H&CP hospital and community psychiatry

HCPCS Health Care Financing Administrators Common Procedure Coding System

HCR heme-controlled repressor; host-cell reactivation; hysterical conversion reaction

HCRE Homeopathic Council for Research and Education

hCRH human corticotropin-releasing hormone

Hcrit hematocrit

HCS Hajdu-Cheney syndrome; Hazard Communication Standard; health care support; hourglass contraction of the stomach; human chorionic somatotropin; human cord serum

17-HCS 17-hydroxycorticosteroid

hCS human chorionic somatomammotropin

HCSD Health Care Studies Division

hCSM human chorionic somatomammotropin

HCSS hypersensitive carotid sinus syndrome

HCT health check test; hematocrit; historic control trial; homocytotrophic; human calcitonin; hydrochlorothiazide; hydroxycortisone

Hct hematocrit

hCT human calcitonin; human chorionic thyrotropin

HCTC Health Care Technology Center

HCTD hepatic computed tomography density

HCTS high cholesterol and tocopherol supplement

HCTU home cervical traction unit

HCTZ hydrochlorothiazide

HCU homocystinuria; hyperplasia cystica uteri

HCV hepatitis C virus

HCVD hypertensive cardiovascular disease

HCW health care worker

Hcy homocysteine

HD Haab-Dimmer [syndrome]; Hajna-

Damon [broth]; Hansen's disease; hearing distance; heart disease; helix destabilizing [protein]; hemidiaphragm; hemodialysis; hemolytic disease; hemolyzing dose; herniated disc; high density; high dose; hip disarticulation; Hirschsprung's disease; Hodgkin's disease; hormone-dependent; house dust; human diploid [cells]; Huntington's disease; hydatid disease; hydroxydopamine
H&D Hunter and Driffield [curve]
HD₅₀ 50% hemolyzing dose of complement
hd at bedtime [Lat. *hora decubitus*]; head
HDA Huntington's Disease Association; hydroxydopamine
HDARAC high dose cytarabine (ARA C)
HDBH hydroxybutyric dehydrogenase
HDC histidine decarboxylase; human diploid cell
HDCS human diploid cell strain
HDCV human diploid cell rabies vaccine
HDD high-dosage depth; Higher Dental Diploma
HDF host defense factor; human diploid fibroblast
HDFP Hypertension Detection and Follow-up Program
HDG high-dose group
HDH heart disease history
HDI hemorrhagic disease of infants; hexamethylene diisocyanate
HDL high-density lipoprotein
HDL-C high-density lipoprotein–cholesterol
HDL-c high-density lipoprotein–cell surface
HDLP high-density lipoprotein
HDLS hereditary diffuse leukoencephalopathy with spheroids
HDLW distance from which a watch ticking is heard by left ear
HDMP high-dose methylprednisolone
HDMTX high-dose methotrexate
HDMTX-CF high-dose methotrexate citrovorum factor

HDMTX-LV high-dose methotrexate leucovorin
HDN hemolytic disease of the newborn
hDNA hybrid deoxyribonucleic acid
HDP hexose diphosphate; high-density polyethylene; hydroxydimethylpyrimidine
HDPAA heparin-dependent platelet-associated antibody
HDRF Heart Disease Research Foundation
HDRS Hamilton Depression Rating Scale
HDRV human diploid rabies vaccine
HDRW distance from which a watch ticking is heard by right ear
HDS Hamilton Depression Scale; Health Data Services; health delivery system; Healthcare Data Systems; herniated disc syndrome; Hospital Discharge Survey
HDU hemodialysis unit
HDV hepatitis delta virus
HDZ hydralazine
HE hard exudate; hektoen enteric [agar]; hemagglutinating encephalomyelitis; hemoglobin electrophoresis; hepatic encephalopathy; hereditary eliptocytosis; high exposure; hollow enzyme; human enteric; hydroxyethyl [cellulose]; hyperextension; hypogonadotropic eunuchoidism
H&E hematoxylin and eosin [stain]; hemorrhage and exudate; heredity and environment
He heart; helium
HEA hexone-extracted acetone; human erythrocyte antigen
HEAL Health Education Assistance Loan
HEAT human erythrocyte agglutination test
HEB hemato-encephalic barrier
hebdom a week [Lat. *hebdomada*]
HEC hamster embryo cell; Health Education Council; human endothelial cell; hydroxyergocalciferol; hydroxyethyl cellulose
HED hereditary ectodermal dysplasia; hydrotropic electron-donor; hypohid-

rotic ectodermal dysplasia; unit skin dose [of x-rays] [Ger. *Haut-Einheits-Dosis*]
HEDH hypohidrotic ectodermal dysplasia with hypothyroidism
HEENT head, ears, eyes, nose, and throat
HEEP health effects of environmental pollutants
HEF hamster embryo fibroblast; human embryo fibroblast
HEG hemorrhagic erosive gastritis
HEHR highest equivalent heart rate
HEI Health Effects Institute; high-energy intermediate; homogenous enzyme immunoassay; human embryonic intestine [cells]
HEIR health effects of ionizing radiation; high-energy ionizing radiation
HEIS high-energy ion scattering
HEK human embryonic kidney
HEL hen egg white lysozyme; human embryonic lung; human erythroleukemia
HeLa Helen Lake [human cervical carcinoma cells]
HELF human embryo lung fibroblast
HELLIS Health, Literature, Library and Information Services
HELLP hemolysis, elevated liver enzymes, and low platelet count [syndrome]
HELP Health Education Library Program; Health Emergency Loan Program; Health Evaluation and Learning Program; heat escape lessening posture; Heroin Emergency Life Project; Hospital Equipment Loan Project
HEM hematology, hematologist; hematuric; hemorrhage; hemorrhoids
HEMA Health Education Media Association
hemat hematology, hematologist
HEMB hemophilia B
hemi hemiparesis, hemiparalysis; hemiplegia
HEMPAS hereditary erythrocytic multinuclearity with positive acidified serum
HEMRI hereditary multifocal relapsing inflammation
HeNe helium neon [laser]

HEP hemolysis end point; high egg passage [virus]; high-energy phosphate; human epithelial cell
Hep hepatic; hepatitis
hEP human endorphin
HEp-1 human cervical carcinoma cells
HEp-2 human laryngeal tumor cells
HEPA high-efficiency particulate air [filter]
HEPES N-2-hydroxyethylpiperazine-N-2-ethanesulfonic [acid]
HEPM human embryonic palatal mesenchymal [cell]
HER hemorrhagic encephalopathy of rats; hernia
hered heredity, hereditary
hern hernia, herniated
HERS Health Evaluation and Referral Service; hemorrhagic fever with renal syndrome
HES health examination survey; hematoxylin-eosin stain; human embryonic skin; human embryonic spleen; hydroxyethyl starch; hypereosinophilic syndrome; hyperprostaglandin E syndrome
HESCA Health Sciences Communications Association
HET Health Education Telecommunications; helium equilibration time
Het heterophil
het heterozygous
HETE hydroxy-eicosatetraenoic [acid]
HETP height equivalent to a theoretical plate; hexaethyltetraphosphate
HEV health and environment; hemagglutinating encephalomyelitis virus; hepato-encephalomyelitis virus; high endothelial venule; human enteric virus
HEW [Department of] Health, Education, and Welfare
HEX hexaminidase; hexosaminidase
Hex hexamethylmelamine
HEX A, hex A hexosaminidase A
HEX B, hex B hexosaminidase B
HEX C, hex C hexosaminidase C
HF Hageman factor; haplotype frequency; hard filled [capsule]; hay fever; head of fetus; head forward; heart fail-

ure; helper factor; hemofiltration; hemorrhagic factor; hemorrhagic fever; Hertz frequency; high fat [diet]; high flow; high frequency; human fibroblast; hydrogen fluoride; hyperflexion

Hf hafnium

hf half; high frequency

HFAK hollow-fiber artificial kidney

HFC hard filled capsule; high-frequency current; histamine-forming capacity

HFD hemorrhagic fever of deer; high-fiber diet; high forceps delivery; hospital field director

HFDK human fetal diploid kidney

HFDL human fetal diploid lung

HFE, HFe hemochromatosis

HFEC human foreskin epithelial cell

HFF human foreskin fibroblast

HFG hand-foot-genital [syndrome]

HFH hemifacial hyperplasia

HFHV high frequency, high volume

HFI hereditary fructose intolerance; human fibroblast interferon

HFIF human fibroblast interferon

HFJV high-frequency jet ventilation

HFL human fetal lung

HFM hemifacial microsomia

HFMA Healthcare Financial Management Association

HFO high-frequency oscillator; high-frequency oscillatory [ventilation]

HFO-A high-frequency oscillatory [ventilation]-active [expiratory phase]

HFOV high-frequency oscillatory ventilation

HFP hexafluoropropylene; high-frequency pulsation; hypofibrinogenic plasma

HFPPV high-frequency positive pressure ventilation

HFR high-frequency recombination

Hfr heart frequency; high frequency

HFRS hemorrhagic fever with renal syndrome

HFS hemifacial spasm; Hospital Financial Support

hfs hyperfine structure

hFSH, HFSH human follicle-stimulating hormone

HFST hearing for speech test

HFT high-frequency transduction; high-frequency transfer

Hft high-frequency transfer

HFU hand-foot-uterus [syndrome]

HFV high-frequency ventilation

HG hand grip; herpes gestationis; Heschl's gyrus; high glucose; human gonadotropin; human growth; hypoglycemia

Hg mercury [Lat. *hydrargyrum*]

hg hectogram; hemoglobin

HGA homogentisic acid

Hgb hemoglobin

HGF hyperglycemic-glucogenolytic factor

Hg-F fetal hemoglobin

HGG herpetic geniculate ganglionitis; human gammaglobulin

HGH, hGH human gamma globulin; human growth hormone

HGHRF human growth hormone releasing factor

HGM hog gastric mucosa; human gene mapping; human glucose monitoring

HGMCR human genetic mutant cell repository

HGO hepatic glucose output; human glucose output

HGP hepatic glucose production; hyperglobulinemic purpura

HGPRT hypoxanthine guanine phosphoribosyl transferase

HGPS hereditary giant platelet syndrome; Hutchinson-Gilford progeria syndrome

hGRH human growth hormone-releasing hormone

HH halothane hepatitis; hard-of-hearing; healthy hemophiliac; healthy human; hiatal hernia; holistic health; home help; hydroxyhexamide; hypergastrinemic hyperchlorhydria; hyperhidrosis; hypogonadotropic hypogonadism; hyporeninemic hypoaldosteronism

H&H hematocrit and hemoglobin

HHA Health Hazard Appraisal; hereditary hemolytic anemia; home health agency; hypothalamo-hypophyseo-adrenal [system]

HHb hypohemoglobinemia; un-ionized hemoglobin

HHC home health care

HHCS high-altitude hypertrophic cardiomyopathy syndrome

HHD high heparin dose; hypertensive heart disease

HHE health hazard evaluation; hemiconvulsion-hemiplegia-epilepsy [syndrome]

HHG hypertrophic hypersecretory gastropathy

HHH hyperornithinemia, hyperammonemia, homocitrillinuria [syndrome]

HHHO hypotonia, hypomentia, hypogonadism, obesity [syndrome]

HHIE Hearing Handicap Inventory for the Elderly

HHIE-S Hearing Handicap Inventory for the Elderly-Screening Version

HHM humoral hypercalcemia of malignancy

H + Hm compound hypermetropic astigmatism

HHNC hyperosmolar nonketotic diabetic coma

HHNK hyperglycemic hyperosmoler nonketotic [coma]

HHNS hyperosmolar hyperglycemic nonketotic syndrome

HHR hydralazine, hydrochlorothiazide, and reserpine

HHRH hereditary hypophosphatemic rickets with hypercalciuria; hypothalamic hypophysiotropic releasing hormone

HHS [Department of] Health and Human Services; Hearing Handicap Scale; hereditary hemolytic syndrome; human hypopituitary serum; hyperglycemic hyperosmolar syndrome; hyperkinetic heart syndrome

HHSSA Home Health Services and Staffing Association

HHT head halter traction; hereditary hemorrhagic telangiectasia; heterotopic heart transplantation; homoharringtonine; hydroxyheptadecatrienoic acid

HHV human herpes virus

HI head injury; health insurance; hearing impaired; heart infusion; hemagglutination inhibition; hepatobiliary imaging; high impulsiveness; histidine; hormone-independent; hormone insensitivity; hospital insurance; humoral immunity; hydroxyindole; hyperglycemic index; hypomelanosis of Ito; hypothermic ischemia

H-I hemagglutination-inhibition

Hi histamine; histidine

HIA Hearing Industries Association; heat infusion agar; hemagglutination inhibition antibody or assay

HIAA Health Insurance Association of America

5-HIAA 5-hydroxyindoleacetic acid

HIB heart infusion broth; hemolytic immune body; *Hemophilus influenzae* type B [vaccine]

HIBAC Health Insurance Benefits Advisory Council

HIC handling-induced convulsions; Heart Information Center

HICA hydroxyisocaproic acid

HiCn cyanomethemoglobin

HID headache, insomnia, depression [syndrome]; herniated intervertebral disc; human infectious dose; hyperkinetic impulse disorder

HIDA Health Industry Distributors Association; hepato-iminodiacetic acid (lidofenin) [nuclear medicine scan]

HIE human intestinal epithelium; hyper-IgE [syndrome]

HIES hyper-IgE syndrome

HIF higher integrative functions

HIFBS heat-inactivated fetal bovine serum

HIFC hog instrinsic factor concentrate

HIFCS heat-inactivated fetal calf serum

HIG, hIG human immunoglobulin

HIg hyperimmunoglobulin

HIH hypertensive intracerebral hemorrhage

HIHA high impulsiveness, high anxiety

HiHb hemiglobin (methemoglobin)

HII Health Industries Institute; Health Insurance Institute; hemagglutination inhibitor immunoassay

HILA high impulsiveness, low anxiety

HIM hepatitis-infectious mononucleosis; hexosephosphate isomerase

HIMA Health Industries Manufacturers Association

HIMC hepatic intramitochondrial crystalloid

HIMP high-dose intravenous methylprednisolone

HIMT hemagglutination inhibition morphine test

Hint Hinton [test]

HIO hypoiodism

HIOMT hydroxyindole-O-methyl transferase

HIOS high index of suspicion

HIP health illness profile; health insurance plan; homograft incus prosthesis; hospital insurance program; hydrostatic indifference point

HIPA heparin-induced platelet activation

HIPE Hospital Inpatient Enquiry

HiPIP high potential iron protein

HIPO hemihypertrophy, intestinal web, preauricular skin tag, and congenital corneal opacity [syndrome]; Hospital Indicator for Physicians Orders

HIR head injury routine

HIS health information system; Health Interview Survey; histidine; hospital information system; hyperimmune serum

His histidine

HISSG Hospital Information Systems Sharing Group

HIST hospital in-service training

hist histamine, history

HISTLINE History of Medicine On-Line

Histo histoplasmin skin test

histol histological, histologist, histology

HIT hemagglutination inhibition test; heparin-induced thrombocytopenia; histamine inhalation test; hypertrophic infiltrative tendonitis

HITB, HiTB *Hemophilus influenzae* type B

HITT heparin-induced thrombocytopenia and thrombosis

HITTS heparin-induced thrombosis-thrombocytopenia syndrome

HIU hyperplasia interstitialis uteri

HIV human immunodeficiency virus

HIV1 human immunodeficiency virus type 1

HIV Ag human immunodeficiency virus antigen

HIVAN human immunodeficiency virus–associated nephropathy

HIV-G human immunodeficiency virus–associated gingivitis

HJ Howell-Jolly [bodies]

HJR hepatojugular reflex

HK hand to knee; heat-killed; heel-to-knee; hexokinase; human kidney

H-K hand to knee

HKAFO hip-knee-ankle-foot orthosis

HKAO hip-knee-ankle orthosis

HKC human kidney cell

HKLM heat-killed *Listeria monocytogenes*

HKS hyperkinesis syndrome

HL hairline; hairy leukoplakia; half life; hearing level; hearing loss; heparin lock; histiocytic lymphoma; histocompatibility locus; Hodgkin's lymphoma; human leukocyte; hyperlipidemia; hypermetropia, latent; hypertrichosis lanuginosa

H&L heart and lung [machine]

H/L hydrophil/lipophil [ratio]

Hl hypermetropia, latent

hl hectoliter

HLA histocompatibility leukocyte antigen; histocompatibility locus antigen; homologous leukocyte antibody; human leukocyte antigen; human lymphocyte antigen

HL-A human leukocyte antigen

HLAA human leukocyte antigen A

HLAB human leukocyte antigen B

HLAC human leukocyte antigen C
HLAD human leukocyte antigen D
HLA-LD human lymphocyte antigen-lymphocyte defined
HLA-SD human lymphocyte antigen-serologically defined
HLB hydrophilic-lipophilic balance; hypotonic lysis buffer
HLBI human lymphoblastoid interferon
HLC heat loss center
HLCL human lymphoblastoid cell line
HLD hepatolenticular degeneration; herniated lumbar disk; Hippel-Lindau disease; hypersensitivity lung disease
HLDH heat-stable lactic dehydrogenase
HLEG hydrolysate lactalbumin Earle's glucose
HLF heat-labile factor
HLH hemophagocytic lymphohistiocytosis
hLH human luteinizing hormone
HLHS hypoplastic left heart syndrome
HLI human leukocyte interferon
H-L-K heart, liver, and kidneys
HLL hypoplastic left lung
HLN hilar lymph node; hyperplastic liver nodules
HLP hepatic lipoperoxidation; hind leg paralysis; hyperkeratosis lenticularis perstans; hyperlipoproteinemia
HLR heart-lung resuscitation
HLS Health Learning System; Hippel-Lindau syndrome
HLT heart-lung transplantation; human lipotropin; human lymphocyte transformation
HLV herpes-like virus
HLVS hypoplastic left ventricle syndrome
HM hand movements; health maintenance; heart murmur; hemifacial microsomia; Holter monitoring; homosexual male; hospital management; human milk; hydatidiform mole; hyperimmune mouse
Hm manifest hypermetropia
hm hectometer
HMA hydroxymethionine analog

HMAC Health Manpower Advisory Council
HMAS hyperimmune mouse ascites
HMB homatropine methobromide
HMBA hexamethylene bisacetamide
HMC hand-mirror cell; health maintenance cooperative; heroin, morphine, and cocaine; histocompatibility complex, major; hospital management committee; hypertelorism-microtia-clefting [syndrome]
HMCCMP human mammary carcinoma cell membrane proteinase
HMD hyaline membrane disease
HME Health Media Education; heat and moisture exchanger; heat, massage, and exercise
HMF hydroxymethylfurfural
HMG high-mobility group; human menopausal gonadotropin; 3-hydroxy-3-methyl-glutaryl
hMG human menopausal gonadotropin
HMG CoA 3-hydroxy-3-methylglutaryl coenzyme A
HMI healed myocardial infarct
HMIS hazardous materials identification system; hospital medical information system
HML human milk lysosome
HMM heavy meromyosin; hexamethyl-melamine
HMMA 4-hydroxy-3-methoxymandelic acid
HMO health maintenance organization; heart minute output
HMP hexose monophosphate pathway; hot moist packs
HMPA hexamethylphosphoramide
HM-PAO hexamethyl-propyleneamine-oxime
HMPG hydroxymethoxyphenylglycol
HMPS hexose monophosphate shunt
HMPT hexamethylphosphorotriamide
HMR histiocytic medullary reticulosis
H-mRNA H-chain messenger ribonucleic acid
HMRTE human milk reverse transcriptase enzyme

HMS hexose monophosphate shunt; hypermobility syndrome

HMSA health manpower shortage area

HMSAS hypertrophic muscular subaortic stenosis

HMSN hereditary motor and sensory neuropathy

HMSS Hospital Management Systems Society

HMT hematocrit; histamine-N-methyltransferase; hospital management team

HMTA hexamethylenetetramine

HMW high-molecular-weight

HMWC high-molecular-weight component

HMWGP high-molecular-weight glycoprotein

HMWK high-molecular-weight kininogen

HMX heat, massage, and exercise

HN head and neck; head nurse; hemagglutinin neuraminidase; hematemesis neonatorum; hemorrhage of newborn; hereditary nephritis; high necrosis; hilar node; histamine-containing neuron; home nursing; human nutrition; hypertrophic neuropathy

H&N head and neck

hn tonight [Lat. *hoc nocte*]

HNA heparin neutralizing activity

HNB human neuroblastoma

HNC hypernephroma cell; hyperosmolar nonketotic coma; hypothalamoneurohypophyseal complex

HNKDS hyperosmolar nonketotic diabetic state

HNL histiocytic necrotizing lymphadenitis

HNP hereditary nephritic protein; herniated nucleus pulposus; human neurophysin

HNPCC hereditary nonpolyposis colorectal cancer

hnRNA heterogeneous nuclear ribonucleic acid

hnRNP heterogeneous nuclear ribonucleoprotein

HNS head and neck surgery; home nursing supervisor

HNSHA hereditary nonspherocytic hemolytic anemia

HNTD highest nontoxic dose

HNV has not voided

HO hand orthosis; high oxygen; hip orthosis; Holt-Oram [syndrome]; house officer; hyperbaric oxygen

H/O history of

Ho holmium; horse

HOA hip osteoarthritis; hypertrophic osteoarthropathy

HoaRhLG horse anti-rhesus lymphocyte globulin

HoaTTG horse anti-tetanus toxoid globulin

HOB head of bed

HOC human ovarian cancer; hydroxycorticoid

HOCM hypertrophic obstructive cardiomyopathy

hoc vesp this evening [Lat. *hoc vespere*]

HOD hyperbaric oxygen drenching

HOF hepatic outflow

HofF height of fundus

HOGA hyperornithinemia with gyrate atrophy

HOH hard of hearing

HOI hospital onset of infection

HoIg horse immunoglobulin

HOME Home Observation for Measurement of the Environment

Homeop homeopathy

HOMO highest occupied molecular orbital; homosexual

homo homosexual

HOOD hereditary onycho-osteodysplasia

HOODS hereditary onycho-osteodysplasia syndrome

HOP high oxygen pressure

HOPE Healthcare Options Plan Entitlement; health-oriented physical education; holistic orthogonal parameter estimation

HOPI history of present illness

HOPP hepatic occluded portal pressure

hor horizontal
hor decub at bedtime [Lat. *hora decubitus*]
hor interm at the intermediate hours [Lat. *horis intermediis*]
hor som at bedtime [Lat. *hori somni*]
hor un spatio at the end of one hour [Lat. *horae unius spatio*]
HOS Holt-Oram syndrome; human osteosarcoma
HoS horse serum
Hosp, hosp hospital
HOST hypo-osmotic shock treatment
HOT human old tuberculin; hyperbaric oxygen therapy
HOTS hypercalcemia–osteolysis–T-cell syndrome
HP halogen phosphorus; handicapped person; haptoglobin; hard palate; Harvard pump; health profession(al); heat production; heel to patella; hemiparkinsonism; hemipelvectomy; hemiplegia; hemoperfusion; *Hemophilus pleuropneumoniae*; heparin; high potency; high power; high pressure; high protein; highly purified; horizontal plane; horsepower; hospital participation; hot pack; house physician; human pituitary; hydrophilic petrolatum; hydrostatic pressure; hydroxypyruvate; hyperparahyroidism; hypersensitivity pneumonitis; hypophoria
H&P history and physical examination
Hp haptoglobin; hematoporphyrin; hemiplegia
HPA *Helix pomatia* agglutinin; hemagglutinating penicillin antibody; *Histoplasma capsulatum* polysaccharide antigen; humeroscapular periarthritis; hypothalamo-pituitary-adrenocortical [system]
HPAA hydroperoxyarachidonic acid; hydroxyphenylacetic acid; hypothalamo-pituitary-adrenal axis
HPAC hypothalamo-pituitary-adrenocortical
HPBC hyperpolarizing bipolar cell
HPBF hepatotrophic portal blood factor

HPBL human peripheral blood leukocyte
HPC hemangiopericytoma; hippocampal pyramidal cell; history of present complaint; holoprosencephaly; hydroxypropylcellulose
HPCA human progenitor cell antigen
HPCHA high red-cell phosphatidylcholine hemolylic anemia
HPD hearing protective device; high-protein diet; home peritoneal dialysis
HPE hepatic portoenterostomy; high-permeability edema; history and physical examination; hydrostatic permeability edema
HPETE hydroxyperoxy-eicosotetranoic [acid]
HPF heparin-precipitable fraction; hepatic plasma flow; high-pass filter; high-power field [microscope]; hypocaloric protein feeding
HPFH hereditary persistence of fetal hemoglobin
hPFSH, HPFSH human pituitary follicle-stimulating hormone
hPG, HPG human pituitary gonadotropin
HPI hepatic perfusion index; history of present illness
HPL human parotid lysozyme; human peripheral lymphocyte; human placental lactogen
hPL human placental lactogen; human platelet lactogen
HPLA hydroxyphenyl lactic acid
HPLAC high-pressure liquid-affinity chromatography
HPLC high-performance liquid chromatography; high-power liquid chromatography; high-pressure liquid chromatography
HPLE hereditary polymorphic light eruption
HPM high-performance membrane
HPMC human peripheral mononuclear cell
HPN home parenteral nutrition; hypertension

hpn hypertension

HPNS high pressure neurological syndrome

HPO high-presure oxygen; hydroperoxide; hydrophilic ointment; hypertrophic pulmonary osteoarthropathy

HPP hereditary pyropoikilocytosis; history of presenting problems

HPP, hPP hydroxyphenylpyruvate; hydroxypyrozolopyrimidine; human pancreatic polypeptide

HPPA hydroxyphenylpyruvic acid

HPPH 5-(4-hydroxyphenyl)-5-phenylhydantoin

HPPO high partial pressure of oxygen; hydroxyphenyl pyruvate oxidase

HPR haptoglobin-related gene

HPr human prolactin

hPRL human prolactin

HPRP human platelet-rich plasma

HPRT hypoxanthine-guanine phosphoribosyltransferase

HPS hematoxylin, phloxin, and saffron; Hermansky-Pudlak syndrome; high-protein supplement; His-Purkinje system; human platelet suspension; hypertrophic pyloric stenosis; hypothalamic pubertal syndrome

HPSL Health Professions Student Loan

HPT histamine provocation test; human placental thyrotropin; hyperparathyroidism; hypothalamo-pituitary-thyroid [system]

HPTH hyperparathyroid hormone

HPTIN human pancreatic trypsin inhibitor

HPU heater probe unit

HPV *Hemophilus pertussis* vaccine; hepatic portal vein; human papillomavirus; human parvovirus; human pulmonary vasoconstriction

HPVD hypertensive pulmonary vascular disease

HPV-DE high-passage virus-duck embryo

HPV-DK high-passage virus-dog kidney

HPVG hepatic portal venous gas

HPW hypergammaglobulinemic purpura of Waldenström

HPX high peroxidase [content]; hypophysectomized

HPZ high pressure zone

[3H]QNB (-)[3H]quinuclidinyl benzilate

HR heart rate; hemorrhagic retinopathy; high resolution; higher rate; hormonal response; hospital record; hospital report; hyperimmune reaction; hypophosphatemic rickets

hr hairless [mouse]; host-range [mutant]; hour

H&R hysterectomy and radiation

HRA health risk appraisal; heart rate audiometry; histamine release activity; Human Resources Administration

HRAE high right atrium electrogram

HRBC horse red blood cell

HRC high-resolution chromatography; horse red cell; human rights committee

HRCT, HR-CT high-resolution computed tomography

HRE hepatic reticuloendothelial [cell]; high-resolution electrocardiography; hormone receptor enzyme

HREH high-renin essential hypertension

HREM high-resolution electron microscopy

HRIG, HRIg human rabies immunoglobulin

HRL head rotation to the left

HRLA human reovirus-like agent

hRNA heterogeneous ribonucleic acid

HRNB Halstead-Reitan Neuropsychological Battery

HRP high-risk patient; high-risk pregnancy; histidine-rich protein; horseradish peroxidase

HRPD Hamburg Rating Scale for Psychiatric Disorders

HRR head rotation to the right; heart rate range

HRRI heart rate retardation index

HRS Hamilton Rating Scale; hepatorenal syndrome; high rate of stimulation;

hormone receptor site; humeroradial synostosis

HRSA Health Resources and Services Administration

HRS-D Hamilton Rating Scale for Depression; Hirschsprung's disease

HRT heart rate; hormone replacement therapy

HRTE human reverse transcriptase enzyme

HRTEM high-resolution transmission electron microscopy

HRV heart rate variability; human reovirus; human rotavirus

HS Haber syndrome; half strength; hamstring; hand surgery; Hartmann's solution; head sling; healthy subject; heart sounds; heat-stable; heavy smoker; Hegglin's syndrome; heme synthetase; Henoch-Schönlein [purpura]; heparan sulfate; hereditary spherocytosis; herpes simplex; hidradenitis suppurativa; homologous serum; horizontally selective; Horner's syndrome; horse serum; hospital ship; hospital staff; hospital stay; hours of sleep; house surgeon; human serum; Hurler's syndrome; hypereosinophilic syndrome; hypersensitivity; hypertonic saline

hs at bedtime [Lat. *hora somni*]

H/S helper-suppressor [ratio]

H&S hemorrhage and shock; hysterectomy and sterilization

HSA Hazardous Substances Act; Health Services Administration; Health Systems Agency; hereditary sideroblastic anemia; horse serum albumin; human serum albumin; hypersomnia-sleep apnea

HSAG N-2-hydroxyethylpiperazine-N-2-ethanesulfonate-saline-albumin-gelatin

HSAN hereditary sensory and autonomic neuropathy

HSAP heat-stable alkaline phosphatase

HSAS hypertrophic subaortic stenosis

HSC Hand-Schüller-Christian [syndrome]; Health and Safety Commission;

health screening center; hematopoietic stem cell; human skin collagenase

HSCL Hopkins Symptom Check List

HS-CoA reduced coenzyme A

HSD honest significant difference; hydroxysteroid dehydrogenase

HSDB Hazardous Substances Data Bank

H(SD) Holtzman Sprague-Dawley [rat]

HSE herpes simplex encephalitis; hemorrhagic shock and encephalopathy

HSES hemorrhagic shock-encephalopathy syndrome

HSF histamine sensitizing factor; human serum esterase; hypothalamic secretory factor

HSG herpex simplex genitalis; hysterosalpingogram, hysterosalpingography

hSGF human skeletal growth factor

HSGP human sialoglycoprotein

HSHC hydrocortisone hemisuccinate

HSI heat stress index; human seminal plasma inhibitor

HSK herpes simplex keratitis

HSL herpes simplex labialis

HSLC high-speed liquid chromatography

HSM hepatosplenomegaly; holosystolic murmur

HSMHA Health Services and Mental Health Administration

HSN hereditary sensory neuropathy

hSOD human superoxide dismutase

h som at bedtime [Lat. *hora somni*]

HSP Health Systems Plan; hemostatic screening profile; Henoch-Schönlein purpura; hereditary spastic paraparesis; Hospital Service Plan; human serum prealbumin; human serum protein

hsp heat shock protein [gene]

HS-PG heparan sulfate-proteoglycan

HSPM hippocampal synaptic plasma membrane

HSPN Henoch-Schönlein purpura nephritis

HSQB Health Standards and Quality Bureau

HSR Harleco synthetic resin; heated

serum reagin; homogeneously staining region

HSRC Health Services Research Center; Human Subjects Review Committee

HSRD hypertension secondary to renal disease

HSRI Health Systems Research Institute

HSRS Health-Sickness Rating Scale

HSRV human spuma retrovirus

HSS Hallermann-Streiff syndrome; Hallervorden-Spatz syndrome; Henoch-Schönlein syndrome; high-speed supernatant; hyperstimulation syndrome; hypertrophic subaortic stenosis

HSSCC hereditary site-specific colon cancer

HSTF human serum thymus factor

HSV herpes simplex virus; high selective vagotomy; hop stunt viroid; hyperviscosity syndrome

HSV-1 herpes simplex virus type 1

HSV-2 herpes simplex virus type 2

HSVE herpes simplex virus encephalitis

HSVtk herpes simplex virus thymidine kinase

HSyn heme synthase

HT Hashimoto's thyroiditis; hearing test; hearing threshold; heart; heart transplantation, heart transplant; hemagglutination titer; hereditary tyrosinemia; high-frequency transduction; high temperature; high tension; histologic technician; home treatment; hospital treatment; Hubbard tank; human thrombin; hydrocortisone test; hydrotherapy; hydroxytryptamine; hypermetropia, total; hypertension; hyperthyroidism; hypertransfusion; hypodermic tablet; hypothalamus; hypothyroidism

H&T hospitalization and treatment

5-HT 5-hydroxytryptamine [serotonin]

Ht height of heart; heterozygote; hyperopia, total; hypothalamus

ht a draft [Lat. *haustus*]; heart; heart tones; height; high tension

HTA heterophil transplantation antigen; human thymocyte antigen; hydroxytryptamine; hypophysiotropic area

HTACS human thyroid adenyl-cyclase stimulator

ht aer heated aerosol

HT(ASCP) Histologic Technician certified by the American Society of Clinical Pathologists

HTB house tube feeding; human tumor bank

HTC hepatoma cell; hepatoma tissue culture; homozygous typing cell

HTCVD hypertensive cardiovascular disease

HTD human therapeutic dose

HTDW heterosexual development of women

HTF heterothyrotropic factor; house tube feeding

HTG hypertriglyceridemia

HTH homeostatic thymus hormone; hypothalamus

HTHD hypertensive heart disease

HTI hemispheric thrombotic infarction

HTIG human tetanus immune globulin

HTK heel to knee

HTL hamster tumor line; hearing threshold level; histotechnologist; human T-cell leukemia; human thymic leukemia

HTLA high-titer, low acidity; human T-lymphocyte antigen

HTL(ASCP) Histotechnologist certified by the American Society of Clinical Pathologists

HTLV human T-cell leukemia/lymphoma virus; human T-lymphotropic virus

HTLV-MA cell membrane antigen associated with the human T-cell leukemia virus

HTLV-I-MA human T-cell leukemia virus-I-associated membrane antigen

HTN Hantaan-[like virus]; hypertension; hypertensive nephropathy

HTO hospital transfer order

HTOR 5-hydroxytryptamine oxygenase regulator

HTP House-Tree-Person [test]; hydroxytryptophan; hypothromboplastinemia

5-HTP 5-hydroxy-L-tryptophan

HtPA hexahydrophthalic anhydride

HTPN home total parenteral nutrition

HTS head traumatic syndrome; human thyroid-stimulating hormone, human thyroid stimulator

HTSAB human thyroid-stimulating antibody

HTSH, hTSH human thyroid-stimulating hormone

HTST high temperature, short time

HTV herpes-type virus

HTVD hypertensive vascular disease

HTX histrionicotoxin

HU heat unit; hemagglutinating unit; hemolytic unit; human urine, human urinary; hydroxyurea; hyperemia unit

Hu human

HUC hypouricemia

HuEPO human erythropoietin

HU-FSH human urinary follicle-stimulating hormone

HUI headache unit index

HUIFM human leukocyte interferon meloy

HuIFN human interferon

HUK human urinary kallikrein

Hum humerus

HUP Hospital Utilization Project

HUR hydroxyurea

HURA health in underserved rural areas

HURT hospital utilization review team

HUS hemolytic uremic syndrome; hyaluronidase unit for semen

HuSA human serum albumin

hut histidine utilization [gene]

HUTHAS human thymus antiserum

HUV human umbilical vein

HV hallux valgus; Hantaan virus; heart volume; hepatic vein; herpesvirus; high voltage; high volume; hospital visit; hyperventilation

H&V hemigastrectomy and vagotomy

HVA homovanillic acid

HVAC heating, ventilating, and air conditioning

HVC Health Visitor's Certificate

HVD hypertensive vascular disease

HVE hepatic venous effluence; high-voltage electrophoresis

HUVEC human umbilical vein endothelial cell

HVG host versus graft [disease]

HVGS high-voltage galvanic stimulation

HVH *Herpesvirus hominis*

HVJ hemagglutinating virus of Japan

HVL, hvl half-value layer

HVLP high volume, low pressure

HVM high-velocity missile

HVPC high-voltage pulsed current

HVPE high-voltage paper electrophoresis

HVPG hepatic venous pressure gradient

HVR hypoxic ventilation response

HVS herpesvirus of Saimiri; herpesvirus sensitivity; hyperventilation syndrome; hyperviscosity syndrome

HVSD hydrogen-detected ventricular septal defect

HVT half-value thickness; herpesvirus of turkeys

HVTEM high-voltage transmission electron microscopy

HVUS hypocomplementemic vasculitis urticaria syndrome

HW healing well

HWB hot water bottle

HWC Health and Welfare, Canada

HWD heartworm disease

HWE healthy worker effect; hot water extract

HWP hot wet pack

HWS hot water-soluble

HX histiocytosis X; hydrogen exchange; hypophysectomized

Hx history; hypoxanthine

HXIS hard x-ray imaging spectrometry

HXM hexamethylmelamine

HXR hypoxanthine riboside

Hy hypermetropia; hyperopia; hypophysis; hypothenar; hysteria

HYD hydralazine; hydration, hydrated; hydrocortisone; hydroxyurea

hydr hydraulic

hydro hydrotherapy

hyg hygiene, hygienic, hygienist

HYL, Hyl hydroxylysine

HYP hydroxyproline; hypnosis
Hyp hydroxyproline; hyperresonance; hypertrophy; hypothalamus
hyp hypophysis, hypophysectomy
hyper-IgE hyperimmunoglobulinemia E
hypn hypertension
hypno hypnosis
Hypo hypodermic, hypodermic injection

hypox hypophysectomized
HypRF hypothalamic releasing factor
Hypro hydroxyproline
hys, hyst hysterectomy; hysteria, hysterical
HZ herpes zoster
Hz hertz
HZO herpes zoster ophthalmicus
HZV herpes zoster virus

I electric current; impression; incisor [permanent]; independent; index; indicated; induction; inertia; inhalation; inhibition, inhibitor; inosine; insoluble; inspiration, inspired; insulin; intake; intensity; intermittent; internal medicine; intestine; iodine; ionic strength; isoleucine; isotope; region of a sarcomere that contains only actin filaments; Roman numeral one

I-131 radioactive iodine

i incisor [deciduous]; insoluble; isochromosome; optically inactive

ι see *iota*

IA ibotenic acid; immune adherence; immunoadsorbent; immunobiologic activity; impedance angle; indolaminergic accumulation; indolic acid; indulin agar; infantile autism; infected area; inferior angle; inhibitory antigen; internal auditory; intra-alveolar; intra-amniotic; intra-aortic; intra-arterial; intra-articular; intra-atrial; intra-auricular; intrinsic activity

I&A irrigation and aspiration

Ia immune response gene-associated antigen

IAA imidazoleacetic acid; indoleacetic acid; infectious agent, arthritis; insulin autoantibody; International Antituberculosis Association; interruption of the aortic arch; iodoacetic acid

IAAR imidazoleacetic acid ribonucleotide

IAB Industrial Accident Board; intraabdominal; intra-aortic balloon

IABA intra-aortic balloon assistance

IABC, IABCP intra-aortic balloon counter-pulsation

IABM idiopathic aplastic bone marrow

IABP intra-aortic balloon pump

IAC ineffective airway clearance; internal auditory canal; intra-arterial catheter; intra-arterial chemotherapy

IACD implantable automatic cardioverter-defibrillator; intra-arterial conduction defect

IACP intra-aortic counterpulsation

IACS International Academy of Cosmetic Surgery

IACV International Association of Cancer Victims and Friends

IAD inactivating dose; internal absorbed dose

IADH inappropriate antidiuretic hormone

IADHS inappropriate antidiuretic hormone syndrome

IADL instrumental activities of daily living

IADR International Association for Dental Research

IAds immunoadsorption

IAEA International Atomic Energy Agency

IAFI infantile amaurotic familial idiocy

IAG International Association of Gerontology; International Academy of Gnathology

IAGP International Association of Geographic Pathology

IAGUS International Association of Genito-Urinary Surgeons

IAH idiopathic adrenal hyperplasia; implantable artificial heart

IAHA idiopathic autoimmune hemolytic anemia; immune adherence hemagglutination

IAHD idiopathic acquired hemolytic disorder

IAHS infection-associated hemophagocytic syndrome; International Association of Hospital Security

IAI intra-abdominal infection

IAIMS Integrated Academic Information Management System

IAIS insulin autoimmune syndrome

IAM Institute of Applied Microbiology

[Japan]; Institute of Aviation Medicine; internal auditory meatus

i am intra-amniotic

IAMM International Association of Medical Museums

IAN idiopathic aseptic necrosis; indole acetonitrile

iANP immunoreactive atrial natriuretic peptide

IAO immediately after onset; intermittent aortic occlusion; International Association of Orthodontists

IAOM International Association of Oral Myology

IAP immunosuppressive acidic protein; inosinic acid pyrophosphorylase; Institute of Animal Physiology; intermittent acute porphyria; International Academy of Pathology; International Academy of Proctology; intra-abdominal pressure; intracisternal A-type particle; islet-activating protein

IAPB International Association for Prevention of Blindness

IAPG interatrial pressure gradient

IAPM International Academy of Preventive Medicine

IAPP International Association for Preventive Pediatrics; islet amyloid polypeptide

IAR immediate asthma reaction; inhibitory anal reflex; iodine-azide reaction

IARC International Agency for Research on Cancer

IARF ischemic acute renal failure

IARSA idiopathic acquired refractory sideroblastic anemia

IAS immunosuppressive acidic substance; infant apnea syndrome; insulin autoimmune syndrome; interatrial septum; interatrial shunting; internal anal sphincter; intra-amniotic saline

IASA interatrial septal aneurysm

IASD interatrial septal defect; interauricular septal defect

IASH isolated asymmetric septal hypertrophy

IASHS Institute for Advanced Study in Human Sexuality

IASL International Association for Study of the Liver

IASP International Association for Study of Pain

IAT instillation abortion time; iodine azide test; invasive activity test

IAV intermittent assisted ventilation; intra-arterial vasopressin

IAVM intramedullary arteriovenous malformation

IB idiopathic blepharospasm; immune body; inclusion body; index of body build; infectious bronchitis; Institute of Biology

ib in the same place [Lat. *ibidem*]

IBAT intravascular bronchoalveolar tumor

IBB intestinal brush border

IBBBB incomplete bilateral bundle branch block

IBC Institutional Biosafety Committee; iodine-binding capacity; iron-binding capacity; isobutyl cyanoacrylate

IBCA isobutyl-2-cyanoacrylate

IBD inflammatory bowel disease; irritable bowel disease

IBE International Bureau for Epilepsy

IBED Inter-African Bureau for Epizootic Diseases

iB-EP immunoreactive beta-endomorphin

IBF immature brown fat; immunoglobulin-binding factor; Insall-Burstein-Freeman [total knee instrumentation]

IBG insoluble bone gelatin

IBI intermittent bladder irrigation; ischemic brain infarction

ibid in the same place [Lat. *ibidem*]

IBK infectious bovine keratoconjunctivitis

IBM inclusion body myositis

IBMP International Board of Medicine and Psychology

IBMX 3-isobutyl-1-methylxanthine

IBP International Biological Program;

intra-aortic balloon pumping; iron-binding protein

IBPMS indirect blood pressure measuring system

IBQ Illness Behavior Questionnaire

IBR infectious bovine rhinotracheitis

IBRO International Brain Research Organization

IBRV infectious bovine rhinotracheitis virus

IBS imidazole buffered saline; immunoblastic sarcoma; irritable bowel syndrome; isobaric solution

IBSA iodinated bovine serum albumin

IBSN infantile bilateral striated necrosis

IBT ink blot test

IBU ibuprofen; international benzoate unit

i-Bu isobutyl

IBV infectious bronchitis vaccine; infectious bronchitis virus

IBW ideal body weight

IC icteric, icterus; immune complex; immunoconjugate; immunocytochemistry; immunocytotoxicity; impedance cardiogram; indirect calorimetry; individual counseling; inferior colliculus; inner canthal [distance]; inorganic carbon; inspiratory capacity; inspiratory center; institutional care; integrated circuit; integrated concentration; intensive care; intercostal; intermediate care; intermittent catheterization; intermittent claudication; internal capsule; internal carotid; internal conjugate; interstitial cell; intracapsular; intracardiac; intracarotid; intracavitary; intracellular; intracerebral; intracisternal; intracranial; intracutaneous; irritable colon; islet cells; isovolumic contraction

IC$_{50}$ inhibitory concentration of 50%

ic between meals [Lat. *inter cibos*]

ICA Institute of Clinical Analysis; internal carotid artery; intracranial aneurysm; islet cell antibody

ICAA International Council on Alcohol and Addictions; Invalid Children's Aid Association

ICAb islet cell antibody

ICAM intercellular adhesion molecule

ICAMI International Committee Against Mental Illness

ICAO internal carotid artery occlusion

ICBF inner cortical blood flow

ICBP intracellular binding protein

ICBR increased chromosomal breakage rate

ICC immunocompetent cells; immunocytochemistry; Indian childhood cirrhosis; intensive coronary care; intercanthal distance; interchromosomal crossing over; interclass correlation coefficient; internal conversion coefficient; International Certification Commission; intracervical device; intraclass correlation coefficient

ICCE intracapsular cataract extraction

iCCK immunoreactive cholecystokinin

ICCM idiopathic congestive cardiomyopathy

ICCR International Committee for Contraceptive Research

ICCU intensive coronary care unit; intermediate coronary care unit

ICD I-cell disease; immune complex disease; implantable cardioverter defibrillator; induced circular dichroism; Institute for Crippled and Disabled; International Center for the Disabled; International Classification of Diseases, Injuries, and Causes of Death; intrauterine contraceptive device; ischemic coronary disease; isocitrate dehydrogenase; isolated conduction defect

ICDA International Classification of Diseases, Adapted

ICDC implantable cardioverter-defibrillator catheter

ICD-9-CM International Classification of Diseases–ninth revision–Clinical Modification

ICDH isocitrate dehydrogenase

ICD-O International Classification of Diseases-Oncology

ICDRC International Contact Dermatitis Research Center

ICDS Integrated Child Development Scheme

ICE ice, compression, elevation; ichthyosis-cheek-eyebrow [syndrome]; iridocorneal endothelial [syndrome]

ICES information collection and evaluation system

ICF indirect centrifugal flotation; intensive care facility; intercellular fluorescence; interciliary fluid; intermediate-care facility; International Cardiology Foundation; intracellular fluid; intravascular coagulation and fibrinolysis

ICFA incomplete Freund's adjuvant; induced complement-fixing antigen

ICF(M)A International Cystic Fibrosis (Mucoviscidosis) Association

ICF-MR intermediate-care facility for the mentally retarded

ICG indocyanine green; isotope cisternography

ICGC indocyanine-green clearance

ICGN immune-complex glomerulonephritis

ICH idiopathic cortical hyperostosis; infectious canine hepatitis; intracerebral hematoma; intracranial hemorrhage; intracranial hypertension

ICHD Inter-Society Commission for Heart Disease Resources

ICHPPC International Classification of Health Problems in Primary Care

ICI intracardiac infection

ICi intracisternal

ICIDH International Classification of Impairments, Disabilities, and Handicaps

ICL idiopathic CD4 T-cell lymphocytopenia; iris-clip lens; isocitrate lyase

ICLA International Committee on Laboratory Animals

ICLH Imperial College, London Hospital

ICM inner cell mass; intercostal margin; International Confederation of Midwives; intracytoplasmic membrane; ion conductance modulator; isolated cardiovascular malformation

ICMI Inventory of Childhood Memories and Imaginings

ICMSF International Commission on Microbiological Specifications for Foods

ICN intensive care nursery; International Council of Nurses

ICNa intracellular concentration of sodium

ICNC intracerebral nuclear cell

ICNND Interdepartmental Committee on Nutrition in National Defense

ICNV International Committee on Nomenclature of Viruses

ICO idiopathic cyclic oedema; impedance cardiac output

ICP incubation period; indwelling catheter program; infection-control practitioner; infectious cell protein; inflammatory cloacogenic polyp; intermittent catheterization protocol; intracranial pressure; intracytoplasmic

ICPA International Commission for the Prevention of Alcoholism

ICPB International Collection of Phytopathogenic Bacteria

ICPEMC International Commission for Protection against Environmental Mutagens and Carcinogens

ICPI Intersociety Committee on Pathology Information

ICR [distance between] iliac crests; Institute for Cancer Research; Institute for Cancer Research [mouse]; intermittent catheter routine; International Congress of Radiology; intracardiac catheter recording; intracavitary radium; intracranial reinforcement; ion cyclotron resonance

ICRC International Committee of the Red Cross

ICRD Index of Codes for Research Drugs

ICRETT International Cancer Research Technology Transfer

ICREW International Cancer Research Workshop

I-CRF immunoreactive corticotropin-releasing factor

ICRF-159 razoxane

ICRP International Commission on Radiological Protection

ICRS Index Chemicus Registry System

ICRU International Commission on Radiation Units and Measurements

ICS ileocecal sphincter; immotile cilia syndrome; impulse-conducting system; intensive care, surgical; intercellular space; intercostal space; International College of Surgeons; intracranial stimulation; irritable colon syndrome

ICSA islet cell surface antibody

ICSC idiopathic central serous choroidopathy

ICSH International Committee for Standardization in Hematology; interstitial cell-stimulating hormone

ICSO intermittent coronary sinus occlusion

ICSP International Council of Societies of Pathology

ICSS intracranial self-stimulation

ICSU International Council of Scientific Unions

ICT icteric, icterus; indirect Coombs' test; inflammation of connective tissue; insulin coma therapy; intensive conventional therapy; intermittent cervical traction; interstitial cell tumor; intracardiac thrombus; intracranial tumor; isovolumic contraction time

Ict icterus

iCT immunoreactive calcitonin

ICTMM International Congress on Tropical Medicine and Malaria

ICTS idiopathic carpal tunnel syndrome

ICTV International Committee for the Taxonomy of Viruses

ICTX intermittent cervical traction

ICU infant care unit; immunologic contact urticaria; intensive care unit; intermediate care unit

ICV intracellular volume; intracerebroventricular

ICVS International Cardiovascular Society

ICW intensive care ward; intracellular water

ICx immune complex

ID identification; iditol dehydrogenase; immunodeficiency; immunodiffusion; immunoglobulin deficiency; inappropriate disability; inclusion disease; index of discrimination; individual dose; infant death; infectious disease; infective dose; inhibitory dose; initial diagnosis; initial dose; initial dyskinesia; injected dose; inside diameter; interdigitating; interhemispheric disconnection; interstitial disease; intradermal; intraduodenal

I-D intensity-duration

I&D incision and drainage

ID$_{50}$ median infective dose

Id infradentale; interdentale

id the same [Lat. *idem*]

i d during the day [Lat. *in diem*]; intradermal

IDA image display and analysis; iminodiacetic acid; insulin-degrading activity; iron deficiency anemia

IDAV immunodeficiency-associated virus

IDBS infantile diffuse brain sclerosis

IDC idiopathic dilated cardiomyopathy; interdigitating cell

IDCI intradiplochromatid interchange

IDD insulin-dependent diabetes; intraluminal duodenal diverticulum; Inventory to Diagnose Depression

IDDF investigational drug data form

IDDM insulin-dependent diabetes mellitus

IDDT immune double diffusion test

IDE investigational device exemption

IDG intermediate dose group

IDI immunologically detectable insulin; induction-delivery interval; inter-dentale inferius

IDIC Internal Dose Information Center

idic isodicentric

IDISA intraoperative digital subtraction angiography

IDK internal derangement of knee

IDL Index to Dental Literature; intermediate density lipoprotein

IDLH immediate danger to life and health

IDM idiopathic disease of myocardium; immune defense mechanism; indirect method; infant of diabetic mother; intermediate-dose methotrexate

ID-MS isotope dilution-mass spectrometry

iDNA intercalary deoxyribonucleic acid

idon vehic in a suitable vehicle [Lat. *idoneo vehiculo*]

IDP immunodiffusion procedure; initial dose period; inosine diphosphate

IDPH idiopathic pulmonary hemosiderosis

IDPN iminodipropionitrile

IDR intradermal reaction

IDS immune deficiency state; inhibitor of DNA synthesis; intraduodenal stimulation; investigational drug service

IdS interdentale superius

IDSA Infectious Disease Society of America

IDSAN International Drug Safety Advisory Network

IDT immune diffusion test; instillation delivery time; intradermal typhoid [vaccine]

IDU idoxuridine; injection or intravenous drug user; iododeoxyuridine

IdUA iduronic acid

IDUR idoxuridine

IdUrd idoxuridine

IDV intermittent demand ventilation

IDVC indwelling venous catheter

Idx cross-reactive idiotype

IE immunizing unit [Ger. *immunitäts Einheit*]; immunoelectrophoresis; infectious endocarditis; inner ear; intake energy; internal elastica; intraepithelial

ie that is [Lat. *id est*]

I/E inspiratory/expiratory [ratio]; internal/external

IEA immediate early antigen; immunoelectroadsorption; immunoelectrophoretic analysis; infectious equine anemia; International Epidemiological Association; intravascular erythrocyte aggregation

IEC injection electrode catheter; intraepithelial carcinoma; ion-exchange chromatography

IECa intraepithelial carcinoma

IED inherited epidermal dysplasia

IEE inner enamel epithelium

IEEE Institute of Electrical and Electronics Engineers

IEF International Eye Foundation; isoelectric focusing

IEI isoelectric interval

IEL internal elastic lamina; intraepithelial lymphocyte

IEM immuno-electron microscopy; inborn error of metabolism

IEMG integrated electromyogram

IEOP immunoelectro-osmophoresis

IEP immunoelectrophoresis; individualized education program; isoelectric point

IF idiopathic fibroplasia; idiopathic flushing; immersion foot; immunofluorescence; indirect fluorescence; infrared; inhibiting factor; initiation factor; interferon; interior facet; intermediate filament; intermediate frequency; internal fixation; interstitial fluid; intrinsic factor; involved field [radiotherapy]

IF1, IF2, IF3 interferon 1, 2, 3

IFA idiopathic fibrosing alveolitis; immunofluorescence assay; immunofluorescent antibody; incomplete Freund's adjuvant; indirect fluorescent antibody; indirect fluorescent assay; International Fertility Association; International Filariasis Association

IFAT indirect fluorescent antibody test

IFC intermittent flow centrifugation; intrinsic factor concentrate

IFCC International Federation of Clinical Chemistry

IFCR International Foundation for Cancer Research

IFCS inactivated fetal calf serum

IFDS isolated follicle-stimulating hormone deficiency syndrome

IFE interfollicular epidermis

IFF inner fracture face

IFFH International Foundation for Family Health

IFGO International Federation of Gynecology and Obstetrics

IFGS interstitial fluid and ground substance

IFHP International Federation of Health Professionals

IFHPMSM International Federation for Hygiene, Preventive Medicine, and Social Medicine

IFL immunofluorescence

IFLrA recombinant human leukocyte interferon A

IFM internal fetal monitor

IFMBE International Federation for Medical and Biological Engineering

IFME International Federation for Medical Electronics

IFMP International Federation for Medical Psychotherapy

IFMSA International Federation of Medical Student Associations

IFMSS International Federation of Multiple Sclerosis Societies

IFN interferon

If nec if necessary

IFO Institute for Fermentation [Japan]

IFP inflammatory fibroid polyp; insulin, compound F [hydrocortisone], prolactin; intermediate filament protein; intrapatellar fat pad

IFPM International Federation of Physical Medicine

IFR infrared; inspiratory flow rate

IFRA indirect fluorescent rabies antibody [test]

IFRP International Fertility Research Program

IFS interstitial fluid space

IFSM International Federation of Sports Medicine

IFSSH Internation Federation of Societies for Surgery of the Hand

IFT immunofluorescence test

IFU interferon unit

IFV interstitial fluid volume; intracellular fluid volume

IG immature granule; immunoglobulin; intragastric; irritable gut

Ig immunoglobulin

IGA infantile genetic agranulocytosis

IgA immunoglobulin A

IgA1, IgA2 subclasses of immunoglobulin A

IgAGN immunoglobulin A glomerulonephritis

IgAN immunoglobulin A nephropathy

IGC immature germ cell; intragastric cannula

IGD idiopathic growth hormone deficiency; interglobal distance; isolated gonadotropin deficiency

IgD immunoglobulin D

IgD1, IgD2 subclasses of immunoglobulin D

IGDM infant of mother with gestational diabetes mellitus

IGE impaired gas exchange

IgE immunoglobulin E

IgE1 subclass of immunoglobulin E

IGF insulin-like growth factor

IGFET insulated gate field effect transistor

IgG immunoglobulin G

IgG1, IgG2, IgG3, IgG4 subclasses of immunoglobulin G

IGH immunoreactive growth hormone

IGHD isolated growth hormone deficiency

IGIV immune globulin intravenous

IgM immunoglobulin M

IgM1 subclass of immunoglobulin M

IgMN immunoglobulin M nephropathy

IGP intestinal glycoprotein

IGR immediate generalized reaction; integrated gastrin response

IGS inappropriate gonadotropin secretion; internal guide sequence

Igs immunoglobulins

IgSC immunoglobulin-secreting cell

IGT impaired glucose tolerance

IGTT intravenous glucose tolerance test

IGV intrathoracic gas volume

IH idiopathic hirsutism; idiopathic hypercalciuria; immediate hypersensitivity; incompletely healed; indirect hemagglutination; industrial hygiene; infantile hydrocephalus; infectious hepatitis; inguinal hernia; inhibiting hormone; in hospital; inner half; inpatient hospital; intermittent heparinization; intracranial hematoma; iron hematoxylin

IHA idiopathic hyperaldosteronism; indirect hemagglutination; indirect hemagglutination antibody

IHAC Industrial Health and Advisory Committee

IHBT incompatible hemolytic blood transfusion

IHC idiopathic hemochromatosis; idiopathic hypercalciuria; inner hair cell; intrahepatic cholestasis

IHCA isocapnic hyperventilation with cold air

IHCP Institute of Hospital and Community Psychiatry

IHD in-center hemodialysis; ischemic heart disease

IHES idiopathic hypereosinophilic syndrome

IHF Industrial Health Foundation; integration host factor; International Hospital Foundation

IHGD isolateral human growth deficiency

IHH idiopathic hypogonadotropic hypogonadism; idiopathic hypothalamic hypogonadism; infectious human hepatitis

IHHS idiopathic hyperkinetic heart syndrome

IHL International Homeopathic League

IHO idiopathic hypertrophic osteoarthropathy

IHP idiopathic hypoparathyroidism; idiopathic hypopituitarism; interhospitalization period; inverted hand position

IHPC intrahepatic cholestasis

IHPH intrahepatic portal hypertension

IHPP Intergovernmental Health Project Policy

IHR intrahepatic resistance; intrinsic heart rate

IHRA isocapnic hyperventilation with room air

IHRB Industrial Health Research Board

IHS idiopathic hypereosinophilic syndrome; inactivated horse serum; Indian Health Service; International Health Society

IHSA iodinated human serum albumin

IHSC immunoreactive human skin collagenase

IHSS idiopathic hypertrophic subaortic stenosis

IHT insulin hypoglycemia test; intravenous histamine test; ipsilateral head turning

I5HT intraplatelet serotonin

Ii incision inferius

II icterus index; image intensifier; Roman numeral two

I&I illness and injuries

II-para secundipara

IID insulin-independent diabetes

IIDM insulin-independent diabetes mellitus

IIE idiopathic ineffective erythropoiesis

IIF immune interferon; indirect immunofluorescence

IIFT itraoperative intraarterial fibrinolytic therapy

IIGR ipsilateral instinctive grasp reaction

III Roman numeral three

III-para tertipara

IIME Institute of International Medical Education

IIP idiopathic interstitial pneumonia; idiopathic intestinal pseudo-obstruction; increased intracranial pressure

IIS intensive immunosuppression; International Institute of Stress

IIT ineffective iron turnover

IJ ileojejunal; internal jugular; intrajejunal; intrajugular

IJD inflammatory joint disease

IJP inhibitory junction potential; internal jugular pressure

IJV internal jugular vein

IK immobilized knee; immune body [Ger. *Immunekörper*]; *Infusoria* killing [unit]; interstitial keratitis

IKE ion kinetic energy

IKU *Infusoria* killing unit

IL ileum; incisolingual; independent laboratory; iliolumbar; independent laboratory; inspiratory load; intensity load; interleukin; intralumbar

Il promethium [*illinium*]

ILA insulin-like activity; International Leprosy Association

ILa incisolabial

ILB infant, low birth [weight]; initial lung burden

ILBBB incomplete left bundle branch block

ILBW infant, low birth weight

ILC ichthyosis linearis circumflex; incipient lethal concentration

ILD interstitial lung disease; ischemic leg disease; ischemic limb disease; isolated lactase deficiency

ILE, ILe, Ileu isoleucine

ILGF insulin-like growth factor

ILH immunoreactive luteinizing hormone

ILL intermediate lymphocytic lymphoma

ILM insulin-like material; internal limiting membrane

ILNR intralobar nephrogenic rest

ILo iodine lotion

ILP inadequate luteal phase; insufficiency of luteal phase; interstitial lymphocytic pneumonia

ILR irreversible loss rate

ILS idiopathic leucine sensitivity; idiopathic lymphadenopathy syndrome; increase in life span; infrared liver scanner; intermittent light stimulation; intralobal sequestration

ILSI International Life Sciences Institute

ILSS integrated life support system; intraluminal somatostatin

ILT iliotibial tract

IM idiopathic myelofibrosis; immunosuppressive method; Index Medicus; indomethacin; industrial medicine; infection medium; infectious mononucleosis; inner membrane; innocent murmur; inspiratory muscles; intermediate; intermediate megaloblast; internal malleolus; internal mammary [artery]; internal medicine; intramedullary; intramuscular; invasive mole

im intramuscular

IMA Industrial Medical Association; inferior mesenteric artery; Interchurch Medical Assistance; internal mammary artery; Irish Medical Association

IMAA iodinated macroaggregated albumin

IMAB internal mammary artery bypass

IMAI internal mammary artery implant

IMB intermenstrual bleeding

IMBC indirect maximum breathing capacity

IMBI Institute of Medical and Biological Illustrators

IMC interdigestive migrating contractions; intestinal mast cell

IMCT Information-Memory-Concentration Test

IMCU intermediate medical care unit

IMD immunologically mediated disease

ImD$_{50}$ immunizing dose sufficient to protect 50% of the animals in a test group

IMDC intramedullary metatarsal decompression

IMDD idiopathic midline destructive disease

IMDG International Maritime Dangerous Goods [code]

IMDP imidocarb diprionate

IME independent medical examination

IMEM improved minimum essential medium

IMET isometric endurance test

IMF idiopathic myelofibrosis; immunofluorescence; intermediate filament

IMG inferior mesenteric ganglion; internal medicine group [practice]; international medical graduate

IMGG intramuscular gammaglobulin

IMH idiopathic myocardial hypertrophy; indirect microhemagglutination [test]

IMHP 1-iodomercuri-2-hydroxypropane

IMHT indirect microhemagglutination test

IMI immunologically measurable insulin; impending myocardial infarction; Imperial Mycological Institute [Great Britain]; inferior myocardial infarction; intermeal interval; intramuscular injection

Imi imipramine

IMIC International Medical Information Center

IMLA intramural left anterior [artery]

IMLAD intramural left anterior descending [artery]

IMLNS idiopathic minimal lesion nephrotic syndrome

ImLy immune lysis

IMM inhibitor-containing minimal medium; internal medial malleolus

immat immaturity, immature

IMMC interdigestive migrating motor complex

immobil immobilization, immobilize

immun immune, immunity, immunization

IMN internal mammary node

IMP idiopathic myeloid proliferation; impression; incomplete male pseudohermaphroditism; individual Medicaid practitioner; inosine 5'-monophosphate; intramembranous particle; intramuscular compartment pressure

imp impacted, impaction

IMPA incisal mandibular plane angle

IMPAC Information for Management, Planning, Analysis and Coordination

IMPC International Myopia Prevention Center

IMPS Inpatient Multidimensional Psychiatric Scale; intact months of patient survival

Impx impacted

IMR individual medical record; infant mortality rate; infant mortality risk; Institute for Medical Research; institution for mentally retarded

IMS incurred in military service; Indian Medical Service; industrial methylated spirit; integrated medical services; international metric system

IMSS in-flight medical support system

IMT indomethacin; induced muscular tension; inspiratory muscle training

IMU Index of Medical Underservice

IMV inferior mesenteric vein; intermittent mandatory ventilation; isophosphamide, methotrexate, and vincristine

IMViC, imvic indole, methyl red, Voges-Proskauer, citrate [test]

IMVP idiopathic mitral valve prolapse

IMVS Institute of Medical and Veterinary Science

IN icterus neonatorum; impetigo neonatorum; incidence; incompatibility number; infundibular nucleus; insulin; interneuron; interstitial nephritis; intranasal; irritation of nociceptors

In index; indium; inion; insulin; inulin

in inch

in² square inch

in³ cubic inch

INA infectious nucleic acid; inferior nasal artery; International Neurological Association

INAA instrumental neutron activation analysis

INAD infantile neuroaxonal dystrophy

INAH isonicotinic acid hydrazide

INB internuclear bridging; ischemic necrosis of bone

inbr inbreeding

INC internodular cortex; inside needle catheter

inc incision; inclusion; incompatibility; incontinent; increase, increased; increment; incurred

IncB inclusion body

INCD infantile nuclear cerebral degeneration

incl inclusion

incr increase, increased; increment

incur incurable

IND indomethacin; industrial medicine; investigational new drug

ind indirect; induction

in d daily [Lat. *in dies*]

indic indication, indicated
indig indigestion
indiv individual
INDM infant of nondiabetic mother
INDO indomethacin
INDOR internuclear double resonance
indust industrial
INE infantile necrotizing encephalo-
myelopathy
INF infant, infantile; infection, infective, infected; inferior; infirmary; infun-
dibulum; infusion; interferon
inf infant, infantile; pour in [Lat. *infunde*]
infect infection, infected, infective
Inflamm inflammation, inflammatory
ING isotope nephrogram
ing inguinal
InGP indolglycerophosphate
INH inhalation; isoniazid; isonicotinic
acid hydrazide
inhal inhalation
inhib inhibition, inhibiting
INI intranuclear inclusion
inj injection; injury, injured, injurious
inject injection
inj enem let an enema be injected [Lat.
injiciatur enema]
INK injury not known
INLSD ichthyosis and neutral lipid storage disease
INN International Nonproprietary Names
innerv innervation, innervated
innom innominate
INO internuclear ophthalmoplegia; inosine
Ino inosine
INOC isonicotinoyloxycarbonyl
inoc inoculation, inoculated
inorg inorganic
Inox inosine, oxidized
INP idiopathic neutropenia
INPAV intermittent negative pressure
assisted ventilation
INPEA isopropyl nitrophenylethan-
olamine
INPH iproniazid phosphate
INPV intermittent negative-pressure
ventilation

INQ interior nasal quadrant
INR international normalized ratio
INREM internal roentgen-equivalent,
man
INS idiopathic nephrotic syndrome;
insurance
Ins insulin; insurance, insured
ins insertion; insulin; insurance, insured
insem insemination
insol insoluble
Insp inspiration
INSR insulin receptor
Inst institute
instab instability
instill instillation
insuf insufflation
insuff insufficient, insufficiency; insufflation
INT intermediate; intermittent; intern,
internship; internal; interval; intestinal;
intima; p-iodonitrotetrazolium
Int international; intestinal
int cib between meals [Lat. *inter cibos*]
INTEG integument
intern internal
Internat international
intes intestine
Intest intestine, intestinal
Int/Ext internal/external
INTH intrathecal
Intmd intermediate
Int Med internal medicine
int noct during the night [Lat. *inter noc-
tem*]
INTOX, Intox intoxication
INTR intermittent
Int Rot internal rotation
Int trx intermittent traction
intub intubation
INV inferior nasal vein
Inv, inv inversion; involuntary
Inv/Ev inversion/eversion
invest investigation
inv ins inverted insertion
invol involuntary
involv involvement, involved
inv(p + q-) pericentric inversion
inv(p-q +) pericentric inversion

IO incisal opening; inferior oblique; inferior olive; internal os; interorbital; intestinal obstruction; intraocular; intraoperative

I&O, I/O in and out; intake/output

Io ionium

IOA inner optic anlage; International Osteopathic Association

IOC International Organizing Committee on Medical Librarianship; intern on call

IOCG intraoperative cholangiogram

IOD injured on duty; integrated optical density; interorbital distance

IOFB intraocular foreign body

IOH idiopathic orthostatic hypotension

IOL intraocular lens

IOM Institute of Medicine

IOMP International Organization for Medical Physics

ION ischemic optic neuropathy

IOP intraocular pressure

IOR index of response

IORT intraoperative radiotherapy

IOS International Organization for Standardization

IOT intraocular tension; intraocular transfer; ipsilateral optic tectum

IOTA information overload testing aid

ι Greek letter *iota*

IOU intensive care observation unit; international opacity unit

IP icterus praecox; immune precipitate; immunoblastic plasma; immunoperoxidase technique; inactivated pepsin; incisoproximal; incisopulpal; incontinentia pigmenti; incubation period; induced potential; induction period; infection prevention; infundibular process; infusion pump; inorganic phosphate; inosine phosphorylase; inpatient; instantaneous pressure; L'Institut Pasteur; International Pharmacopoeia; interpeduncular; interphalangeal; interpupillary; intestinal pseudo-obstruction; intraperitoneal; intrapulmonary; ionization potential; isoelectric point; isoproterenol

ip intraperitoneal

IPA immunoperoxidase assay; incontinentia pigmenti achromians; independent practice association; individual practice association; infantile papular acrodermatitis; International Pediatric Association; International Pharmaceutical Association; International Psychoanalytical Association; isopropyl alcohol

IPAA International Psychoanalytical Association

I-para primipara

IPAT Iowa Pressure Articulation Test

IPC intermittent pneumatic compression; International Poliomyelitis Congress; ion pair chromatography; isopropyl carbamate; isopropyl chlorophenyl

IPCS intrauterine progesterone contraception system

IPD idiopathic Parkinson's disease; idiopathic protracted diarrhea; immediate pigment darkening; increase in pupillary diameter; incurable problem drinker; inflammatory pelvic disease; intermittent peritoneal dialysis; intermittent pigment darkening; interpupillary distance; Inventory of Psychosocial Development

IPE infectious porcine encephalomyelitis; interstitial pulmonary emphysema

IPEH intravascular papillary endothelial hyperplasia

IPF idiopathic pulmonary fibrosis; infection-potentiating factor; interstitial pulmonary fibrosis

IPG impedance plethysmography; inspiration-phase gas

iPGE immunoreactive prostaglandin E

IPH idiopathic portal hypertension; idiopathic pulmonary hemosiderosis; inflammatory papillary hyperplasia; interphalangeal; intraparenchymal hemorrhage

IPHR inverted polypoid hamartoma of the rectum

IPI interpulse interval

IPIA immunoperoxidase infectivity assay

IPJ interphalangeal joint

IPK intractable plantar keratosis

IPKD infantile polycystic kidney disease

IPL inner plexiform layer; intrapleural

IPM impulses per minute; inches per minute

IPMS inhibited power motive syndrome

IPN infantile polyarteritis nodosa; infectious pancreatic necrosis [of trout]; intern progress note; interpeduncular nucleus; interstitial pneumonitis

IPNA isopropyl noradrenalin

IPO improved pregnancy outcome

IPOF immediate postoperative fitting

IPOP immediate postoperative prosthesis

IPP independent practice plan; inflatable penile prosthesis; inorganic pyrophosphate; intermittent positive pressure; intrahepatic partial pressure

IPPA inspection, palpation, percussion, and auscultation

IPPB intermittent positive-pressure breathing

IPPB-I intermittent positive-pressure breathing-inspiration

IPPI interruption of pregnancy for psychiatric indication

IPPO intermittent positive-pressure inflation with oxygen

IPPR integrated pancreatic polypeptide response; intermittent positive-pressure respiration

IPPV intermittent positive-pressure ventilation

IPQ intimacy potential quotient

IPR insulin production rate; intraparenchymal resistance

i-Pr isopropyl

IPRL isolated perfused rat liver or lung

IPRT interpersonal reaction test

IPS idiopathic postprandial syndrome; inches per second; infundibular pulmonary stenosis; initial prognostic score; intrapartum stillbirth; intraperitoneal shock; ischiopubic synchondrosis

ips inches per second

IPSC inhibitory postsynaptic current

IPSC-E Inventory of Psychic and Somatic Complaints in the Elderly

IPSF immediate postsurgical fitting

IPSID immunoproliferative small intestine disease

IPSP inhibitory postsynaptic potential

IPT immunoperoxidase technique; immunoprecipitation; isoproterenol

IPTG isopropyl thiogalactose

iPTH immunoreactive parathyroid hormone

IPTX intermittent pelvic traction

IPU inpatient unit

IPV inactivated poliomyelitis vaccine or virus; infectious pustular vaginitis; infectious pustular vulvovaginitis; intrapulmonary vein

IPW interphalangeal width

IPZ insulin protamine zinc

IQ intelligence quotient

IQB individual quick blanch

IQ&S iron, quinine, and strychnine

IR drop of voltage across a resistor produced by a current; ileal resection; immune response; immunization rate; immunoreactive; immunoreagent; index of response; individual reaction; inferior rectus [muscle]; inflow resistance; information retrieval; infrared; infrarenal; inside radius; insoluble residue; inspiratory reserve; inspiratory resistance; insulin resistance; internal resistance; internal rotation; intrarectal; intrarenal; inversion recovery; inverted repeat; irritant reaction; isovolumic relaxation

I-R Ito-Reenstierna [reaction]

Ir immune response [gene]; iridium

ir immunoreactive; intrarectal; intrarenal

IRA immunoradioassay; immunoregulatory alpha-globulin; inactive renin activity

IR-ACTH immunoreactive adrenocorticotropic hormone

IrANP immunoreactive atrial natriuretic peptide

IR-AVP immunoreactive arginine-vasopressin

IRB Institutional Review Board

IRBBB incomplete right bundle branch block

IRBC immature or infected red blood cell

IRC inspiratory reserve capacity; instantaneous resonance curve; International Red Cross; International Research Communications System

IRCA intravascular red cell aggregation

IRCC International Red Cross Committee

IRCU intensive respiratory care unit

IRD infantile Refsum's syndrome; isorhythmic dissociation

IRDP insulin-related DNA polymorphism

IRDS idiopathic respiratory distress syndrome; infant respiratory distress syndrome

IRE internal rotation in extension

IRF idiopathic retroperitoneal fibrosis; internal rotation in flexion

IRG immunoreactive gastrin; immunoreactive glucagon

IRGH immunoreactive growth hormone

IRGl immunoreactive glucagon

IRH Institute for Research in Hypnosis; Institute of Religion and Health; intrarenal hemorrhage

IRHCS immunoradioassayable human chorionic somatomammotropin

IRhGH immunoreactive human growth hormone

IRhPL immunoreactive human placental lactogen

IRI immunoreactive insulin; insulin resistance index

IRIA indirect radioimmunoassay

IRIg insulin-reactive immunoglobulin

IRIS Integrated Risk Information System; interleukin regulation of immune system; International Research Information Service

IRM innate releasing mechanism; Institute of Rehabilitation Medicine

IRMA immunoradiometric assay; intraretinal microvascular abnormalities

iRNA immune ribonucleic acid; informational ribonucleic acid

IROS ipsilateral routing of signal

IRP immunoreactive plasma; immunoreactive proinsulin; incus replacement prosthesis; insulin-releasing polypeptide; interstitial radiation pneumonitis

IRR intrarenal reflux

Irr irradiation; irritation

IRRD Institute for Research in Rheumatic Diseases

irreg irregularity, irregular

irrig irrigation, irrigate

IRS immunoreactive secretion; infrared spectrophotometry; insulin receptor species; internal resolution site; International Rhinologic Society

IRSA idiopathic refractory sideroblastic anemia; iodinated rat serum albumin

IRT immunoreactive trypsin; interresponse time

IRTO immunoreactive trypsin output

IRTU integrating regulatory transcription unit

IRU industrial rehabilitation unit; interferon reference unit

IRV inferior radicular vein; inspiratory reserve volume; inverse ratio ventilation

IS ileal segment; immediate sensitivity; immune serum; immunosuppression; impingement syndrome; incentive spirometer; index of sexuality; infant size; infantile spasms; information system; insertion sequence; in situ; insulin secretion; intercellular space; intercostal space; interictal spike; interstitial space; intracardial shunt; intraspinal; intrasplenic; intrastriatal; intraventricular septum; invalided from service; ischemic score; isoproterenol

Is incision superius

is in situ; island; islet; isolated

ISA Instrument Society of America; intracarotid sodium amytal; intrinsic simulating activity; intrinsic sympathomimetic activity; iodinated serum albumin; irregular spiking activity

ISADH inappropriate secretion of antidiuretic hormone

ISB incentive spirometry breathing

ISBI International Society for Burn Injuries

ISBP International Society for Biochemical Pharmacology

ISBT International Society for Blood Transfusion

ISC immunoglobulin-secreting cells; insoluble collagen; International Society of Cardiology; International Society of Chemotherapy; intensive supportive care; intershift coordination; interstitial cell; irreversibly sickled cell

ISCF interstitial cell fluid

ISCLT International Society for Clinical Laboratory Technology

ISCM International Society of Cybernetic Medicine

ISCN International System for Human Cytogenetic Nomenclature

ISCO immunostimulating complex [vaccine]

ISCP infection surveillance and control program; International Society of Comparative Pathology

ISD immunosuppressive drug; Information Services Division; inhibited sexual desire; interventricular septal defect; isosorbide dinitrate

ISDN isosorbide dinitrate

ISE inhibited sexual excitement; International Society of Endocrinology; International Society of Endoscopy; ion-selective electrode

ISEK International Society of Electromyographic Kinesiology

ISEM immunosorbent electron microscopy

ISF interstitial fluid

ISFV interstitial fluid volume

ISG immune serum globulin

ISGE International Society of Gastroenterology

ISH icteric serum hepatitis; International Society of Hematology

ISI infarct size index; initial slope index;

injury severity index; Institute for Scientific Information; insulin sensitivity index; interstimulus interval

ISIH interspike interval histogram

ISIS International Study of Infarct Survival

ISKDC International Study of Kidney Diseases in Childhood

ISL inner scapular line; interspinous ligament; isoleucine

ISM International Society of Microbiologists; intersegmental muscle

ISMED International Society on Metabolic Eye Disorders

ISMH International Society of Medical Hydrology

ISMHC International Society of Medical Hydrology and Climatology

ISN International Society of Nephrology; International Society of Neurochemistry

ISO International Standards Organization

iso isoproterenol; isotropic

isol isolation, isolated

isom isometric

ISP distance between iliac spines; interspace; intraspinal; isoproterenol

ISPO International Society for Prosthetics and Orthotics

ISPT interspecies ovum penetration test

isq unchanged [Lat. *in status quo*]

ISR information storage and retrieval; Institute for Sex Research; Institute of Surgical Research; insulin secretion rate

ISRM International Society of Reproductive Medicine

ISS Index-Injury Severity Score; International Society of Surgery; ion-scattering spectroscopy; ion surface scattering

ISSN International Standard Serial Number

IST inappropriate sinus tachycardia; insulin sensitivity test; insulin shock therapy; International Society on Toxicology; isometric systolic tension

ISTD International Society of Tropical Dermatology

ISU International Society of Urology

I-sub inhibitor substance

ISW interstitial water

ISWI incisional surgical wound infection

ISY intrasynovial

IT immunological test; immunotherapy; implantation test; individual therapy; inhalation test; inhalation therapy; insulin therapy; intensive therapy; intentional tremor; intermittent traction; interstitial tissue; intradermal test; intratesticular; intrathecal; intrathoracic; intratracheal; intratracheal tube; intratumoral; ischial tuberosity; isomeric transition

I/T intensity/time

I&T intolerance and toxicity

ITA inferior temporal artery; internal thoracic artery; International Tuberculosis Association

ITB iliotibial band

ITC imidazolyl-thioguanine chemotherapy; Interagency Testing Committee

ITc International Table calorie

ITCP idiopathic thrombocytopenic purpura

ITCVD ischemic thrombotic cerebrovascular disease

ITD intensely transfused dialysis

ITE insufficient therapeutic effect; in the ear; in-training examination; intrapulmonary interstitial emphysema

ITET isotonic endurance test

ITF interferon

ITFS iliotibial tract friction syndrome; incomplete testicular feminization syndrome

ITh, ith intrathecal

IThP intrathyroidal parathyroid

ITI intertrial interval

ITLC instant thin-layer chromatography

ITM improved Thayer-Martin [medium]; intrathecal methotrexate; Israel turkey meningoencephalitis

ITOU intensive therapy observation unit

ITP idiopathic thrombocytopenic purpura; immunogenic thrombocytopenic purpura; inosine triphosphate; islet-cell tumor of the pancreas; isotachophoresis

ITPA Illinois Test of Psycholinguistic Abilities; inosine triphosphatase

ITQ inferior temporal quadrant

ITR intraocular tension recorder; intratracheal

ITS infective toxic shock

ITSHD isolated thyroid-stimulating hormone deficiency

ITT insulin tolerance test; internal tibial torsion

ITU intensive therapy unit

ITV inferior temporal vein

IU immunizing unit; international unit; intrauterine; in utero; 5-iodouracil

iu infectious unit

IUA intrauterine adhesions

IUB International Union of Biochemistry

IUBS International Union of Biological Sciences

IUC idiopathic ulcerative colitis

IUCD intrauterine contraceptive device

IUD intrauterine death; intrauterine device

IUDR idoxuridine

IUF isolated ultrafiltration

IUFB intrauterine foreign body

IUG infusion urogram; intrauterine growth

IUGR intrauterine growth rate; intrauterine growth retardation

IU/l international units per liter

IUM internal urethral meatus; intrauterine [fetus] malnourished; intrauterine membrane

IU/min international units per minute

IUP intrauterine pregnancy; intrauterine pressure

IUPAC International Union of Pure and Applied Chemistry

IUPAP International Union of Pure and Applied Physics

IUPD intrauterine pregnancy delivered

IUPHAR International Union of Pharmacology

IUPS International Union of Physiological Sciences

IUPTB intrauterine pregnancy, term birth
IURES International Union of Reticuloendothelial Societies
IUT intrauterine transfusion
IUVDT International Union against Venereal Diseases and the Treponematoses
IV ichthyosis vulgaris; initial visit; interventricular; intervertebral; intravaginal; intravascular; intravenous; intraventricular; intravertebral; invasive; in vivo; in vitro; iodine value; Roman numeral four; symbol for class 4 controlled substances
iv intravascular; intravenous
IVAP in-vivo adhesive platelet
IVB intraventricular block; intravitrial blood
IVBAT intravascular bronchioalveolar tumor
IVBC intravascular blood coagulation
IVC inferior vena cava; inspiratory vital capacity; integrated vector control; intravascular coagulation; intravenous cholangiogram, intravenous cholangiography; intraventricular catheter
IVCC intravascular consumption coagulopathy
IVCD intraventricular conduction defect
IVCH intravenous cholangiography
IVCP inferior vena cava pressure
IVCR inferior vena cava reconstruction
IVCT inferior vena cava thrombosis; intravenously enhanced computed tomography
IVCV inferior venocavography
IVD intervertebral disc
IVDA/IVDU intravenous drug abuse/abuser; intravenous drug use/user
IVF interventricular foramen; intervertebral foramen; intravascular fluid; in vitro fertiliztion
IVGG intravenous gammaglobulin

IVGTT intravenous glucose tolerance test
IVH intravenous hyperalimentation; intraventricular hemorrhage; in vitro hyperploidy
IVIG intravenous immunoglobulin
IVJC intervertebral joint complex
IVM intravascular mass
IVMP intravenous methylprednisolone
IVN intravenous nutrition
IVOTTS Irvine viable organ-tissue transport system
IVP intravenous push; intravenous pyelogram, intravenous pyelography; intraventricular pressure
IVPB intravenous piggyback
IVPF isovolume pressure flow curve
IVR idioventricular rhythm; intravaginal ring; isolated volume responder
IVRT isovolumic relaxation time
IVS inappropriate vasopressin secretion; intervening sequence; interventricular septum; intervillous space
IVSA International Veterinary Students Association
IVSD interventricular septal defect
IVT index of vertical transmission; intravenous transfusion; intraventricular; in vitro tetraploidy; isovolumetric time
IVTTT intravenous tolbutamide tolerance test
IVU intravenous urography
IVV influenza virus vaccine; intravenous vasopressin
IW inner wall
IWGMT International Working Group on Mycobacterial Taxonomy
IWI inferior wall infarction; interwave interval
IWL insensible water loss
IWMI inferior wall myocardial infarct
IWS Index of Work Satisfaction
i (Xq) long arm isochromosome
IZ infarction zone
IZS insulin zinc suspension

J dynamic movement of inertia; electric current density; flux density; joint; joule; journal; juvenile; juxtapulmonary-capillary receptor; magnetic polarization; a polypeptide chain in polymeric immunoglobulins; a reference point following the QRS complex, at the beginning of the ST segment, in electrocardiography; sound intensity

J flux [density]

j jaundice [rat]

JA judgment analysis; juvenile atrophy; juxta-articular

JAI juvenile amaurotic idiocy

JAMG juvenile autoimmune myasthenia gravis

JAS Jenkins Activity Survey

jaund jaundice

JBE Japanese B encephalitis

JBS Johanson-Blizzard syndrome

JC Jakob-Creutzfeldt; joint contracture

J/C joules per coulomb

jc juice

JCA juvenile chronic arthritis

JCAE Joint Committee on Atomic Energy

JCAH Joint Commission on Accreditation of Hospitals

JCAHO Joint Commission on Accreditation of Healthcare Organizations

JCAI Joint Council of Allergy and Immunology

JCC Joint Committee on Contraception

JCF juvenile calcaneal fracture

JCM Japanese Collection of Microorganisms

JCML juvenile chronic myelogenous leukemia

JCP juvenile chronic polyarthritis

jct junction

JCV Jamestown Canyon virus

JD jejunal diverticulitis; juvenile delinquent; juvenile diabetes

JDF Juvenile Diabetes Foundation

JDM juvenile diabetes mellitus

JE Japanese encephalitis; junctional escape

JEBL junctional epidermolysis bullosa letalis

JEE Japanese equine encephalitis

Jej, jej jejunum

JEMBEC agar plates for transporting cultures of gonococci

jentac breakfast [Lat. *jentaculum*]

JER junctional escape rhythm

JEV Japanese encephalitis virus

JF joint fluid; jugular foramen; junctional fold

JFET junction field effect transistor

JFS jugular foramen syndrome

JG, jg juxtaglomerular

JGA juxtaglomerular apparatus

JGC juxtaglomerular cell

JGCT juvenile granulosa cell tumor; juxtaglomerular cell tumor

JGI jejunogastric intussusception; juxtaglomerular granulation index

JGP juvenile general paresis

JH juvenile hormone

J$_H$ heat transfer factor

JHA juvenile hormone analog

JHMO Junior Hospital Medical Officer

JHR Jarisch-Herxheimer reaction

JI jejunoileal; jejunoileitis; jejunoileostomy

JIB jejunoileal bypass

JIH joint interval histogram

JIS juvenile idiopathic scoliosis

JJ jaw jerk; jejunojejunostomy

J/kg joules per kilogram

JLP juvenile laryngeal papilloma

JMD juvenile macular degeneration

JMS junior medical student

JN Jamaican neuropathy

JNA Jena Nomina Anatomica

JND just noticeable difference

jnt joint

JOD juvenile-onset diabetes

JODM juvenile-onset diabetes mellitus

jour journal
JP Jackson-Pratt [drain]; joining peptide; juvenile periodontitis
JPB junctional premature beat
JPC junctional premature contraction
JPD juvenile plantar dermatosis
JPI Jackson Personality Inventory
JPS joint position sense
JR Jolly reaction; junctional rhythm
JRA juvenile rheumatoid arthritis
JROM joint range of motion
JRT junctional recovery time
JS jejunal segment; Job syndrome; junctional slowing
J/s joules per second
JSV Jerry-Slough virus
JT jejunostomy tube

J/T joules per tesla
jt joint
JTPS juvenile tropical pancreatitis syndrome
Ju jugale
JUA joint underwriting association
jug jugular
junct junction
juv juvenile
JV jugular vein; Junin virus
JVC jugular venous catheter
JVD jugular venous distention
JVP jugular vein pulse; jugular venous pressure
JVPT jugular venous pulse tracing
juxt near [Lat. *juxta*]
Jx junction
JXG juvenile xanthogranuloma

K absolute zero; capsular antigen [Ger. *Kapsel*, capsule]; carrying capacity; cathode; coefficient of heat transfer; in electroencephalography, a burst of diphasic slow waves in response to stimuli during sleep; electron capture; electrostatic capacity; equilibrium constant; ionization constant; kallikrein inhibiting unit; kanamycin; Kell factor; kelvin; kerma; kidney; killer [cell]; kilo-; kinetic energy; *Klebsiella;* knee; lysine; modulus of compression; the number 1024 in computer core memory; potassium [Lat. *kalium*]; vitamin K

°K degree on the Kelvin scale

K_1 phylloquinone

17-K 17-ketosteroid

k Boltzmann constant; constant; kilo; kilohm

κ see *kappa*

KA alkaline phosphatase; kainic acid; keratoacanthoma; keto acid; ketoacidosis; King-Armstrong [unit]

K/A ketogenic/antiketogenic ratio

Ka cathode

K_a acid ionization constant

kA kiloampere

ka cathode

KAAD kerosene, alcohol, acetic acid, and dioxane

KABC Kaufman Assessment Battery for Children

KAF conglutinogen-activating factor; killer-assisting factor; kinase activating factor

KAFO knee-ankle-foot orthosis

KAL Kallmann syndrome

Kal potassium [Lat. *Kalium*]

KAO knee-ankle orthosis

KAP knowledge, aptitude, and practice

κ Greek letter *kappa*; magnetic susceptibility

kappa a light chain of human immunoglobulins [chain]

KAS Katz Adjustment Scales; Kennedy-Alter-Sung [syndrome]

KAT kanamycin acetyltransferase

kat katal

kat/l katals per liter

KAU King-Armstrong unit

KB human oral epidermoid carcinoma cells; Kashin-Bek [disease]; ketone body; kilobyte; Kleihauer-Betke [test]; knee brace

K_b base ionization constant

kb kilobase

KBG syndrome of multiple abnormalities designated with the original patient's initials

kbp kilobase pair

kBq kilobecquerel

KBS Klüver-Bucy syndrome

KC cathodal closing; keratoconus; keratoconjunctivitis; knee-to-chest; Kupffer cell

kC kilocoulomb

kc kilocycle

K Cal, Kcal, kcal kilocalorie

KCC cathodal closing contraction; Kulchitzky cell carcinoma

KCCT kaolin-cephalin clotting time

K cell killer cell

KCG kinetocardiogram

kCi kilocurie

kcps kilocycles per second

KCS keratoconjunctivitis sicca

kc/s kilocycles per second

KCT, KCTe cathodal closing tetanus

KD cathodal duration; Kawasaki disease; killed

K_d dissociation constant; distribution coefficient; partition coefficient

kd, kDa kilodalton

KDA known drug allergies

KDC kidney disease treatment center

KDNA kinetoblast deoxyribonucleic acid

KDO ketodeoxyoctonate

KDS Kaufman Developmental Scale;

King-Denborough syndrome; Kocher-Debré-Semelaigne [syndrome]
KDT cathodal duration tetanus
kdyn kilodyne
KE Kendall compound E; kinetic energy
K$_e$ exchangeable body potassium
KED Kendrick extrication device
Kera keratitis
KERV Kentucky equine respiratory virus
keV kiloelectron volt
KF Kenner-fecal medium; kidney function; Klippel-Feil [syndrome]
KF, K-F Kayser-Fleischer [rings]
kf flocculation rate in antigen-antibody reaction
KFAB kidney-fixing antibody
KFAO knee-foot-ankle orthosis
KFD Kyasanur forest disease
KFR Kayser-Fleischer ring
KFS Klippel-Feil syndrome
KG ketoglutarate
kG kilogauss
kg kilogram
KG-1 Koeffler Golde-1 [cell line]
kg-cal kilocalorie
kg/cm^2 kilogram per square centimeter
kgf kilogram-force
kg/l kilograms per liter
kg-m kilogram-meter
kg/m kilograms per meter
kg-m/s^2 kilogram-meter per second squared
Kgn kininogen
kgps kilograms per second
KGS ketogenic steroid
17-KGS 17-ketogenic steroid
KH Krebs-Henseleit [buffer]
K24H potassium, urinary 24-hour
KHB Krebs-Henseleit buffer
KHb potassium hemoglobinate
KHC kinetic hemolysis curve
KHD kinky hair disease
KHF Korean hemorrhagic fever
KHM keratoderma hereditaria mutilans
KHN Knoop hardness number
KHP King's Honorary Physician
KHS King's Honorary Surgeon; kinky hair syndrome; Krebs-Henseleit solution

kHz kilohertz
KI karyopyknotic index; Krönig's isthmus
KIA Kligler iron agar
KIC ketoisocaproate; keto isocaproic acid
KICB killed intracellular bacteria
KID keratitis, ichthyosis, and deafness [syndrome]
kilo kilogram
KIMSA Kirsten murine sarcoma
KIMSV, Ki-MSV Kirsten murine sarcoma virus
KIP key intermediary protein
KISS key integrative social system; saturated solution of potassium iodide
KIT Kahn Intelligence Test
KIU kallikrein inactivation unit
KIVA keto isovaleric acid
KJ, kj knee jerk
kJ kilojoule
KK knee kick
kkat kilokatal
KKS kallikrein-kinin system
KL kidney lobe; Klebs-Loeffler [bacillus]; Kleine-Levin [syndrome]
kl kiloliter
Klebs *Klebsiella*
KLH keyhole limpet hemocyanin
KLS kidneys, liver, and spleen; Kreuzbein's lipomatous syndrome
KM kanamycin
km kilometer
km^2 square kilometer
K$_m$ Michaelis-Menten constant
kMc kilomegacycle
K-MCM potassium-containing minimum capacitation medium
kMc/s kilomegacycles per second
KMEF keratin, myosin, epidermin, and fibrin
kmps kilometers per second
KMS kwashiorkor-marasmus syndrome
KMV killed measles virus vaccine
Kn knee; Knudsen number
kN kilonewton
kn knee
K nail Küntscher nail

KNRK Kirsten sarcoma virus in normal rat kidney

KO keep on; keep open; killed organism; knee orthosis; knock out

KOC cathodal opening contraction

kΩ kilohm

KP Kaufmann-Peterson [base]; keratitic precipitate; keratitis punctata; kidney protein; killed parenteral [vaccine]; *Klebsiella pneumoniae*

K-P Kaiser-Permanente [diet]

kPa kilopascal

kPa·s/l kilopascal seconds per liter

KPB ketophenylbutazone; potassium phosphate buffer

KPE Kelman pharmacoemulsification

KPI kallikrein-protease inhibitor; karyopyknotic index

KPR key pulse rate

KPS Karnofsky Performance Status

KPT kidney punch test

KPTI Kunitz pancreatic trypsin inhibitor

KPTT kaolin partial thromboplastin time

KPV key process variable; killed parenteral vaccine

KQC key quality characteristics

KR key-ridge; Kopper Reppart [medium]

Kr krypton

kR kiloroentgen

KRB Krebs-Ringer buffer

KRBG Krebs-Ringer bicarbonate buffer with glucose

KRBS Krebs-Ringer bicarbonate solution

KRP Kolmer test with Reiter protein [antigen]; Krebs-Ringer phosphate

KRRS kinetic resonance Raman spectroscopy

KS Kallmann syndrome; Kaposi's sarcoma; Kartagener syndrome; Kawasaki syndrome; keratan sulfate; ketosteroid; Klinefelter syndrome; Korsakoff syndrome; Kveim-Siltzbach [test]

17-KS 17-ketosteroid

ks kilosecond

KSC cathodal closing contraction

KS/OI Kaposi's sarcoma with opportunistic infection

K$_{sp}$ solubility product

KSP Karolinska Scales of Personality; kidney-specific protein

KSS Kearns-Sayre syndrome; Kearns-Sayre-Shy [syndrome]

KST cathodal closing tetanus

KT kidney transplant, kidney transplantation

KTI kallikrein-trypsin inhibitor

KTSA Kahn test of symbol arrangement

KTW, KTWS Klippel-Trenaunay-Weber [syndrome]

KU kallikrein unit; Karmen unit

Ku kurchatovium; Peltz factor

KUB kidneys and upper bladder; [x-ray examination of the] kidneys, ureter, and bladder

KUS, kidney, ureter, spleen

KV kanamycin and vancomycin; killed vaccine

kV, kv kilovolt

kVA kilovolt-ampere

kvar kilovar

KVBA kanamycin-vancomycin blood agar

kV̄cp, kvcp kilovolt constant potential

KVE Kaposi's varicelliform eruption

KVLBA kanamycin-vancomycin laked blood agar

KVO keep vein open

kVp, kvp kilovolt peak

KW Keith-Wagener [ophthalmoscopic finding]; Kimmelstiel-Wilson [syndrome]; Kugelberg-Welander [syndrome]

Kw weighted kappa

K$_w$ dissociation constant of water

kW, kw kilowatt

KWB Keith-Wagener-Barker [hypertension classification]

kWh, kW-hr, kw-hr kilowatt-hour

K wire Kirschner wire

KZ ketoconazole

L angular momentum; Avogadro's constant; boundary [Lat. *limes*]; coefficient of induction; diffusion length; inductance; *Lactobacillus*; lambda; lambert; latent heat; latex; Latin; leader sequence; left; *Legionella; Leishmania*; length; lente insulin; lethal; leucine; levo-; lidocaine; ligament; light; light sense; lingual; *Listeria;* liter; liver; low; lower; lumbar; luminance; lymph; lymphocyte; outer membrane layer of cell wall of gram-negative bacteria [layer]; pound [Lat. *libra*]; radiance; self-inductance; syphilis [Lat. *lues*]; threshold [Lat. *limen*]

L-variant a defective bacterial variant that can multiply on hypertonic medium

L_0 limes zero [*limes nul*]

L_+ limes tod

L1, L2, L3, L4, L5 first, second, third, fourth, and fifth lumbar vertebrae

LI, LII, LIII first, second, third stage of syphilis

L/3 lower third

l azimuthal quantum number; left; length; lethal; levorotatory; liter; long; longitudinal; specific latent heat

Λ see *lambda*

λ see *lambda*

LA lactic acid; large amount; late abortion; late antigen; latex agglutination; left angle; left arm; left atrium; left auricle; leucine aminopeptidase; leukemia antigen; leukoagglutination; leuprolide acetate; levator ani; linguo-axial; linoleic acid; lobuloalveolar; local anesthesia; long-acting [drug]; long arm; low anxiety; Ludwig's angina; lupus anticoagulant; lymphocyte antibody

L&A light and accommodation; living and active

LA50 total body surface area of burn that will kill 50% of patients (lethal area)

La labial; lambda; lambert; lanthanum

la according to the art [Lat. *lege artis*]

LAA left atrial appendage; leukemia-associated antigen; leukocyte ascorbic acid

LAAO L-amino acid oxidase

LA/Ao left atrial/aortic [ratio]

LAB, lab laboratory

LABV left atrial ball valve

LAC La Crosse [virus]; left atrial contraction; linguoaxiocervical; long-arm cast; low-amplitude contraction; lung adenocarcinoma cells; lupus anticoagulant

LaC labiocervical

lac laceration; lactation

LACN local area communications network

lacr lacrimal

lact lactate, lactating, lactation; lactic

lact hyd lactalbumin hydrolysate

LAD lactic acid dehydrogenase; left anterior descending [artery]; left axis deviation; leukocyte adhesion deficiency; ligament augmentation device; linoleic acid depression; lipoamide dehydrogenase; lymphocyte-activating determinant

LADA laboratory animal dander allergy; left acromio-dorso-anterior [position]

LADCA left anterior descending coronary artery

LADD lacrimoauriculodentodigital [syndrome]; left anterior descending diagonal [coronary artery]

LADH lactic acid dehydrogenase; liver alcohol dehydrogenase

LAD-MIN left axis deviation, minimal

LADP left acromio-dorso-posterior [position]

LAE left atrial enlargement

LAEDV left atrial volume in end diastole

LAEI left atrial emptying index

LAESV left atrial volume in end systole

laev left [Lat. *laevus*]

LAF laminar air flow; Latin American female; leukocyte-activating factor; lymphocyte-activating factor

LAFB left anterior fascicular block

LAFR laminar air flow room

LAFU laminar air flow unit

LAG linguo-axiogingival; lymphangiogram

LaG labiogingival

lag flask [Lat. *lagena*]

LAH lactalbumin hydrolysate; left anterior hemiblock; left atrial hypertrophy; Licentiate of Apothecaries Hall; lithium, aluminum, hydroxide

LAHB left anterior hemiblock

LAHC low affinity–high capacity

LAHV leukocyte-associated herpesvirus

LAI latex particle agglutination inhibition; leukocyte adherence inhibition

LaI labioincisal

LAIF leukocyte adherence inhibition factor

LAIT latex agglutination inhibition test

LAK lymphokine-activated killer [cells]

LAL left axillary line; *Limulus* amebocyte lysate; low air loss; lysosomal acid lipase

LaL labiolingual

LALB low air-loss bed

LALI lymphocyte antibody-lymphocytolytic interaction

LAM laminectomy; late ambulatory monitoring; Latin American male; left anterior measurement; left atrial myxoma; lymphangioleiomyomatosis

lam laminectomy

LAMB lentigines, atrial myxoma, mucocutaneous myxomas, blue nevi [syndrome]

λ Greek lower case letter *lambda*; craniometric point; decay constant; an immunoglobulin light chain; mean free path; microliter; thermal conductivity; wavelength

LAMMA laser microprobe mass analyzer

LAN local area network; long-acting neuroleptic [agent]

LANC long-arm navicular cast

LANV left atrial neovascularization

LAO left anterior oblique; left atrial overload; Licentiate of the Art of Obstetrics

LAP laparoscopy; laparotomy; left arterial pressure; left atrial pressure; leucine aminopeptidase; leukocyte alkaline phosphatase; low atmospheric pressure; lyophilized anterior pituitary

lap laparoscopy; laparotomy

lapid of stone [Lat. *lapideus*]

LAPW left atrial posterior wall

LAR laryngology; late asthmatic response; late reaction; left arm recumbent

lar larynx; left arm reclining

LARC leukocyte automatic recognition computer

LARD lacrimoauriculoradiodental [syndrome]

Laryngol laryngology

LAS laboratory automation system; lateral amyotrophic sclerosis; laxative abuse syndrome; left anterior-superior; leucine acetylsalicylate; linear alkylsulfonate; local adaptation syndrome; long arm splint; lower abdominal surgery; lymphadenopathy syndrome

LASER light amplification by stimulated emission of radiation

LASH left anterior superior hemiblock

L-ASP L-asparaginase

LASS labile aggregation stimulating substance

LAT lateral; latex agglutination test; left atrial thrombus; lysolecithin acyltransferase

Lat Latin

lat latent; lateral

lat admov let it be applied to the side [Lat. *lateri admoveatum*]

lat bend lateral bending

LATCH literature attached to charts

lat dol to the painful side [Lat. *lateri dolenti*]

l·atm liter atmosphere

LATP left atrial transmural pressure

LATPT left atrial transesophageal pacing test

LATS long-acting thyroid stimulator

LATS-P long-acting thyroid stimulator-protector

LATu lobulo-alveolar tumor

LAV leafhopper A virus; lymphadenopathy-associated virus

lav lavoratory

LAW left atrial wall

lax laxative; laxity

LB lamellar body; large bowel; left breast; left bundle; left buttock; leiomyoblastoma; lipid body; live birth; liver biopsy; loose body; low back [pain]; lung biopsy

L&B left and below

Lb pound force

lb pound [Lat. *libra*]

LBA left basal artery

LBB left bundle branch; low back bending

LBBB left bundle branch block

LBBsB left bundle branch system block

LBC lidocaine blood concentration; lymphadenosis benigna cutis

LBCD left border of cardiac dullness

LBCF Laboratory Branch complement fixation [test]

LBD large bile duct; left border of dullness

LBF *Lactobacillus bulgaricus* factor; limb blood flow; liver blood flow

lbf pound force

lbf-ft pound force foot

LBH length, breadth, height

LBI low back injury; low serum–bound iron

lb/in² pounds per square inch

LBL labeled lymphoblast; lymphoblastic lymphoma

LBM lean body mass; loose bowel movement; lung basement membrane

LBNP lower body negative pressure

LBO large bowel obstruction

LBP low back pain; low blood pressure

LBPF long bone or pelvic fracture

LBPQ Low Back Pain Questionnaire

LBRF louse-borne relapsing fever

LBS low back syndrome

LBSA lipid-bound sialic acid

LBT low back tenderness or trouble

LBTI lima bean trypsin inhibitor

lb tr pound troy

LBV left brachial vein; lung blood volume

LBW lean body weight; low birth weight

LBWI low-birth-weight infant

LBWR lung-body weight ratio

LC Laennec's cirrhosis; Langerhans' cell; late clamped; large chromophobe; lecithin cholesterol acyltransferase; lethal concentration; Library of Congress; life care; light chain; linguocervical; lipid cytosomes; liquid chromatography; liver cirrhosis; living children; locus ceruleus; long chain; low calorie; lung cancer; lung cell

LC₅₀ median lethal concentration

LCA left circumflex artery; left coronary artery; leukocyte common antigen; lithocholic acid; lymphocyte chemotactic activity

LCAO linear combination of atomic orbitals

LCAR late cutaneous anaphylactic reaction

LCAT lecithin cholesterol acyltransferase

LCB Laboratory of Cancer Biology; left costal border; lymphomatosis cutis benigna

LCBF local cerebral blood flow

LCC lactose coliform count; left circumflex coronary (artery); left common carotid; left coronary cusp; lipid-containing cell; liver cell carcinoma

LCCA late cortical cerebellar atrophy; leukoclastic angiitis

LCCME Liaison Committee on Continuing Medical Education

LCCS lower cervical cesarean section

LCCSCT large-cell calcifying Sertoli cell tumor

LCD coal tar solution [liquor carbonis detergens]; liquid crystal diode; localized collagen dystrophy

LCDD light chain deposition disease

LCF least common factor; lymphocyte culture fluid

LCFA long-chain fatty acid

LCFU leukocyte colony-forming unit

LCG Langerhans cell granule

LCGL large-cell granulocytic leukemia

LCGME Liaison Committee on Graduate Medical Education

LCGU local cerebral glucose utilization

LCH Langerhans cell histiocytosis

LCh Licentiate in Surgery

LCI length complexity index

LCL Levinthal-Coles-Lillie [body]; lower confidence limit; lymphoblastoid cell line; lymphocytic lymphosarcoma; lymphoid cell line

LCM latent cardiomyopathy; left costal margin; leukocyte-conditioned medium; lowest common multiple; lymphatic choriomeningitis; lymphocytic choriomeningitis

LCME Liaison Committee on Medical Education

LCMG long-chain monoglyceride

L/cm H₂O liters per centimeter of water

LCMV lymphocytic choriomeningitis virus

LCN lateral cervical nucleus; left caudate nucleus

LCO low cardiac output

LCOS low cardiac output syndrome

LCP long-chain polysaturated [fatty acid]

LCPD Legg-Calvé-Perthes disease

LCPS Licentiate of the College of Physicians and Surgeons

LCS cerebrospinal fluid [Lat. *liquor cerebrospinalis*]; left coronary sinus; life care service; low constant suction; low continuous suction; lymphocyte culture supernatants

LCSB Liaison Committee for Specialty Boards

LCT liver cell tumor; long-chain triglyceride; lymphocytotoxicity; lymphocytotoxin

LCTA lymphocytotoxic antibody

LCU life change unit

LCV lecithovitellin

LCx left circumflex artery

LD labor and delivery; laboratory data; labyrinthine defect; lactate dehydrogenase; learning disability; learning disorder; left deltoid; Legionnaires' disease; lethal dose; light differentiation; limited disease; linear dichroism; linguodistal; lipodystrophy; liver disease; living donor; loading dose; Lombard-Dowell [agar]; longitudinal diameter; low density; low dose; lymphocyte-defined; lymphocyte depletion

L-D Leishman-Donovan [body]

L/D light/darkness [ratio]

L&D labor and delivery

LD₁ isoenzyme of lactate dehydrogenase found in the heart, erythrocytes, and kidneys

LD₂ isoenzyme of lactate dehydrogenase found in the lungs

LD₃ isoenzyme of lactate dehydrogenase found in the lungs

LD₄ isoenzyme of lactate dehydrogenase found in the liver

LD₅ isoenzyme of lactate dehydrogenase found in the liver and muscles

LD₅₀ median lethal dose

LD₅₀/₃₀ a dose that is lethal for 50% of test subjects within 30 days

LD₁₀₀ lethal dose in all exposed subjects

Ld *Leishmania donovani*

LDA laser Doppler anemometry; left dorso-anterior [fetal position]; linear discriminant analysis; lymphocyte-dependent antibody

LDAC low-dose cytosine arabinoside

LDAR latex direct agglutination reaction

LDB lamb dysentery bacillus; Legionnaires' disease bacillus

LDC lymphoid dendritic cell; lysine decarboxylase

LDCC lectin-dependent cellular cytotoxicity

LDCI low-dose continuous infusion

LDCT late distal cortical tubule

LDD late dedifferentiation; light-darkness discrimination

LDER lateral-view dual-energy radiography

LD-EYA Lombard-Dowell egg yolk agar

LDF laser Doppler flux, laser Doppler fluxometry; limit dilution factor

LDG lactic dehydrogenase; lingual developmental groove

LDH lactate dehydrogenase; low-dose heparin

LDHA lactic dehydrogenase A

LDHB lactic dehydrogenase-B

LDHC lactic dehydrogenase-C

LDHK lactic dehydrogenase-K

LDIH left direct inguinal hernia

LDL loudness discomfort level; low density lipoprotein

LDLA low-density lipoprotein apheresis

LDLC low-density lipoprotein cholesterol

LDLP low-density lipoprotein

LDM lactate dehydrogenase, muscle

LD-NEYA Lombard-Dowell neomycin egg yolk agar

L-DOPA, L-dopa levodopa, levo-3, 4-dihydroxyphenylalanine

LDP left dorsoposterior [fetal position]

LDS Licentiate in Dental Surgery

LDSc Licentiate in Dental Science

LDT left dorsotransverse [fetal position]

LDUB long double upright brace

LDV lactic dehydrogenase virus; large dense-cored vesicle; laser Doppler velocimetry; lateral distant view

LE left ear; left eye; leukocyte elastase; leukoerythrogenic; live embryo; Long Evans [rat]; low exposure; lower extremity; lupus erythematosus

LEA lower extremity amputation

LEC leukoencephalitis; lower esophageal contractility

LECP low-energy charged particle

LED light-emitting diode; lowest emitting dose; lupus erythematosus disseminatus

LEED low-energy electron diffraction

LEEDS low-energy electron diffraction spectroscopy

LEEP left end-expiratory pressure

LEF leukokinesis-enhancing factor; lupus erythematosus factor

leg legislation; legal

LeIF leukocyte interferon

LEIS low-energy ion scattering

LEL lower explosive limit; lowest effect level

LEM lateral eye movement; Leibovitz-Emory medium; leukocyte endogenous mediator; light emission microscopy

LEMO lowest empty molecular orbital

LEMS Lambert-Eaton myasthenic syndrome

lenit lenitive

LEOPARD lentigines, EKG abnormalities, ocular hypertelorism, pulmonary stenosis, abnormalities of genitalia, retardation of growth, and deafness [syndrome]

LEP lethal effective phase; lipoprotein electrophoresis; low egg passage; lower esophagus

L$_{EPN}$ effective perceived noise level

Leq loudness equivalent

LER lysozomal enzyme release

LERG local electroretinogram

LES Lambert-Eaton syndrome; Lawrence Experimental Station [agar]; local excitatory state; Locke egg serum; low excitatory state; lower esophageal sphincter; lupus erythematosus, systemic

les lesion

LESP lower esophageal sphincter pressure

LESS lateral electrical spine stimulation

LET linear or low energy transfer

LETD lowest effective toxic dose

LETS large external transformation–sensitive [protein]

LEU leucine; leucovorin; leukocyte equivalent unit

Leu leucine

leuc leukocyte

lev light [Lat. *levis*]

LEW Lewis [rat]
l/ext lower extremity
LF labile factor; lactoferrin; laryngofissure; Lassa fever; latex fixation; left foot; left forearm; lethal fctor; leukotactic factor; ligamentum flavum; limit of flocculation; low fat [diet]; low forceps; low frequency
Lf limit of flocculation
lf lactoferrin; low frequency
LFA left femoral artery; left frontal craniotomy; left fronto-anterior [fetal position]; leukocyte function associated antigen; leukotactic factor activity; low-friction arthroplasty
LFC living female child; low fat and cholesterol [diet]
LFD lactose-free diet; large for date [fetus]; late fetal death; lateral facial dysplasia; least fatal dose; low-fat diet; low-fiber diet; low forceps delivery
LFER linear free-energy relationship
LFH left femoral hernia
LFL left frontolateral; leukocyte feeder layer; lower flammable limit
LFN lactoferrin
L-[form] a defective bacterial variant that can multiply on hypertonic medium
LFP left frontoposterior [fetal position]
LFPPV low-frequency positive pressure ventilation
LFPS Licentiate of the Faculty of Physicians and Surgeons
LFR lymphoid follicular reticulosis
LFS lateral facet syndrome; limbic forebrain structure; liver function series
LFT latex fixation test; latex flocculation test; left fronto-transverse [fetal position]; liver function test; low-frequency tetanus; low-frequency transduction; low-frequency transfer
LFU lipid fluidity unit
LFV Lassa fever virus; low-frequency ventilation
LFx linear fracture
LG lactoglobulin; lamellar granule; laryngectomy; left gluteal; Lennox-Gastaut [syndrome]; leucylglycine; linguogingi-

val; lipoglycopeptide; liver graft; low glucose; lymphatic gland
lg large; leg
LGA large for gestational age; left gastric artery
LGB Landry-Guillain-Barré [syndrome]; lateral geniculate body
LGBS Landry-Guillain-Barré syndrome
LGE Langat encephalitis
LGF lateral giant fiber
LGH lactogenic hormone
LGI large glucagon immunoreactivity
LGL large granular leukocyte; large granular lymphocyte; Lown-Ganong-Levine [syndrome]
LGL-NK large granular lymphocyte-natural killer
LGMD limb-girdle muscular dystrophy
LGN lateral geniculate nucleus; lateral glomerulonephritis
LGS Lennox-Gastaut syndrome; limb girdle syndrome
LGT late generalized tuberculosis
LGV large granular vesicle; lymphogranuloma venereum
LGVHD lethal graft-versus-host disease
LgX lymphogranulomatosis X
LH late healing; lateral hypothalamic [syndrome]; left hand; left heart; left hemisphere; left hyperphoria; liver homogenate; lower half; lues hereditaria; lung homogenate; luteinizing hormone
LHA lateral hypothalamic area; left hepatic artery
LHBV left heart blood volume
LHC Langerhans cell histiocytosis; left heart catheterization; left hypochondrium; light-harvesting complex; Local Health Council
LHF left heart failure
LHFA lung Hageman factor activator
LHG left hand grip; localized hemolysis in gel
LHI lipid hydrocarbon inclusion
LHL left hepatic lobe
LHM lysuride hydrogen maleate
LHMP Life Health Monitoring Program
LHN lateral hypothalamic nucleus

LHPZ low high-pressure zone
LHR leukocyte histamine release
l-hr lumen-hour
LHRF luteinizing hormone-releasing factor
LHRH, LH-RH luteinizing hormone-releasing hormone
LHS left hand side; left heart strain; left heelstrike; lymphatic/hematopoietic system
LHT left hypertropia
LI labeling index; lactose intolerance; lacunar infarct; lamellar ichthyosis; large intestine; *Leptospira icterohaemorrhagica;* linguoincisal; lithogenic index; low impulsiveness
L&I liver and iron
Li a blood group system; labrale inferius; lithium
LIA Laser Institute of America; leukemia-associated inhibitory activity; lock-in amplifier; lymphocyte-induced angiogenesis; lysine iron agar
LIAFI late infantile amaurotic familial idiocy
lib a pound [Lat. *libra*]
LIBC latent iron-binding capacity
LIC left internal carotid [artery]; limiting isorrheic concentration; local intravascular coagulation
Lic licentiate
LICA left internal carotid artery
LICM left intercostal margin
LicMed Licentiate in Medicine
LICS left intercostal space
LID late immunoglobulin deficiency; lymphocytic infiltrative disease
LIF laser-induced fluorescence; left iliac fossa; left index finger; leukemia-inhibiting factor; leukocyte inhibitory factor; leukocytosis-inducing factor
LIFE lung imaging fluorescence endoscope
LIFO last in, first out
LIFT lymphocyte immunofluorescence test
lig ligament; ligation
LIH left inguinal hernia

LIHA low impulsiveness, high anxiety
LILA low impulsiveness, low anxiety
LIM line isolation monitor
lim limit, limited
LIMA left internal mammary artery
Linim, lin liniment
LIO left inferior oblique
LIP lithium-induced polydipsia; lymphoid interstitial pneumonitis
Lip lipoate
lipoMM lipomyelomeningocele
LIQ low inner quadrant
liq liquid [Lat. *liquor*]
liq dr liquid dram
liq oz liquid ounce
liq pt liquid pint
liq qt liquid quart
LIR left iliac region; left inferior rectus
LIRBM liver, iron, red bone marrow
LIS laboratory information system; lateral intercellular space; left intercostal space; lobular *in situ*; locked-in syndrome; low intermittent suction; low ionic strength
LISA Library and Information Science Abstracts
LISP List Processing Language
LISS low-ionic-strength saline
LIV left innominate vein
liv live, living
LIV-BP leucine, isoleucine, and valine-binding protein
LIVC left inferior vena cava
LIVEN linear inflammatory verrucous epidermal nevus
LJI List of Journals Indexed
LJM limited joint mobility; Lowenstein-Jensen medium
LK left kidney; lichenoid keratosis; lymphokine
LKKS liver, kidneys, spleen
LKM liver-kidney microsomal [antibody]
LKP lamellar keratoplasty
LKS Landau-Kleffner syndrome; liver, kidneys, spleen
LKSB liver, kidney, spleen, bladder
LKV laked kanamycin vancomycin [agar]

LL large lymphocyte; lateral leminiscus; left lateral; left leg; left lower; left lung; lepromatous leprosy; lipoprotein lipase; loudness level; lower [eye]lid; lower limb; lower lip; lower lobe; lumbar length; lymphocytic lymphoma; lymphoid leukemia; lysolecithin

LLA limulus lysate assay

L lat left lateral

LLB left lateral border; long-leg brace

LLBCD left lower border of cardiac dullness

LLC Lewis lung carcinoma; liquid-liquid chromatography; long-leg cast; lymphocytic leukemia

LLCC long-leg cylinder cast

LLC-MK1 rhesus monkey kidney cells

LLC-MK2 rhesus monkey kidney cells

LLC-MK3 *Cercopithecus* monkey kidney cells

LLC-RK1 rabbit kidney cells

LLD left lateral decubitus [muscle]; leg length discrepancy; long-lasting depolarization

LLE left lower extremity

LLF Laki-Lóránd factor; left lateral femoral; left lateral flexion

LLL left lower [eye]lid; left liver lobe; left lower leg; left lower lobe

LLM localized leukocyte mobilization

LLN lower limit of normal

LLO *Legionella*-like organism

LLP late luteal phase; long-lasting potentiation

LLQ left lower quadrant

LLR large local reaction; left lateral rectus [muscle]; left lumbar region

LLS lazy leukocyte syndrome; long-leg splint

LLSB left lower scapular border; left lower sternal border

LLT left lateral thigh; lysolecithin

LLV lymphatic leukemia virus

LLV-F lymphatic leukemia virus, Friend associated

LLVP left lateral ventricular preexcitation

LLWC long-leg walking cast

LLX left lower extremity

LM lactic acid mineral [medium]; lactose malabsorption; laryngeal muscle; lateral malleolus; left median; legal medicine; lemniscus medialis; Licentiate in Medicine; Licentiate in Midwifery; light microscope, light microscopy; light minimum; lincomycin; lingual margin; linguomesial; lipid mobilization; liquid membrane; *Listeria monocytogenes;* localized movement; longitudinal muscle; lower motor [neuron]

Lm *Listeria monocytogenes*

lm lumen

l/m liters per minute

LMA left mentoanterior [fetal position]; limbic midbrain area; liver cell membrane autoantibody

LMB leiomyoblastoma

LMBB Laurence-Moon-Bardet-Biedl [syndrome]

LMBS Laurence-Moon-Biedl syndrome

LMC large motile cell; lateral motor column; left main coronary [artery]; left middle cerebral [artery]; living male child; lymphocyte-mediated cytotoxicity; lymphomyeloid complex

LMCA left main coronary artery; left middle cerebral artery

LMCAD left main coronary artery disease

LMCC Licentiate of the Medical Council of Canada

LMCL left midclavicular line

LMD lipid-moiety modified derivative; local medical doctor; low molecular weight dextran

LMDX low-molecular-weight dextran

LME left mediolateral episiotomy; leukocyte migration enhancement

LMed&Ch Licentiate in Medicine and Surgery

LMF left middle finger; lymphocyte mitogenic factor

lm/ft² lumens per square foot

LMG lethal midline granuloma

LMH lipid-mobilizing hormone

lmh lumen hour

LMI leukocyte migration inhibition

LMIF leukocyte migration inhibition factor

l/min liters per minute

LML large and medium lymphocytes; left mediolateral; left middle lobe

LMM *Lactobacillus* maintenance medium; lentigo maligna melanoma; light meromyosin

lm/m² lumens per square meter

LMN lower motor neuron

LMNL lower motor neuron lesion

LMO localized molecular orbital

LMP last menstrual period; latent membrane potential; left mentoposterior [fetal position]; lumbar puncture

LMR left medial rectus [muscle]; lymphocytic meningpolyradiculitis

LMRCP Licentiate in Midwifery of the Royal College of Physicians

LMS lateral medullary syndrome; leiomyosarcoma; Licentiate in Medicine and Surgery

lms lumen-second

LMSSA Licentiate in Medicine and Surgery of the Society of Apothecaries

LMT left mentotransverse [fetal position]; leukocyte migration technique

LMV larva migrans visceralis

LMW low molecular weight

lm/W lumens per watt

LMWD low-molecular-weight dextran

LN Lesch-Nyhan [syndrome]; lipoid nephrosis; low necrosis; lupus nephritis; lymph node

L/N letter/numerical [system]

ln natural logarithm

LNAA large neutral amino acid

LNC lymph node cell

LNE lymph node enlargement

LNH large number hypothesis

LNKS low natural killer syndrome

LNL lymph node lymphocyte

LNLS linear-nonlinear least squares

LNMP last normal menstrual period

LNNB Luria-Nebraska Neuropsychological Battery

LNP large neuronal polypeptide

LNPF lymph node permeability factor

LNS lateral nuclear stratum; Lesch-Nyhan syndrome

LO linguo-occlusal

LOA leave of absence; Leber's optic atrophy; left occipitoanterior [fetal position]

LOC laxative of choice; level of consciousness; liquid organic compound; locus of control; loss of consciousness

lo cal low calorie

lo calc low calcium

loc dol to the painful spot [Lat. *loco dolenti*]

lo CHO low carbohydrate

lo chol low cholesterol

LOD line of duty

LOF lofexidine

log logarithm

LOH loop of Henle; loss of heterozygosity

LOI level of incompetence; limit of impurities

LOIH left oblique inguinal hernia

lo k low potassium

LOL left occipitolateral [fetal position]

LOM left otitis media; limitation of motion; loss of motion

LOMSA left otitis media suppurativa acuta

LOMSC, LOMSCh left otitis media suppurativa chronica

lo Na low sodium

long longitudinal

LOP leave on pass; left occipitoposterior [fetal position]

LOPS length of patient's stay

LOQ lower outer quadrant

LOR long open reading frame; lorazepam; loss of righting reflex

Lord lordosis, lordotic

LOS length of stay; Licentiate in Obstetrical Science; lipo-oligosaccharide; low cardiac output syndrome; lower [o]esophageal sphincter

LOS(P) lower [o]esophageal sphincter (pressure)

LOT lateral olfactory tract; left occipitotransverse [fetal position]
lot lotion
LOV large opaque vesicle
LOWBI low-birth-weight infant
LP labile peptide; labile protein; laboratory procedure; lactic peroxidase; lamina propria; laryngopharyngeal; latent period, latency period; lateral plantar; lateral posterior; lateral pylorus; *Legionella pneumophila;* leukocyte poor; leukocytic pyrogen; lichen planus; light perception; lingua plicata; linguopulpal; lipoprotein; liver plasma [concentration]; loss of privileges; low potency; low power; low pressure; low protein; lumbar puncture; lumboperitoneal; lung parenchyma; lymphoid plasma; lymphomatoid papulosis
L/P lactate/pyruvate [ratio]; liver plasma [concentration]; lymph/plasma [ratio]
Lp lipoprotein; sound pressure level
LPA latex particle agglutination; left pulmonary artery; lysophosphatidic acid
LPAM L-phenylalanine mustard
LPB lipoprotein B
LPBP low-profile bioprosthesis
LPC late positive component; lysophosphatidylcholine
LPCM low-placed conus medullaris
LPCT late proximal cortical tubule
LPD low-protein diet; luteal phase defect
LPDF lipoprotein-deficient fraction
LPE lipoprotein electrophoresis
LPF leukocytosis-promoting factor; leukopenia factor; lipopolysaccharide factor; localized plaque formation; low-power field; lymphocytosis-promoting factor
lpf low-power field
LPFB left posterior fascicular block
LPFN low-pass filtered noise
LPFS low-pass filtered signal
LPH left posterior hemiblock; lipotropic pituitary hormone
LPI left posterior-inferior; lysinuric protein intolerance

LPIFB left posteroinferior fascicular block
LPIH left posteroinferior hemiblock
LPK liver pyruvate kinase
LPL lichen planus-like lesion; lipoprotein lipase
LPLA lipoprotein lipase activity
LPM lateral pterygoid muscle; liver plasma membrane
lpm lines per minute; liters per minute
LPN Licensed Practical Nurse
LPO left posterior oblique; light perception only; lipid peroxidation
LPP lateral pterygoid plate
LPPH late postpartum hemorrhage
LPR lactate-pyruvate ratio
LPS levator palpebrae superioris [muscle]; linear profile scan; lipase; lipopolysaccharide
lps liters per second
LPSR lipopolysaccharide receptor
LPT lipotropin
LPV left portal view; left pulmonary veins
LPVP left posterior ventricular preexcitation
LPW lateral pharyngeal wall
lpw lumens per watt
LPX, Lp-X lipoprotein-X
LQ longevity quotient; lordosis quotient; lower quadrant
LQTS long QT syndrome
LQTS long QT syndrome
LR labeled release; laboratory references; laboratory report; labor room; lactated Ringer's [solution]; large reticulocyte; latency reaction; latency relaxation; lateral rectus [muscle]; lateral retinaculum; left rotation; light reaction; light reflex; limb reduction [defect]; limit of reaction; logistic regression; low renin; lymphocyte recruitment
L/R left-to-right [ratio]
L&R left and right
Lr lawrencium; Limes reacting dose of diphtheria toxin
LRA low right atrium
LRC lower rib cage

LRCP Licentiate of the Royal College of Physicians

LRCS Licentiate of the Royal College of Surgeons

LRCSE Licentiate of the Royal College of Surgeons, Edinburgh

LRD living related donor

LRDT living related donor transplant

LRE lamina rara externa; leukemic reticuloendotheliosis; lymphoreticuloendothelial

LREH low renin essential hypertension

LRF latex and resorcinol formaldehyde; liver residue factor; luteinizing hormone-releasing factor

LRH luteinizing hormone-releasing hormone

LRI lamina rara interna; lower respiratory [tract] illness; lower respiratory [tract] infection; lymphocyte reactivity index

LRM left radical mastectomy

LRMP last regular menstrual period

LRN lateral reticular nucleus

LROP lower radicular obstetrical paralysis

LRP lichen ruber planus; long-range planning

LRQ lower right quadrant

LRR labyrinthine righting reflex; lymph return rate

LRS lactated Ringer's solution; lateral recess syndrome; low rate of stimulation; lumboradicular syndrome

LRSF lactating rat serum factor; liver regenerating serum factor

LRSS late respiratory systemic syndrome

LRT local radiation therapy; long terminal repeat; lower respiratory tract

LRTI lower respiratory tract illness; lower respiratory tract infection

LRV left renal vein

LS lateral suspensor; left sacrum; left septum; left side; legally separated; leiomyosarcoma; length of stay; Leriche syndrome; Licentiate in Surgery; life sciences; light sensitive, light-sensitivity; light sleep; liminal sensation; linear scleroderma; lipid synthesis; liver and spleen; long sleep; low-sodium [diet]; lower strength; lumbar spine; lumbosacral; lung surfactant; lymphosarcoma

L/S lactase/sucrase [ratio]; lecithin/sphingomyelin [ratio]; lipid/saccharide [ratio]

L&S liver and spleen

LSA left sacro-anterior [fetal position]; left subclavian artery; leukocyte-specific activity; lichen sclerosus et atrophicus; lymphosarcoma

LS&A lichen sclerosus et atrophicus

LSANA leukocyte-specific antinuclear antibody

LSA/RCS lymphosarcoma-reticulum cell sarcoma

LSB least significant bit; left sternal border; left scapular border; long spike burst

LS-BMD lumbar spine bone mineral density

LSC late systolic click; left side colon cancer; lichen simplex chronicus; liquid scintillation counting; liquid-solid chromatography

LSc local scleroderma

LScA left scapulo-anterior [fetal position]

LSCL lymphosarcoma cell leukemia

LScP left scapulo-posterior [fetal position]

LSCS lower segment cesarean section

LSD least significant difference; least significant digit; low-sodium diet; lysergic acid diethylamide

LSD-25 lysergic acid diethylamide

LSEP left somatosensory evoked potential; lumbosacral somatosensory evoked potential

LSF lymphocyte-stimulating factor

LSG labial salivary gland

LSH lutein-stimulating hormone; lymphocyte-stimulating hormone

LSHTM London School of Hygiene and Tropical Medicine

LSI large-scale integration; lumbar spine index

LSK liver, spleen, kidneys

LSKM liver-spleen-kidney-megalia

LSL left sacrolateral [fetal position]; left short leg; lymphosarcoma [cell] leukemia

LSM late systolic murmur; lymphocyte separation medium; lysergic acid morpholide

LSN left substantia nigra

LSO lateral superior olive; left salpingo-oophorectomy; left superior oblique; lumbosacral orthosis

LSP left sacroposterior [fetal position]; liver-specific protein

LSp life span

L-Spar asparaginase (Elspar)

LSSA lipid-soluble secondary antioxidant

LSR lanthanide shift reagent; lecithin/sphingomyelin ratio; left superior rectus [muscle]

LSRA low septal right atrium

LSS life support station

LST lateral spinothalamic tract; left sacrotransverse [fetal position]; life-sustaining treatment

LSTL laparoscopic tubal ligation

LSU lactose-saccharose-urea [agar]; life support unit

LSV lateral sacral vein; left subclavian vein

LSVC left superior vena cava

LSWA large amplitude slow wave activity

LT heat-labile toxin; laminar tomography; left; left thigh; less than; lethal time; leukotriene; Levin tube; levothyroxine; light; long-term; low temperature; lymphocytotoxin; lymphotoxin; syphilis [lues] test

L-T3 L-triiodothyronine

L-T4 L-thyroxine

lt left; light; low tension

LTA leukotriene A; lipoate transacetylase; lipotechoic acid; local tracheal anesthesia

LTAS lead tetra-acetate Schiff

LTB laryngotracheobronchitis; leukotriene B

LTC large transformed cell; leukotriene C; lidocaine tissue concentration; long-term care

LTCF long-term care facility

LTCS low transverse cervical section

LTD Laron-type dwarfism; leukotriene D; long-term disability

LTE laryngotracheoesophageal; leukotriene E

LT-ECG long-term electrocardiography

LTF lactotransferrin; lipotropic factor; lymphocyte-transforming factor

LTH lactogenic hormone; local tumor hyperthermia; low temperature holding; luteotropic hormone

LTI lupus-type inclusions

lt lat left lateral

LTM long-term memory

LTP leukocyte thromboplastin; long-term potentiation; L-tryptophan

LTPP lipothiamide pyrophosphate

LTR long terminal repeat

LTS long-term survival

LTT lactose tolerance test; leucine tolerance test; limited treadmill test; lymphocyte transformation test

LTV lung thermal volume

LTW Leydig-cell tumor in Wistar rat

LU left upper [limb]; loudness unit; lytic unit

Lu lutetium

L&U lower and upper

LUC large unstained cell

LUE left upper extremity

LUF luteinized unruptured follicle

LUFS luteinized unruptured follicle syndrome

LUL left upper eyelid; left upper limb; left upper lobe; left upper lung

lumb lumbar

LUMD lowest usual maintenance dose

LUMO lowest unoccupied molecular orbital

LUO left ureteral orifice

LUOQ left upper outer quadrant

LUP left ureteropelvic

LUQ left upper quadrant

LUSB left upper scapular border; left upper sternal border

lut yellow [Lat. *luteus*]
LUV large unilamellar vesicle
LV laryngeal vestibule; lateral ventricle; lecithovitellin; left ventricle, left ventricular; leucovorin; leukemia virus; live vaccine; live virus; low volume; lumbar vertebra; lung volume
Lv brightness or luminance
lv leave
LVA left ventricular aneurysm; left vertebral artery
LVAD left ventricular assist device
LVAS left ventricular assist system
LVBP left ventricular bypass pump
LVC low-viscosity cement
LVCS low vertical cesarean section
LVD left ventricular dysfunction
LVDd left ventricular dimension in end-diastole
LVDI left ventricular dimension
LVDP left ventricular diastolic pressure
LVDV left ventricular diastolic volume
LVE left ventricular ejection; left ventricular enlargement
LVED left ventricular end-diastole
LVEDC left ventricular end-diastolic circumference
LVEDD left ventricular end-diastolic diameter
LVEDP left ventricular end-diastolic pressure
LVEDV left ventricular end-diastolic volume
LVEF left ventricular ejection fraction
LVEP left ventricular end-diastolic pressure
LVESD left ventricular end-systolic dimension
LVESV left ventricular end-systolic volume
LVET left ventricular ejection time
LVETI left ventricular ejection time index
LVF left ventricular failure; left ventricular function; left visual field; low-voltage fast; low-voltage foci
LVFP left ventricular filling pressure
LVH large vessel hematocrit; left ventricular hypertrophy

LVI left ventricular insufficiency; left ventricular ischemia
LVID left ventricular internal dimension
LVIV left ventricular infarct volume
LVL left vastus lateralis
LVLG left ventrolateral gluteal
LVM left ventricular mass
LVMF left ventricular minute flow
LVN lateral ventricular nerve; lateral vestibular nucleus; Licensed Visiting Nurse; Licensed Vocational Nurse
LVOT left ventricular outflow tract
LVP large volume parenteral [infusion]; left ventricular pressure; levator veli palatini; lysine-vasopressin
LVPFR left ventricular peak filling rate
LVPW left ventricular posterior wall
LVS left ventricular strain
LVSEMI left ventricular subendocardial ischemia
LVSI left ventricular systolic index
LVSO left ventricular systolic output
LVSP left ventricular systolic pressure
LVST lateral vestibulospinal tract
LVSV left ventricular stroke volume
LVSW left ventricular stroke work
LVSWI left ventricular stroke work index
LVT left ventricular tension; lysine vasotonin
LVV left ventricular volume; Le Veen valve; live varicella vaccine; live varicella virus
LVW left ventricular wall; left ventricular work
LVWI left ventricular work index
LVWM left ventricular wall motion
LVWT left ventricular wall thickness
LW lacerating wound; lateral wall; Lee-White [method]
L&W, L/W living and well
Lw lawrencium
LWCT Lee-White clotting time
LWK large white kidney
LWP lateral wall pressure
LX local irradiation; lower extremity
Lx latex
lx larynx; lower extremity; lux
LXT left exotopia

LY lactoalbumin and yeastolate [medium]; lymphocyte

Ly a T-cell antigen used for grouping T-lymphocytes into different classes

LYDMA lymphocyte-detected membrane antigen

LYES liver yang exuberance syndrome

LYG lymphomatoid granulomatosis

lym, lymph lymphocyte, lymphocytic

LyNeF lytic nephritic factor

lyo lyophilized

LYP lactose, yeast, and peptone [agar]; lower yield point

LYS, Lys lysine; lytes electrolytes

LySLk lymphoma syndrome leukemia

LZM, Lzm lysozyme

M blood factor in the MNS blood group system; chin [Lat. *mentum*]; concentration in moles per liter; death [Lat. *mors*]; dullness [of sound] [Lat. *mutitas*]; handful [Lat. *manipulus*]; macerate, macerated [Lat. *macerare*]; macroglobulin; magnetization; male; malignant; married; masculine; mass; massage; maternal contribution; matrix; mature; maximum; mean; meatus; median; mediator; medical, medicine; medium; mega-; megohm; membrane; memory; mental; mesial; metabolite; metanephrine; metastases; meter; methionine; methotrexate; *Micrococcus*; *Microspora*; minim; minute; mitochondria; mitosis; mix, mixed, mixture; molar [permanent tooth]; molar [solution]; molarity; mole; molecular; moment of force; monkey; monocyte; month; morgan; morphine; mother; motile; mouse; mucoid [colony]; mucous; multipara; murmur [cardiac]; muscle; muscular response to an electrical stimulation of its motor nerve [wave]; *Mycobacterium*; *Mycoplasm*; myeloma or macroglobulinemia [component]; myopia; strength of pole; thousand [Lat. *mille*]

M-I first meiotic metaphase

M_1 mitral first [sound]; myeloblast; slight dullness

M-II second meiotic metaphase

M_2 dose per square meter of body surface; marked dullness; promyelocyte

2-M 2-microglobulin

M_3 absolute dullness; myelocyte at the 3rd stage of maturation

3-M [syndrome] initials for Miller, McKusick, and Malvaux, who first described the syndrome

M/3 middle third

M_4 myelocyte at the 4th stage of maturation

M_5 metamyelocyte

M_6 band form in the 6th stage of myelocyte maturation

M_7 polymorphonuclear neutrophil

M/10 tenth molar solution

M/100 hundredth molar solution

m electron rest mass; electromagnetic moment; in the morning [Lat. *mane*]; magnetic moment; magnetic quantum number; mass; median; melting [temperature]; meter; milli-; minim; minimum; minute; molality; molar [deciduous tooth]; send [Lat. *mitte*]

m^2 square meter

m^3 cubic meter

m_8 spin quantum number

μ see mu

MA malignant arrhythmia; mandelic acid; masseter; Master of Arts; mean arterial; medical assistance; medical audit; medical authorization; mega-ampere; megaloblastic anemia; membrane antigen; menstrual age; mental age; mentum anterior [fetal position]; metatarsus adductus; meter-angle; microadenoma; microagglutination; microaneurysm; microscopic agglutination; Miller-Abbott [tube]; milliampere; mitochondrial antibody; mitogen activation; mitotic apparatus; mixed agglutination; moderately advanced; monoamine; monoclonal antibody; multiple action; mutagenic activity; myelinated axon

M/A male, altered [animal]; mood and/or affect

MA-104 embryonic rhesus monkey kidney cells

MA-111 embryonic rabbit kidney cells

MA-163 human embryonic thymus cells

MA-184 newborn human foreskin cells

Ma mass of atom

mA, ma milliampere; meter-angle

mÅ milliångström

ma milliampere

MAA macroaggregated albumin; Medical Assistance for the Aged; melanoma-associated antigen; moderate aplastic anemia; monoarticular arthritis

MAACL Multiple Affect Adjective Check List

MAAGB Medical Artists Association of Great Britain

MAB, MAb monoclonal antibody

m-AB m-aminobenzamide

MABP mean arterial blood pressure

Mabs monoclonal antibodies

MAC MacConkey's [broth]; malignancy-associated changes; maximum allowable concentration; maximum allowable cost; medical alert center; membrane attack complex; midarm circumference; minimum alveolar concentration; minimum antibiotic concentration; mitral anular calcium; modulator of adenylate cyclase; monitored anesthesia care; *Mycobacterium avium* complex

mac macerate [Lat. *macerare*]

m accur mix very accurately [Lat. *misce accuratissime*]

MACDP Metropolitan Atlanta Congenital Defects Program

macer maceration

mAChR muscarinic acetylcholine receptor

MACR mean axillary count rate

macro macrocyte, macrocytic; macroscopic

MAD maximum allowable dose; methylandrostenediol; mind-altering drug; minimum average dose; myoadenylate deaminase

mAD, MADA muscle adenylate deaminase

MADD multiple acyl-CoA dehydrogenase deficiency

MADRS Montgomery Asberg Depression Rating Scale

MADU methylaminodeoxyuridine

MAE medical air evacuation; moves all extremities

MAF macrophage activation factor; macrophage agglutinating factor; maximum atrial fragmentation; minimum audible field; mouse amniotic fluid

MAFH macroaggregated ferrous hydroxide

MAG myelin-associated glycoprotein

Mag magnesium

mag, magn large [Lat. *magnus*]; magnification

mag cit magnesium citrate

MAGF male accessory gland fluid

MAggF macrophage agglutination factor

MAGIC microprobe analysis generalized intensity correction

mAH, mA-h milliampere-hours

MAHA microangiopathic hemolytic anemia

MAHH malignancy-associated humoral hypercalcemia

MAI microscopic aggregation index; movement assessment of infants; *Mycobacterium avium intracellulare*

MAIDS mouse acquired immunodeficiency syndrome

MAKA major karyotypic abnormality

MAL midaxillary line

Mal malate; malfunction; malignancy

mal malaise; malposition

Mal-BSA maleated bovine serum albumin

MALG Minnesota antilymphoblast globulin

MALiMET Master List of Medical Indexing Terms

MALT male, altered [animal]; mucosa-associated lymphoid tissue; Munich Alcoholism Test

MAM methylazoxymethanol

mam milliampere-minute; myriameter

M + Am compound myopic astigmatism

MAMA monoclonal anti-malignin antibody

MAM Ac methylazoxymethanol acetate

MAMC mean arm muscle circumference

ma-min milliampere-minute

MAN, Man mannose

MAN-6-P mannose-6-phosphate

man handful [Lat. *manipulus*]; manipulate; morning [Lat. *mane*]

mand mandible, mandibular
manifest manifestation
manip handful [Lat. *manipulus*]; manipulation
MANOVA multivariate analysis of variance
man pr early in the morning [Lat. *mane primo*]
MAO Master of the Art of Obstetrics; maximal acid output; monoamine oxidase
MAOA monoamine oxidase A
MAOB monoamine oxidase B
MAOI monoamine oxidase inhibitor
MAP malignant atrophic papulosis; maximal aerobic power; mean airway pressure; mean aortic pressure; mean arterial pressure; Medical Audit Program; megaloblastic anemia of pregnancy; mercapturic acid pathway; methyl acceptor protein; methylacetoxy-progesterone; methylaminopurine; microtubule-associated protein; minimum audible pressure; monophasic action potential; motor [nerve] action potential; mouse antibody production; muscle action potential
MAPA muscle adenosine phosphoric acid
MAPC migrating action potential complex
MAPF microatomized protein food
MAPI microbial alkaline protease inhibitor; Millon Adolescent Personality Inventory
MAPS Make a Picture Story [test]
MAR main admissions room; marasmus; marrow; maximal aggregation ratio; medication administration record; minimal angle resolution; mixed antiglobulin reaction
mar margin; marker [chromosome]
MARC multifocal and recurrent choroidopathy
MARS mouse antirat serum
MAS Manifest Anxiety Scale; McCune-Albright syndrome; meconium aspiration syndrome; medical advisory service; mesoatrial shunt; milk-alkali syndrome;

milliampere-second; minor axis shortening; mobile arm support; monoclonal antibodies; Morgagni-Adams-Stokes [syndrome]; motion analysis system
mA-s, mas milliampere-second
MASA Medical Association of South Africa
masc masculine; mass concentration
MASER microwave amplification by stimulated emission of radiation
MASH mobile Army surgical hospital; multiple automated sample harvester
mas pil pill mass [Lat. *massa pilularum*]
mass massage
massc mass concentration
MAST military antishock trousers; Michigan Alcohol Screening Test
mast mastectomy; mastoid
MASU mobile Army surgical unit
MAT manual arts therapist; mean absorption time; medical assistance team (emergency medicine); methionine adenosyltransferase; microagglutination test; multifocal atrial tachycardia; multiple agent therapy
Mat, mat maternal [origin]; mature
mat gf maternal grandfather
mat gm maternal grandmother
MATSA Marek-associated tumor-specific antigen
matut in the morning [Lat. *matutinus*]
MAV mechanical auditory ventricle; minimum apparent viscosity; movement arm vector; myeloblastosis-associated virus
MAVIS mobile artery and vein imaging system
MAVR mitral and aortic valve replacement
max maxilla, maxillary; maximum
MaxEP maximum esophageal pressure
MB Bachelor of Medicine [Lat. *Medicinae Baccalaureus*]; buccal margin; isoenzyme of creatine kinase containing M and B subunits; mammillary body; Marsh-Bender [factor]; maximum breathing; medulloblastoma; megabyte; mesiobuccal; methyl bromide; methylene blue;

microbiological assay; muscle balance; myocardial band

Mb mouse brain; myoglobin

mb millibar; mix well [Lat. *misce bene*]

MBA methylbenzyl alcohol; methyl bovine albumin

MBAC Member of the British Association of Chemists

MBAR myocardial beta adrenergic receptor

mbar millibar

MBAS methylene blue active substance

MBB modified barbiturate buffer

MBC male breast cancer; maximal bladder capacity; maximal breathing capacity; metastatic breast cancer; methylthymol blue complex; microcrystalline bovine collagen; minimum bactericidal concentration

MB-CK creatine kinase isoenzyme containing M and B subunits

MBCL monocytoid B-cell lymphoma

MbCO carbon monoxide myoglobin

MBD Marchiafava-Bignami disease; Mental Deterioration Battery; methylene blue dye; minimal brain damage; minimal brain dysfunction; Morquio-Brailsford disease

MBDG mesiobuccal developmental groove

MBF medullary blood flow; muscle blood flow; myocardial blood flow

MBFC medial brachial fascial compartment

MBFLB monaural bifrequency loudness balance

MBG mean blood glucose; morphine-benzedrine group [scale]

MBH medial basal hypothalamus

MBH₂ reduced methylene blue

MBI Maslach Burnout Inventory; maximum blink index

MBK methyl butyl ketone

MBL Marine Biological Laboratory; menstrual blood loss; minimum bactericidal level

MBLA methylbenzyl linoleic acid;

mouse-specific bone-marrow-derived lymphocyte antigen

MBM mineral basal medium

MBNOA Member of the British Naturopathic and Osteopathic Association

MBO mesiobucco-occlusal

MBO₂ oxymyoglobin

MBP major basic protein; maltose-binding protein; mean blood pressure; melitensis, bovine, porcine [antigen from *Brucella bovis, B. melitensis,* and *B. suis*]; mesiobuccopulpal; myelin basic protein

MBPS multigated blood pool scanning

MBq megabecquerel

MBR methylene blue, reduced

MBRT methylene blue reduction time

MBS Martin-Bell syndrome

MBSA methylated bovine serum albumin

MBT mercaptobenzothiazole; mixed bacterial toxin

MBTE meningeal tick-borne encephalitis

MBTH 3-methyl-2-benzothiazoline hydrazone

MC mass casualties; mast cell; Master of Surgery [Lat. *Magister Chirurgiae*]; maximum concentration; Medical Corps; medium chain; medullary cavity; medullary cyst; megacoulomb; melanoma cell; menstrual cycle; Merkel's cell; mesiocervical; mesocaval; metacarpal; methyl cellulose; microcephaly; microcirculation; midcapillary; mineralocorticoid; minimal change; mitomycin C; mitotic cycle; mitral commissurotomy; mixed cellularity; mixed cryoglobulinemia; monkey cell; mononuclear cell; mucous cell; myocarditis

M/C male, castrated [animal]

M-C mineralocorticoid

M&C morphine and cocaine

Mc megacurie; megacycle

mC millicoulomb

mc millicurie

MCA major coronary artery; Maternity Center Association; medical care administration; methylcholanthrene; middle cerebral artery; monoclonal antibody;

multichannel analyzer; multiple congenital abnormalities

MCAB monoclonal antibody

MCAD medium chain acyl-CoA dehydrogenase

MCA/MR multiple congenital anomalies/mental retardation [syndrome]

MCAR mixed cell agglutination reaction

MCAS middle cerebral artery syndrome

MCAT Medical College Admission Test; middle cerebral artery thrombosis

m caute mix with caution [Lat. *misce caute*]

MCB membranous cytoplasmic body

McB McBurney's [point]

mCBF mean cerebral blood flow

MCBM muscle capillary basement membrane

MCBR minimum concentration of bilirubin

MCC mean corpuscular hemoglobin concentration; medial cell column; metacerebral cell; metastatic cord compression; microcrystalline collagen; minimum complete–killing concentration; mucocutaneous candidiasis

MCCD minimum cumulative cardiotoxic dose

MCCU mobile coronary care unit

MCD magnetic circular dichroism; mastcell degranulation; mean cell diameter; mean of consecutive differences; mean corpuscular diameter; medullary collecting duct; medullary cystic disease; metacarpal cortical density; minimal cerebral dysfunction; minimal change disease; multiple carboxylase deficiency; muscle carnitine deficiency

MCDI Minnesota Child Development Inventory

MCE medical care evaluation; multicystic encephalopathy; multiple cartilaginous exostosis

MCES multiple cholesterol emboli syndrome

MCF macrophage chemotactic factor; median cleft face; medium corpuscular

fragility; microcomplement fixation; mononuclear cell factor; myocardial contraction force

MCFA medium-chain fatty acid; miniature centrifugal fast analyzer

MCFP mean circulating filling pressure

MCG magnetocardiogram; membrane coating granule; monoclonal gammopathy

mcg microgram

MCGC metacerebral giant cell

MCGF mast cell growth factor

MCGN mesangiocapillary glomerulonephritis; minimal change glomerulonephritis; mixed cryoglobulinemia with glomerulonephritis

MCH Maternal and Child Health; mean corpuscular hemoglobin

MCh Master of Surgery [Lat. *Magister Chirurgiae*]

mc-h, mch millicurie-hour

MCHC maternal/child health care; mean corpuscular hemoglobin concentration; mean corpuscular hemoglobin count

MChD Master of Dental Surgery

MCHgb mean corpuscular hemoglobin

MChir Master in Surgery [Lat. *Magister Chirurgiae*]

MChOrth Master of Orthopaedic Surgery

MChOtol Master of Otology

MCHR Medical Committee for Human Rights

mc-hr millicurie-hour

MCHS Maternal and Child Health Service

MCI mean cardiac index; methicillin; mucociliary insufficiency

MCi megacurie

mCi millicurie

MCICU medical coronary intensive care unit

MCi-hr millicurie-hour

MCINS minimal change idiopathic nephrotic syndrome

MCKD multicystic kidney disease

MCL maximum containment laboratory; medial collateral ligament; midclavicular line; midcostal line; minimal change lesion; mixed culture, leukocyte; modified chest lead; most comfortable loudness

MCLNS, MCLS mucocutaneous lymph node syndrome

MClSci Master of Clinical Science

MCM minimum capacitation medium

MCMI Millon Clinical Multiaxial Inventory

MCMV murine cytomegalovirus

MCN minimal change nephropathy; mixed cell nodular [lymphoma]

MCNS minimal change nephrotic syndrome

MCO medical care organization; multicystic ovary

MCommH Master of Community Health

mcoul millicoulomb

MCP maximum closure pressure; maximum contraction pattern; melphalan, cyclophosphamide, and prednisone; metacarpophalangeal; metoclopramide; mitotic-control protein; mucin clot prevention

MCPa Member of the College of Pathologists, Australasia

MCPH metacarpophalangeal

MCPP metacarpophalangeal pattern profile; meta-chlorophenylpiperazine

MCPPP metacarpophalangeal pattern profile plot

MCPS Member of the College of Physicians and Surgeons

Mcps megacycles per second

MCR Medical Corps Reserve; message competition ratio; metabolic clearance rate

MCRA Member of the College of Radiologists, Australasia

MCRE mother-child relationship evaluation

MCRI Multifactorial Cardiac Risk Index

MCS malignant carcinoid syndrome; massage of the carotid sinus; mesocaval shunt; methylcholanthrene [induced] sarcoma; microculture and sensitivity; moisture-control system; multiple chem-

ical sensitivity; multiple combined sclerosis; myocardial contraction state

mc/s megacycles per second

MCSA Moloney cell surface antigen

MCSDS Marlowe-Crowne Social Desirability Scale

MCSF macrophage colony-stimulating factor

MCSP Member of the Chartered Society of Physiotherapists

MCT manual cervical traction; mean cell thickness; mean cell threshold; mean circulation time; mean corpuscular thickness; medium-chain triglyceride; medullary carcinoma of thyroid; medullary collecting tubule; microtoxicity test; multiple compressed tablet

MCTC metrizamide computed tomography cisternography

MCTD mixed connective tissue disease

MCTF mononuclear cell tissue factor

MCU malaria control unit; maximum care unit; micturating cystourethrography; motor cortex unit

MCUG micturating cystogram

MCV mean cell volume; mean clinical value; mean corpuscular volume; median cell volume; motor conduction velocity

MD Doctor of Medicine [Lat. *Medicinae Doctor*]; magnesium deficiency; main duct; maintenance dose; major depression; malate dehydrogenase; malignant disease; malrotation of duodenum; manic-depressive; Mantoux diameter; Marek disease; maternal deprivation; maximum dose; mean deviation; Meckel's diverticulum; mediastinal disease; medical department; Medical Design [brace]; mediodorsal; medium dosage; Ménière disease; mental deficiency; mental depression; mesiodistal; Minamata disease; minimum dose; mitral disease, mixed diet; moderate disability; monocular deprivation; movement disorder; multiple deficiency; muscular dystrophy; myelodysplasia; myocardial damage; myocardial disease; myotonic dystrophy

Md mendelevium

md median

MDA malondialdehyde; manual dilation of anus; methylene dianiline; 3,4-methylenedioxyamphetamine; minimal deviation adenocarcinoma; monodehydroascorbate; motor discriminative acuity; multivariant discriminant analysis; right mentoanterior [fetal position] [Lat. *mentodextra anterior*]

MDa megadalton

MDAD mineral dust airway disease

MDAP Machover Draw-A-Person [test]

MDBDF March of Dimes Birth Defect Foundation

MDBK Madin-Darby bovine kidney [cell]

MDC major diagnostic categories; minimum detectable concentration; moncyte-depleted mononuclear cell

MDCK Madin-Darby canine kidney

MDCR Miller-Dieker chromosome region

MDD major depressive disorder; mean daily dose

MDE major depressive episode

MDEBP mean daily erect blood pressure

MDentSc Master of Dental Science

MDF mean dominant frequency; myocardial depressant factor

MDG mean diastolic gradient

MDGF macrophage-derived growth factor

MDH malate dehydrogenase; medullary dorsal horn

MDHR maximum determined heart rate

MDHV Marek's disease herpesvirus

MDI manic-depressive illness; metered dose inhaler; multiple daily injection; Multiscore Depression Inventory

m dict as directed [Last. *more dicto*]

MDIPT Multicenter Diltiazem Postinfarction Trial

MDIT mean disintegration time

MDM medical decision making; middiastolic murmur; minor determinant mix [penicillin]

MDMA methylenedioxymethamphetamine

mdn median

MDNB mean daily nitrogen balance; metadinitrobenzene

MDOPA, mdopa methyldopa

MDP manic-depressive psychosis; maximum digital pulse; methylene diphosphate; muramyldipeptide; muscular dystrophy, progressive; right mentoposterior [fetal position] [Lat. *mento-dextra posterior*]

MDPD maximum daily permissible dose

MDQ memory deviation quotient; Menstrual Distress Questionnaire; minimum detectable quantity

MDR median duration of response; medical device reporting; minimum daily requirement; multidrug resistance

MDRS Mattis Dementia Rating Scale

MDR TB multidrug-resistant tuberculosis

MDS Master of Dental Surgery; maternal deprivation syndrome; medical data screening; medical data system; mesonephric duct system; micro-dilution system; milk drinker's syndrome; Miller-Dieker syndrome; myelodysplastic syndrome; myocardial depressant substance

MDSBP mean daily supine blood pressure

MDSO mentally disturbed sex offender

MDT mast [cell] degeneration test; mean dissolution time; median detection threshold; multidisciplinary team; right mentotransverse [fetal position] [Lat. *mento-dextra transversa*]

MDTP multidisciplinary treatment plan

MDTR mean diameter-thickness ratio

MDUO myocardial disease of unknown origin

MDV Marek disease virus; mean dye [bolus] velocity; mucosal disease virus

MDY month, date, year

Mdyn megadyne

ME macular edema; malic enzyme; manic episode; maximum effort; median eminence; medical education; medical examiner; meningoencephalitis; mercaptoethanol; metabolic energy; metabolism; microembolism; middle ear; mouse embryo; mouse epithelial [cell]; myoepithelial

M/E myeloid/erythroid [ratio]

2-ME 2-mercaptoethanol

Me menton; methyl

MEA Medical Exhibition Association; mercaptoethylamine; monoethanolamine; multiple endocrine adenomatosis

MEA-I multiple endocrine adenomatosis type I

mEAD monophasic action potential early afterdepolarization

meas measurement

MEB Medical Evaluation Board; muscle-eye-brain [disease]

MeB methylene blue

ME-BH medial eminence of basal hypothalamus

MeBSA methylated bovine serum albumin

MEC median effective concentration; middle ear canal; middle ear cell; minimum effective concentration

mec meconium

MeCCNU methylchloroethylcyclohexylnitrosourea [semustine]

MECG mixed essential cryoglobulinemia

MECTA mobile electroconvulsive therapy apparatus

MECY methotrexate and cyclophosphamide

MED median erythrocyte diameter; medical, medication, medicine; minimum effective dose; minimum erythema dose; multiple epiphyseal dysplasia

med medial; median; medication; medicine, medical; medium

MEDAC multiple endocrine deficiency, Addison's disease, and candidiasis [syndrome]

MED-ART Medical Automated Records Technology

MEDEX, Medex extension of physician [Fr. *médicin extension*]

medic military medical corpsman [Lat. *medicus*]

MEDICO Medical International Cooperation

MEDIHC Military Experience Directed Into Health Careers

MEDLARS Medical Literature Analysis and Retrieval System

MEDLINE MEDLARS On-Line

MEDPAR Medical Provider Analysis and Review

MEdREP Medical Education Reinforcement and Enrichment Program

MEDScD Doctor of Medical Science

Med-surg medicine and surgery

Med Tech medical technology, medical technologist

MEE measured energy expenditure; methylethyl ether; middle ear effusion

MEF maximal expiratory flow; middle ear fluid; midexpiratory flow; migration enhancement factor; mouse embryo fibroblast

MEF$_{50}$ mean maximal expiratory flow

MEFR maximal expiratory flow rate

MEFV maximal expiratory flow volume

MEG magnetoencephalogram, magnetoencephalography; megakaryocyte; mercaptoethylguanidine; multifocal eosinophilic granuloma

meg megacycle; megakaryocyte; megaloblast

MEGD minimal euthyroid Graves' disease

mEGF mouse epidermal growth factor

MEGX monoethylglycinexylidide

MEK methylethylketone

MEL metabolic equivalent level; mouse erythroleukemia

mel melena; melanoma

MELAS mitochondrial encephalomyopathy–lactic acidosis–and stroke-like symptoms [syndrome]

MEL B melarsoprol

MELC murine erythroleukemia cell

MEM macrophage electrophoretic mobility; malic enzyme, mitochondrial; minimal essential medium

memb membrane, membranous
MEMR multiple exostoses-mental retardation [syndrome]
MEN multiple endocrine neoplasia
men meningeal; meningitis; meniscus; menstruation
MEND Medical Education for National Defense
MEN-I multiple endocrine neoplasia, type I
ment mental, mentality
MEO malignant otitis media
5-MeODMT 5-methoxy-N,N-dimethyltryptamine
MeOH methyl alcohol
MEOS microsomal ethanol oxidizing system
MEP maximum expiratory pressure; mean effective pressure; mepiridine; mitochondrial encephalopathy; motor endplate
mep meperidine
MEPC miniature end-plate current
MEPP miniature end-plate potential
mEQ, mEq, meq milliequivalent
mEq/l milliequivalents per liter
MER mean ejection rate; methanol extraction residue
MERB Medical Examination and Review Board
MERG macular electroretinogram
MERRF myoclonus epilepsy with ragged red fibers [syndrome]
MES maintenance electrolyte solution; maximal electroshock; maximal electroshock seizures; myoelectric signal; multiple endocrine syndrome
Mes mesencephalon, mesencephalic
MESA myoepithelial sialadenitis
Mesc mescaline
MESCH Multi-Environment Scheme
MeSH Medical Subject Headings
MesPGN mesangial proliferative glomerulonephritis
MET metabolic equivalent of the task; metastasis, metastatic; methionine; mid-expiratory time; multistage exercise test
Met methionine

met metallic [chest sounds]
metab metabolic, metabolism
metas metastasis, metastatic
Met-Enk methionine-enkephalin
METH methicillin
Meth methedrine
meth methyl
Met-Hb methemoglobin
MeTHF methyltetrahydrofolic acid
MetMb metmyoglobin
m et n morning and night [Lat. *mane et nocte*]
METS metabolic equivalents [of oxygen consumption]
mets metastases
m et sig mix and write a label [Lat. *misce et signa*]
METT maximum exercise tolerance test
MEU maximum expected utility
MEV maximum exercise ventilation; murine erythroblastosis virus
MeV, mev megaelectron volts
MEWD, MEWDS multiple evanescent white dot [syndrome]
MF meat free; medium frequency; megafarad; membrane filler; merthiolate-formaldehyde [solution]; microfibril; microfilament; microflocculation; microscopic factor; midcavity forceps; mitochondrial fragments; mitogenic factor; mitomycin-fluorouracil; mitotic figure; mucosal fluid; multifactorial; multiplication factor; mutation frequency; mycosis fungoides; myelin figure; myelofibrosis; myocardial fibrosis; myofibrillar
M/F male/female [ratio]
M& F male and female; mother and father
Mf maxillofrontale
mF millifarad
mf microfilaria
MFA monofluoroacetate; multifocal functional autonomy; multiple factor analysis
MFAT multifocal atrial tachycardia
MFB medial forebrain bundle; metallic foreign body
MFC minimal fungicidal concentration

MFCM Master, Faculty of Community Medicine

MFCV muscle fiber conduction velocity

MFD mandibulofacial dysostosis; mid-forceps delivery; milk-free diet; minimum fatal dose

mfd microfarad

MFH malignant fibrous histiocytoma

MFHom Member of the Faculty of Homeopathy

MFID multielectrode flame ionization detector

m flac membrana flaccida [Lat.]

MFO mixed function oxidase

MFOM Master, Faculty of Occupational Medicine

MFP monofluorophosphate; myofascial pain

MFR mean flow rate; mucus flow rate

MFSS Medical Field Service School

MFST Medical Field Service Technician

MFT multifocal atrial tachycardia; muscle function test

m ft let a mixture be made [Lat. *mistura fiat*]

MFW multiple fragment wounds

MG Marcus Gunn [pupil]; margin; medial gastrocnemius [muscle]; membranous glomerulonephritis; menopausal gonadotropin; mesiogingival; methylglucoside; methylguanidine; monoclonal gammopathy; monoglyceride; mucous granule; muscle group; myasthenia gravis; myoglobin

Mg magnesium

M3G morphine-3-glucuronide

m⁷G 7-methylguanosine

mg milligram

MGA medical gas analyzer; melengestrol acetate

MgATP magnesium adenosine triphosphate

mγ milligamma

MGB medial geniculate body

MGBG methylglyoxal-bis-(guanylhydrazone)

MGC minimal glomerular change

MgC magnocellular neuroendocrine cell

MGCE multifocal giant cell encephalitis

MGD maximal glucose disposal; mixed gonadal dysgenesis

mg/dl milligrams per deciliter

MGDS Member in General Dental Surgery

MGES multiple gated equilibrium scintigraphy

MGF macrophage growth factor; maternal grandfather

MGG May-Grünwald-Giemsa [staining]; molecular and general genetics; mouse gammaglobulin; multinucleated giant cell

MGGH methylglyoxal guanylhydrazone

MGH Massachusetts General Hospital

mgh milligram-hour

mg/kg milligrams per kilogram

MGL minor glomerular lesion

Mgl myoglobin

mg/l milligrams per liter

MGM maternal grandmother

mgm milligram

MGMA Medical Group Management Association

MGN medial geniculate nucleus; membranous glomerulonephritis

MGP marginal granulocyte pool; membranous glomerulonephropathy; mucin glycoprotein

MGPS hereditary giant platelet syndrome

MGR modified gain ratio; multiple gas rebreathing

mgr milligram

MGS metric gravitational system

MGT multiple glomus tumors

MGUS monoclonal gammopathies of undetermined significance

MGW magnesium sulfate, glycerin, and water

mGy milligray

MH malignant histiocytosis; malignant hyperpyrexia; malignant hypertension; malignant hyperthermia; mammotropic hormone; mannoheptulose; marital history; medial hypothalamus; medical history; melanophore-stimulating hormone; menstrual history; mental health; mental hygiene; moist heat; monosymptomatic hypochondriasis; murine hepatitis; mutant hybrid; myohyoid

mH millihenry

MHA major histocompatibility antigen; May-Hegglin anomaly; Mental Health Association; methemalbumin; microangiopathic hemolytic anemia; microhemagglutination; middle hepatic artery; mixed hemadsorption; Mueller-Hinton agar

MHA-TP microhemagglutination-*Treponema pallidum*

MHB maximum hospital benefit; Mueller-Hinton base

MHb methemoglobin; myohemoglobin

MHBSS modified Hank's balanced salt solution

MHC major histocompatibility complex; mental health care

MHCS Mental Hygiene Consultation Service

MHCU mental health care unit

MHD maintenance hemodialysis; mean hemolytic dose; mental health department; minimum hemolytic dilution; minimum hemolytic dose

MHDPS Mental Health Demographic Profile System

mHg millimeter of mercury

MHI malignant histiocytosis of intestine; Mental Health Index

MHL medial hypothalamic lesion

MHLC Multidimensional Health Locus of Control

MHLS metabolic heat load stimulator

MHN massive hepatic necrosis; Mohs hardness number; morbus hemolyticus neonatorum

MHO microsomal heme oxygenase

mho reciprocal ohm, siemens unit [ohm spelled backwards]

MHP maternal health program; maternal health program; 1-mercuri-2-hydroxy-propane; monosymptomatic hypochondriacal psychosis

MHPA mild hyperphenylalaninemia

MHPG 3-methoxy-4-hydroxyphenylglycol

MHR major histocompatibility region; malignant hyperthermia resistance; maternal heart rate; maximal heart rate; methemoglobin reductase

MHRI Mental Health Research Institute

MHS major histocompatibility system; malignant hyperthermia in swine; malignant hyperthermia syndrome; malignant hypothermia susceptibility; multiple health screening

MHSA microaggregated human serum albumin

MHT mixed hemagglutination test

MHTS Multiphasic Health Testing Services

MHV magnetic heart vector; mouse hepatitis virus

MHW mental health worker

MHx medical history

MHyg Master of Hygiene

MHz megahertz

MI maturation index; medical inspection; melanophore index; menstruation induction; mental illness; mental institution; mercaptoimidazole; mesioincisal; metabolic index; migration index; migration inhibition; mild irritant; mitotic index; mitral incompetence; mitral insufficiency; mononucleosis infectiosa; morphology index; motility index; myocardial infarction; myocardial ischemia; myoinositol

mi mile

MIA Medical Library Association; missing in action

MIAs multi-institutional arrangements; medically indigent adults

MIB Medical Impairment Bureau

MIBG metaiodobenzylguanidine

MIBiol Member of the Institute of Biology

MIBK methylisobutyl ketone

MIBT methyl isatin-beta-thiosemicarbazone

MIC maternal and infant care; medical intensive care; Medical Interfraternity Conference; microscopy; minimal inhibitory concentration; minimal isorrheic concentration; minocycline; model immune complex; mononuclear inflammatory cell

MICC mitogen-induced cellular cytotoxicity

MICG macromolecular insoluble cold globulin

MICR methacholine inhalation challenge response

micro microcyte, microcytic; microscopic

microbiol microbiology

MICU medical intensive care unit; mobile intensive care unit

MID maximum inhibiting dilution; mesioincisodistal; minimum infective dose; minimum inhibitory dose; minimum irradiation dose; multi-infarct dementia; multiple ion detection

mid middle

MIDAS Multicenter Isradipine Diuretic Arteriosclerosis [study]

MIDS Management Information Decision System

midsag midsagittal

MIF macrophage inhibitory factor; melanocyte[-stimulating hormone]-inhibiting factor; maximum inspiratory flow; merthiolate-iodine-formaldehyde [method]; microimmunofluorescence; midinspiratory flow; migration-inhibiting factor; mixed immunofluorescence; müllerian inhibiting factor

MIFC merthiolate-iodine-formaldehyde concentration

MIFR maximal inspiratory flow rate

MIG measles immune globulin; Medicare Insured Groups

MIg malaria immunoglobulin; measles immunoglobulin; membrane immunoglobulin

MIGT multiple inert gas elimination technique

MIH Master of Industrial Health; migraine with interval headache; minimal intermittent heparin [dose]

MIHA minor histocompatibility antigen

MIKA minor karyotype abnormalities

MIKE mass-analyzed ion kinetic energy

MILP mitogen-induced lymphocyte proliferation

MILS medication information leaflet for seniors

MIMR minimal inhibitor mole ratio

MIMS medical information management system; medical inventory management system

MIN medial interlaminar nucleus

min mineral; minim; minimum, minimal; minor; minute

MINA monoisonitrosoacetone

MINIA monkey intranuclear inclusion agent

MIO minimum identifiable odor

MiO microorchidism

MIP maximum inspiratory pressure; mean incubation period; mean intravascular pressure; middle interphalangeal [joint]; minimal inspiratory pressure

MIR multiple isomorphous replacement

MIRC microtubuloreticular complex

MIRD medical internal radiation dose

MIRP myocardial infarction rehabilitation program

MIRU myocardial infarction research unit

MIS management information system; medical information service; meiosis-inducing substance; müllerian inhibiting substance

misc miscarriage; miscellaneous

MISG modified immune serum globulin

MISHAP microcephalus–imperforate anus–syndactyly–hamartoblastoma–abnormal lung lobulation–polydactyly [syndrome]

MISS Modified Injury Severity Scale

MIST Medical Information Service by Telephone

mist mixture [Lat. *mistura*]

MIT male impotence test; marrow iron turnover; metabolism inhibition test; miracidial immobilization test; mitomycin; monoiodotyrosine

mit mitral; send [Lat. *mitte*]

mitt tal send such [Lat. *mitte tales*]

mIU milli-International unit; one-thousandth of an International unit

mix, mixt mixture

MJ Machado-Joseph [disease]; marijuana; megajoule

mJ, mj millijoule

MJA mechanical joint apparatus

MJAD Machado-Joseph Azorean disease

MJD Machado-Joseph disease; Mseleni joint disease

MJRT maximum junctional recovery time

MJT Mead Johnson tube

MK megakaryocyte; monkey kidney; myokinase

Mk monkey

mkat millikatal

mkat/l millikatals per liter

MKB megakaryoblast

MKC monkey kidney cell

m-kg meter-kilogram

MKHS Menkes' kinky hair syndrome

MkK monkey kidney

MkL megakaryoblastic leukemia

MKP monobasic potassium phosphate

MKS, mks meter-kilogram-second

MKSAP Medical Knowledge Self-Assessment Program

MKTC monkey kidney tissue culture

MKV killed measles vaccine

ML Licentiate in Medicine; Licentiate in Midwifery; malignant lymphoma; marked latency; maximum likelihood; medial leminiscus; mesiolingual; middle lobe; midline; molecular layer; motor latency; mucolipidosis; multiple lentiginosis; muscular layer; myeloid leukemia

ML I, II, III, IV mucolipidosis I, II, III, IV

M/L monocyte/lymphocyte [ratio]

M-L Martin-Lewis [medium]

mL millilambert, milliliter

ml milliliter

MLA left mentoanterior [fetal position] [Lat. *mento-laeva anterior*]; Medical Library Association; mesiolabial; monocytic leukemia, acute

mLa millilambert

MLAB Multilingual Aphasia Battery

MLaI mesiolabioincisal

MLAP mean left atrial pressure

MLaP mesiolabiopulpal

MLB monoaural loudness balance

MLb macrolymphoblast

MLBP mechanical low back pain

MLC minimum lethal concentration; mixed leukocyte culture; mixed ligand chelate; mixed lymphocyte concentration; mixed lymphocyte culture; morphine-like compound; multilamellar cytosome; myelomonocytic leukemia, chronic; myosin light chain

MLCK myosin light chain kinase

MLCO Member of the London College of Osteopathy

MLCP myosin light-chain phosphatase

MLCT metal-to-ligand charge transfer

MLD median lethal dose; metachromatic leukodystrophy; minimal lesion disease; minimum lethal dose

MLD$_{50}$ median lethal dose

ml/dl milliliters per deciliter

MLE maximum likelihood estimation

MLF medial longitudinal fasciculus; morphine-like factor

MLG mesiolingual groove; mitochondrial lipid glycogen

MLGN minimal lesion glomerulonephritis

ML-H malignant lymphoma, histiocytic

MLI mesiolinguoincisal; mixed lymphocyte interaction

ml/l milliliters per liter

MLN manifest latent nystagmus; membranous lupus nephropathy; mesenteric lymph node

MLNS minimal lesion nephrotic syndrome; mucocutaneous lymph node syndrome

MLO mesiolinguo-occlusal; *Mycoplasma*-like organism

MLP left mentoposterior [fetal position] [Lat. *mento-laeva posterior*]; mesiolinguopulpal; microsomal lipoprotein

ML-PDL malignant lymphoma, poorly differentiated lymphocytic

MLR mean length response; middle latency response; mixed lymphocyte reaction

MLS mean lifespan; median life span; median longitudinal section; middle lobe syndrome; mouse leukemia virus; myelomonocytic leukemia, subacute

MLSB migrating long spike burst

MLT left mentotransverse [fetal position] [Lat. *mento-laeva transversa*]; mean latency time; median lethal time; Medical Laboratory Technician

MLT(ASCP) Medical Laboratory Technician certified by the American Society of Clinical Pathologists

MLTC mixed leukocyte-trophoblast culture; mixed lymphocyte tumor cell

MLTI mixed lymphocyte target interaction

MLU mean length of utterance

MLV Moloney's leukemogenic virus; multilaminar vesicle; murine leukemia virus

MLVDP maximum left ventricular developed pressure

mlx millilux

MM macromolecule; major medical [insurance]; malignant melanoma; manubrium to malleus; Marshall-Marchetti; Master of Management; medial malleolus; megamitochondria; melanoma metastasis; meningococcal meningitis; menstrually-related migraine; metastatic melanoma; methadone maintenance; minimal medium; mismatched; morbidity and mortality; mucous membrane; multiple myeloma; muscularis mucosae; myeloid metaplasia; myelomeningocele

M&M morbidity and mortality

mM millimolar; millimole

mm methylmalonyl; millimeter; mucous membrane; muscles

mm² square millimeter

mm³ cubic millimeter

MMA mastitis-metritis-agalactia [syndrome]; medical materials account; methylmalonic acid; minor morphologic aberration; monomethyladenosine

MMAD mass median aerodynamic diameter

MMATP methadone maintenance and aftercare treatment program

MMC migrating myoelectric complex; minimum medullary concentration; mitomycin C; mucosal mast cell

MMD mass median diameter; minimum morbidostatic dose; moyamoya disease; myotonic muscular dystrophy

MME M-mode echocardiography; mouse mammary epithelium

MMED Master of Medicine

MMEF maximum midexpiratory flow

MMEFR maximum midexpiratory flow rate

MMF maximum midexpiratory flow; mean maximum flow; Member of the Medical Faculty

MMFR maximum midexpiratory flow rate; maximal midflow rate

MMFV maximum midrespiratory flow volume

MMG mean maternal glucose

MMH monomethylhydrazine

mmHg millimeters of mercury

mmH₂O millimeters of water

MMI macrophage migration inhibition; methylmercaptoimidazole; mucous membrane irritation

MMIHS megacystis-microcolon-intestinal hypoperistalsis syndrome

MMIS Medicaid Management Information System

MML Moloney murine leukemia; monomethyllysine; myelomonocytic leukemia

mM/l millimoles per liter

MMLV Moloney murine leukemia virus

MMM see 3-M [syndrome]; microsome-mediated mutagenesis; Minnesota Mining and Manufacturing Company [3M]; myelofibrosis with myeloid metaplasia; myelosclerosis with myeloid metaplasia

MMMF man-made mineral fibers

MMMT malignant mixed müllerian tumor

MMN morbus maculosus neonatorum; multiple mucosal neuroma

MMNC marrow mononuclear cell

MMO methane monooxygenase

MMOA maxillary mandibular odontectomy alveolectomy

MMoL myelomonoblastic leukemia

mmol millimole

mmol/l millimoles per liter

MMPI Minnesota Multiphasic Personality Inventory

MMPNC Medical Maternal Program for Nuclear Casualties

mmpp millimeters partial pressure

MMPR methylmercaptopurine riboside

MMR mass miniature radiography; maternal mortality rate; measles-mumps-rubella [vaccine]; mild mental retardation; mobile mass x-ray; mono-methylorutin; myocardial metabolic rate

MMS Master of Medical Science; methyl methanesulfonate; Mini-Mental State

MMSA Master of Midwifery, Society of Apothecaries

MMSc Master of Medical Science

MMSE Mini-Mental State Exam

mm/sec millimeters per second

mm st muscle strength

MMT alpha-methyl-m-tyrosine; manual muscle test; mouse mammary tumor

MMTA methylmetatyramine

MMTP methadone maintenance treatment program

MMTV mouse mammary tumor virus

MMU medical maintenance unit; mercaptomethyl uracil

mmu millimass unit

mμ millimicron

mμc millimicrocurie

mμg millimicrogram

MMuLV Moloney murine leukemia virus

mμs millimicrosecond

μmμ meson

MMWR Morbidity and Mortality Weekly Report

MN a blood group in the MNSs blood group system; malignant nephrosclerosis; Master of Nursing; meganewton; melena neonatorum; melanocytic nevus; membranous nephropathy; membranous neuropathy; mesenteric node; metanephrine; midnight; mononuclear; motor neuron; multinodular; myoneural

M&N morning and night

Mn manganese

mN micronewton; millinormal

mn modal number

MNA maximum noise area

MNAP mixed nerve action potential

MNB murine neuroblastoma

5-MNBA 5-mercapto-2-nitrobenzoic acid

MNBCCS multiple nevoid basal-cell carcinoma syndrome

MNC mononuclear cell

MNCV motor nerve conduction velocity

MND minimum necrosing dose; minor neurological dysfunction; modified neck dissection; motor neuron disease

mng morning

MNGIE myo-, neuro-, gastrointestinal encephalopathy

MNJ myoneural junction

MNL marked neutrophilic leukocytosis; maximum number of lamellae; mononuclear leukocyte

MN/m² meganewtons per square meter

MNMS myonephropathic metabolic syndrome

MNNG N-methyl N'-nitro-N-nitrosoguanidine

MNP mononuclear phagocyte

MNR marrow neutrophil reserve

MNS medial nuclear stratum; Melnick-Needles syndrome

Mn-SOD manganese-superoxide dismutase

MNSs a blood group system consisting of groups M, N, and MN

MNU N-methyl-N-nitrosourea

MO macroorchidism; manually operated; Master of Obstetrics; Master of Osteopathy; medical officer; mesio-occlusal; metastases, zero; mineral oil; minute output; molecular orbital; mono-oxygenase; morbid obesity

MO₂ myocardial oxygen [utilization]

Mo Moloney [strain]; molybdenum; monoclonal

mo mode; month; morgan

MoA mechanism of action

MoAb monoclonal antibody

mob, mobil mobility, mobilization

MOC maximum oxygen consumption; multiple ocular coloboma

MOD maturity onset diabetes; Medical Officer of the Day; mesio-occlusodistal

mod moderate, moderation; modification

modem modulator/demodulator

MODM maturity-onset diabetes mellitus

mod praesc in the way directed [Lat. *modo praescripto*]

MODS medically oriented data system

MODY maturity onset diabetes of the young

MOF marine oxidation/fermentation; methotrexate, Oncovin, and fluorouracil; multiple organ failure

MOFS multiple organ failure syndrome

MO&G Master of Obstetrics and Gynaecology

MOH Medical Officer of Health

MΩ megohm

mΩ milliohm

MOI maximum oxygen intake; multiplicity of infection

MOIVC membranous obstruction of the inferior vena cava

MOL molecular

mol mole, molecular, molecule

molc molar concentration

molfr mole fraction

mol/kg moles per kilogram

mol/l moles per liter

moll soft [Lat. *mollis*]

mol/m³ moles per meter cubed

mol/s moles per second

mol wt molecular weight

MOM milk of magnesia; mucoid otitis media

MoM multiples of the median

MOMA methylhydroxymandelic acid

MO-MOM mineral oil and milk of magnesia

MOMS multiple organ malrotation syndrome

Mo-MSV Moloney murine sarcoma virus

MOMX macroorchidism-marker X chromosome [syndrome]

MON Mongolian [gerbil]

mono monocyte; mononucleosis

MOOW Medical Officer of the Watch

MOP major organ profile; medical outpatient

8-MOP 8-methoxypsoralen

MOPEG 3-methoxy-4-hydroxyphenyl-glycol

MOPV monovalent oral poliovirus vaccine

Mor, mor morphine

MORC Medical Officers Reserve Corps

MORD magnetic optical rotatory dispersion

mor dict in the manner directed [Lat. *more dicto*]

morphol morphology

mor sol in the usual way [Lat. *more solito*]

mort, mortal mortality

MOS medial orbital sulcus; Medical Outcome Study; microsomal ethanol-oxidizing system; Moloney murine sarcoma; myelofibrosis osteosclerosis

mOs milliosmolal

MOSF multiple organ system failure

MOSFET metal oxide semiconductor field effect transistor

mOsm, MOsm milliosmole

mOsm/kg milliosmoles per kilogram

MOT mouse ovarian tumor

Mot, mot motor

MOTT mycobacteria other than tuberculosis

MOUS multiple occurrence of unexplained symptoms

MOVC membranous obstruction of inferior vena cava

MOX moxalactam

MP as directed [Lat. *modo prescripto*]; macrophage; matrix protein; mean pressure; melphalan and prednisone; melting point; membrane potential; menstrual period; mentum posterior; mercaptopurine; mesial pit; mesiopulpal; metacarpophalangeal; metaphalangeal; metatarsophalangeal; methylprednisolone; Mibelli's porokeratosis; middle phalanx; moist pack; monophosphate; mouth piece; mucopolysaccharide; multiparous; multiprogrammable pacemaker; muscle potential; mycoplasmal pneumonia

6-MP mercaptopurine

8-MP 8-methylpsoralen

mp in the manner prescribed [Lat. *modo prescripto*]; millipond; melting point

MPA main pulmonary artery; medial preoptic area; Medical Procurement Agency; medroxyprogesterone acetate; methylprednisolone acetate; microscopic polyarteritis; minor physical anomaly

MPa megapascal

MPAP mean pulmonary arterial pressure

MPAS mild perioxic acid Schiff [reaction]

MPB male pattern baldness; meprobamate

MPC marine protein concentrate; maximum permissible concentration; mean plasma concentration; meperidine, promethazine, and chlorpromazine; metallophthalocyanine; minimum mycoplasmacidal concentration

MPCO micropolycystic ovary syndrome

MPCUR maximum permissible concentration of unidentified radionucleotides

MPD main pancreatic duct; maximum permissible dose; mean population doubling; membrane potential difference; minimal perceptible difference; minimal phototoxic dose; multiple personality disorder; myeloproliferative disease; myofascial pain dysfunction

MPDS mandibular pain dysfunction syndrome; myofascial pain dysfunction syndrome

MPE maximum permissible exposure; maximum possible error

MPEC monopolar electrocoagulation

MPED minimum phototoxic erythema dose

MPEH methylphenylethylhydantoin

MPF maturation promoting factor; mean power frequency

MPG magnetopneumography; mercaptopropionylglycine; methyl green pyronine

MPGM monophosphoglycerate mutase

MPGN membranoproliferative glomerulonephritis

MPH male pseudohermaphroditism; Master of Public Health; milk protein hydrolysate

MPharm Master of Pharmacy

MPHD multiple pituitary hormone deficiencies

mphot milliphot

MPhysA Member of Physiotherapists' Association

MPI mannose phosphate isomerase; master patient index; maximum permitted intake; maximum point of impulse; Multiphasic Personality Inventory; myocardial perfusion imaging

MPJ metacarpophalangeal joint

MPL maximum permissible level; melphalan; mesiopulpolingual

MPLa mesiopulpolabial

MPM malignant papillary mesothelioma; medial pterygoid muscle; minor psychiatric morbidity; multiple primary malignancy; multipurpose meal

MPME (5R,8R)-8-(4-p-methoxyphenyl)-1-piperazynylmethyl-6-methylergolene

MPMP 10[(1-methyl-3-piperidinyl)-methyl]-1OH-phenothiazine

MPMT Murphy punch maneuver test

MPMV Mason-Pfizer monkey virus

MPN most probable number

MPO maximum power output; minimal perceptible odor; myeloperoxidase

MPOA medial preoptic area

MPOD myeloperoxidase deficiency

MPP massive peritoneal proliferation; methyl phenylpyridinium; medical personnel pool; mercaptopyrazide pyrimidine; metacarpophalangeal profile

mppcf millions of particles per cubic foot of air

MPPEC mean peak plasma ethanol concentration

MPPG microphotoelectric plethysmography

MPPH p-tolylphenylhydantoin

MPPN malignant persistent positional nystagmus

MPPT methylprednisolone pulse therapy

MPQ McGill Pain Questionnaire

MPR marrow production rate; massive preretinal retraction; maximum pulse rate; myeloproliferative reaction

MPS meconium plug syndrome; Member of the Pharmaceutical Society; microbial profile system; mononuclear phagocyte system; Montreal platelet syndrome; movement-produced stimulus; mucopolysaccharide, mucopolysaccharidosis; multiphasic screening; myocardial perfusion scintigraphy; myofascial pain syndrome

MPSoSIS mucopolysaccharidosis

MPSS methylprednisolone sodium succinate

MPSV myeloproliferative sarcoma virus

MPsyMed Master of Psychological Medicine

MPT Michigan Picture Test

MPTP 1-methyl-4-phenyl-1,2,3,6-tetrahydropyridine

MPT-R Michigan Picture Test, Revised

MPU Medical Practitioners Union

MPV mean platelet volume; mitral valve prolapse

mpz millipièze

MQ memory quotient

MQC microbiologic quality control

MQL Medical Query Language [computer]

MR Maddox rods; magnetic resistance; magnetic resonance; mandibular reflex; mannose-resistant; may repeat; measles and rubella; medial raphe; medial rectus [muscle]; medical record; medical release; medium range; megaroentgen; mental retardation; metabolic rate; methemoglobin reductase; methyl red; mitral reflux; mitral regurgitation; modulation rate; mortality rate; mortality ratio; multicentric reticulohistiocytosis; muscle receptor; muscle relaxant

M_r relative molecular mass

mR, mr milliroentgen

MRA main renal artery; marrow repopulation activity; medical records administrator; multivariate regression analysis

mrad millirad

MRAP maximal resting anal pressure; mean right atrial pressure

MRAS main renal artery stenosis

MRBC monkey red blood cell; mouse red blood cell

MRBF mean renal blood flow

MRC maximum recycling capacity; Medical Registration Council; Medical Research Council; Medical Reserve Corps; methylrosaniline chloride

MRD maximum rate of depolarization; measles–rindenpest–distemper [virus group]; medical records department; minimal reacting dose; minimal renal disease; minimal residual disease

mrd millirutherford

MRE maximal resistive exercise; maximal respiratory effectiveness

MREI mean rate ejection index

mrem millirem

mrep milliroentgen equivalent physical

MRF medical record file; melanocyte-[stimulating hormone]-releasing factor;

mesencephalic reticular formation; midbrain reticular formation; mitral regurgitant flow; moderate renal failure; monoclonal rheumatoid factor; müllerian regression factor

mRF monoclonal rheumatoid factor

MRFC mouse rosette-forming cell

MRFIT Multiple Risk Factor Intervention Trial

MRFT modified rapid fermentation test

MRH melanocyte-stimulating hormone-releasing hormone

MRHA mannose-resistant hemagglutination

mrhm milliroentgens per hour at one meter

MRI machine-readable identifier; magnetic resonance imaging; medical records information; Medical Research Institute; moderate renal insufficiency

MRIF melanocyte[-stimulating hormone] release-inhibiting factor

MRIH melanocyte[-stimulating hormone] release-inhibiting hormone

MRIPHH Member of the Royal Institute of Public Health and Hygiene

MRK Mayer-Rokitansky-Küster [syndrome]

MRL medical records librarian; Medical Research Laboratory

MRM modified radical mastectomy

MRN malignant renal neoplasm

mRNA messenger ribonucleic acid

mRNP messenger ribonucleoprotein

MRO minimal recognizable odor; muscle receptor organ

MROD Medical Research and Operations Directorate

MRP mean resisting potential; medical reimbursement plan

MRR marrow release rate; maximum relation rate

MRS Mania Rating Scale; medical receiving station; Melkersson-Rosenthal syndrome

MRSA methicillin-resistant *Staphylococcus aureus*

MRSH Member of the Royal Society of Health

MRT magnetic resonance tomography; maximum relaxation time; median range score; median reaction time; median recognition threshold; median relapse time; medical records technology; milk ring test; muscle response test

MRU mass radiography unit; minimal reproductive unit

MRV minute respiratory volume; mixed respiratory vaccine

MRVI mixed virus respiratory infection

MRVP mean right ventricular pressure; methyl red, Voges-Proskauer [medium]

MS Maffuci syndrome; maladjustment score; Marfan syndrome; Marie-Strümpell [syndrome]; mass spectrometry; Master of Science; Master of Surgery; mean square [statistics]; mechanical stimulation; Meckel syndrome; mediastinal shift; medical services; medical student; medical supplies; medical survey; Menkes syndrome; menopausal syndrome; mental status; Meretoja syndrome; microscope slide; minimal support; mitral sounds; mitral stenosis; mobile surgical [unit]; modal sensitivity; molar solution; Mongolian spot; morphine sulfate; motile sperm; mucosubstance; Münchausen syndrome; multiple sclerosis; muscle shortening; muscle strength; musculoskeletal

MS I, II, III, IV medical student–first, second, third, and fourth year

Ms murmurs

ms millisecond; morphine sulfate

m/s meters per second

m/s² meters per second squared

MSA major serologic antigen; male-specific antigen; mannitol salt agar; Medical Services Administration; membrane stabilizing action; metropolitan statistical area; mouse serum albumin; multiple system atrophy; muscle sympathetic activity

MSAA multiple sclerosis-associated agent

MSAFP, MS-AFP maternal serum alpha-fetoprotein

MSAN medical student's admission note

MSAP mean systemic arterial pressure

MSB Master of Science in Bacteriology; mid-small bowel; most significant bit

MSBC maximum specific binding capacity

MSBLA mouse-specific B lymphocyte antigen

MSC marrow stromal cell; Medical Service Corps; Medical Staff Corps

MSc Master of Science

MScD Master of Dental Science

MScMed Master of Science in Medicine

MScN Master of Science in Nursing

MSCP mean spherical candle power

MSCU medical special care unit

MSD mean square deviation; mild sickle cell disease; most significant digit; multiple sulfatase deficiency

MSDC Mass Spectrometry Data Centre

MSDI Martin Suicide Depression Inventory

MSDS material safety data sheet

MSE medical support equipment; mental status examination; muscle-specific enolase

mse mean square error

MSEA Medical Society Executives Association

msec millisecond

m/sec meters per second

MSEL myasthenic syndrome of Eaton-Lambert

MSER mean systolic ejection rate

MSES medical school environmental stress

MSF macrophage slowing factor; macrophage spreading factor; Mediterranean spotted fever; melanocyte-stimulating factor; modified sham feeding

MSG monosodium L-glutamate

MSGV mouse salivary gland virus

MSH medical self-help; melanocyte-stimulating hormone; melanophore-stimulating hormone

MSHA mannose-sensitive hemagglutination; Mine Safety and Health Administration

MSHIF melanocyte-stimulating hormone-inhibiting factor

MSHRF melanocyte-stimulating hormone-releasing factor

MSHRH melanocyte-stimulating hormone-releasing hormone

MSHSC multiple self-healing squamous carcinoma

MSHyg Master of Science in Hygiene

MSI magnetic source imaging; medium-scale integration

MSIS multi-state information system

MSK medullary sponge kidney

MSKCC Memorial Sloan-Kettering Cancer Center

MSKP Medical Sciences Knowledge Profile

MSL midsternal line; multiple symmetric lipomatosis

MSLA mouse-specific lymphocyte antigen

MSLR mixed skin cell-leukocyte reaction

MSLT multiple sleep latency test

MSM medium-size molecule; mineral salts medium

MSN main sensory nucleus; Master of Science in Nursing; mildly subnormal

MSO medial superior olive

MSOF multiple systems organ failure

MSP maximum squeeze pressure; Münchausen syndrome by proxy

msp muscle spasm

MSPGN mesangial proliferative glomerulonephritis

MSPH Master of Science in Public Health

MSPhar Master of Science in Pharmacy

MSPN medical student's progress note

MSPQ Modified Somatic Perception Questionnaire

MSPS myocardial stress perfusion scintigraphy

MSQ mental status questionnaire

MSR Member of the Society of Radiographers; monosynaptic reflex; muscle stretch reflex

MSRPP Multidimensional Scale for Rating Psychiatric Patients

MSRT Minnesota Spatial Relations Test

MSS Marshall-Smith syndrome; massage; Medical Superintendents' Society; Medicare Statistical System; mental status schedule; minor surgery suite; motion sickness susceptibility; mucus-stimulating substance; multiple sclerosis susceptibility; muscular subaortic stenosis

mss massage

MSSc Master of Sanitary Science

MSSE Master of Science in Sanitary Engineering

MSSG multiple sclerosis susceptibility gene

MSSVD Medical Society for the Study of Venereal Diseases

MST mean survival time; mean swell time

MSTh mesothorium

MSTI multiple soft tissue injuries

MSU maple sugar urine; maple syrup urine; medical studies unit; mid-stream urine; monosodium urate; myocardial substrate uptake

MSUD maple syrup urine disease

MSurg Master of Surgery

MSV maximum sustained level of ventilation; mean scale value; Moloney sarcoma virus; murine sarcoma virus

MSVC maximal sustained ventilatory capacity

MSW Master of Social Welfare; Master of Social Work; medical social worker; multiple stab wounds

MSWYE modified sea water yeast extract

MT malaria therapy; malignant teratoma; mammary tumor; mammilothalamic tract; manual traction; Martin-Thayer [plate, medium]; mastoid tip; maximal therapy; medial thalamus; medial thickness; medical technologist; medical therapy; melatonin; membrana tympani; mesangial thickening; metallothionein; metatarsal; methoxytryptamine; meth-

yltyrosine; microtome; microtubule; midtrachea; minimum threshold; Monroe tidal drainage; more than; movement time; multiple tics; Muir-Torre [syndrome]; multitest [plate]; muscles and tendons; muscle test; music therapy

M-T macroglobulin-trypsin

M&T *Monilia* and *Trichomonas*

Mt megatonne; *Mycobacterium tuberculosis*

mt mitochondrial

3-MT 3-methoxytyramine

MTA malignant teratoma, anaplastic; medical technical assistant; metatarsus adductus; myoclonic twitch activity

mTA meta-tyramine

MTAC mass transfer area coefficient

MT(ASCP) Medical Technologist certified by the American Society of Clinical Pathologists

MTAD membrana tympana auris dextrae

MTAL medullary thick ascending limb

MTAS membrana tympana auris sinistrae

MTB methylthymol blue

Mtb *Mycobacterium tuberculosis*

MTBE meningeal tick-borne encephalitis; methyl *tert*-butyl ester

MTBF mean time between (or before) failures

MTC mass transfer coefficient; maximum tolerated concentration; maximum toxic concentration; medical test cabinet; medical training center; medullary thyroid carcinoma; mitomycin C

MTD maximum tolerated dose; mean total dose; metastatic trophoblastic disease; Midwife Teacher's Diploma; Monroe tidal drainage; multiple tic disorder

mtd send such doses [Lat. *mitte tales doses*]

MTDDA Minnesota Test for Differential Diagnosis of Aphasia

MT-DN multitest, dermatophytes and *Nocardia* [plate]

mtDNA mitochondrial deoxyribonucleic acid

MTDT modified tone decay test

MTET modified treadmill exercise test

MTF maximum terminal flow; medical treatment facility; modulation transfer function

MTg mouse thyroglobulin

MTH mithramycin

5-MTHF 5-methyl-tetrahydrofolate

MTI malignant teratoma, intermediate; minimum time interval; moving target indicator

MTLP metabolic toxemia of late pregnancy

MTM Thayer-Martin, modified [agar]

MT-M multitest, mycology [plate]

MTO Medical Transport Officer; methoxyhydroxyphenylalanine

MTOC microtubule organizing center; mitotic organizing center

MTP maximum tolerated pressure; medial tibial plateau; median time to progression; metatarsophalangeal; microtubule protein

MTPJ metatarsophalangeal joint

MTQ methaqualone

MTR Meinicke turbidity reaction; 5-methylthioribose

MTS multicellular tumor spheroid

MTST maximal treadmill stress test

MTT malignant teratoma, trophoblastic; maximal treadmill test; meal tolerance test; mean transit time

MTU malignant teratoma, undifferentiated; medical therapy unit; methylthiouracil

MTV mammary tumor virus; metatarsus varus; mouse mammary tumor virus

MTX methotrexate

MT-Y multitest yeast [plate]

MU megaunit; mescaline unit; methyluric [acid]; Montevideo unit; motor unit; mouse unit

Mu Mache unit

mU milliunit

mu mouse unit

μ Greek letter *mu*; chemical potential; electrophoretic mobility; heavy chain of immunoglobulin M; linear attenuation coefficient; magnetic moment; mean; micro; micrometer; micron; mutation rate; permeability

μₒ permeability of vacuum

μA microampere

MUA middle uterine artery; motor unit activity

MUAP motor unit action potential

μb microbar

μ_B Bohr magneton

μbar microbar

MUC maximum urinary concentration; mucilage; mucosal ulcerative colitis

muc mucilage; mucous, mucus

μC microcoulomb

μc microcurie

μch microcurie-hour

μC-hr microcurie-hour

μCi microcurie

μCi-hr microcurie-hour

μcoul microcoulomb

MUD minimum urticarial dose

MUE motor unit estimated

μF, μf microfarad

MUG MUMPS (see p. 204) Users' Group

μg microgram

MUGA multiple gated acquisition [blood pool scan]

μγ microgamma

MUGEx multigated blood pool image during exercise

μg/kg micrograms per kilogram

μg/l micrograms per liter

MUGR multigated blood pool image at rest

μGy microgray

μH microhenry

μHg micron of mercury

μin microinch

μIU one-millionth of an International Unit

μkat microkatal

μL, μl microliter

mult multiple

multip multiparous

MuLV, MuLv murine leukemia virus

μM micromolar

μm micrometer; micromilli-

μmg micromilligram [nanogram]

μmHg micrometer of mercury

μmm micromillimeter [nanometer]

μmol micromole

MUMPS Massachusetts General Hospital Utility Multi-Programming System

MuMTv murine mammary tumor virus

μμC micromicrocurie [picocurie]

μμF micromicrofarad [picofarad]

μμg micromicrogram [picogram]

μN nuclear magneton

MUN(WI) Munich Wistar [rat]

MUO myocardiopathy of unknown origin

μΩ microhm

MUP major urinary protein; maximal urethral pressure; motor unit potential

μP microprocessor

μPa micropascal

μR, μr microroentgen

μ/ρ mass attenuation coefficient

MURC measurable undesirable respiratory contaminants

MurNAc N-acetylmuramate

MURP Master of Urban and Regional Planning

MUS mouse urologic syndrome

μs microsecond

musc muscle, musculature, muscular

μsec microsecond

MUST medical unit, self-contained and transportable

MUT mutagen

MUU mouse uterine unit

μU microunit

μV microvolt

μW microwatt

MUWU mouse uterine weight unit

MV measles virus; mechanical ventilation; megavolt; microvascular; microvillus; minute volume; mitral valve; mixed venous; multivessel; veterinary physician [Lat. *Medicus Veterinarius*]

Mv mendelevium

mV, mv millivolt

MVA mechanical ventricular assistance; mevalonic acid; mitral valve area; motor vehicle accident

MV·A megavolt-ampere

mV·A millivolt-ampere

mval millival

MVB multivesicular body

MVC maximum voluntary contraction; myocardial vascular capacity

MVD Doctor of Veterinary Medicine; microvascular decompression; mitral valve disease; multivessel coronary disease

MVE mitral valve excursion; Murray Valley encephalitis

MVH massive vitreous hemorrhage

MVI multivalvular involvement; multivitamin infusion

MVL mitral valve leaflet

MVLS mandibular vestibulolingual sulcoplasty

MVM microvillose membrane; minute virus of mice

MVMT movement

MVN medial ventromedial nucleus

MVO maximum venous outflow

MVO2, MVO$_2$ myocardial oxygen consumption

mVO$_2$ minute venous oxygen consumption

MVOA mitral valve orifice area

MVOS mixed venous oxygen saturation

MVP microvascular pressure; mitral valve prolapse

MVPP mustine, vinblastine, procarbazine, and prednisone

MVPS Medicare Volume Performance Standards; mitral valve prolapse syndrome

MVP-SC mitral valve prolapse–systolic click [syndrome]

MVPT Motor-Free Visual Perception Test

MVR massive vitreous reaction; microvitreoretinal; minimal vascular resistance; mitral valve replacement

mV·s millivolt-second

mvt movement

MVV maximal voluntary ventilation

MW Mallory-Weiss [syndrome]; mean weight; megawatt; microwave; Minot-von Willebrand [syndrome]; molecular weight

mW milliwatt

mWb milliweber
MWD microwave diathermy; molecular weight distribution
MWP mean wedge pressure
MWS Marden-Walker syndrome; Moersch-Woltman syndrome
MWT myocardial wall thickness
MX matrix
Mx maxwell; MEDEX (see p. 189)
M_{xy} transverse magnetization
My myopia; myxedema
my mayer
Myco *Mycobacterium*
Mycol mycology, mycologist

MyD myotonic dystrophy
MYEL myelogram
Myel myelocyte
myel myelin, myelinated
MyG myasthenia gravis
MyMD myotonic muscular dystrophy
MYO myoglobin
MYX myoxoma
MZ mantle zone; meziocillin; monozygotic
M_z longitudinal magnetization
m/z mass-to-charge ratio
MZA monozygotic twins raised apart
MZT monozygotic twins raised together

N asparagine; Avogadro's number; blood factor in the MNS blood group system; loudness; nasal; nasion; negative; neomycin; neper; nerve; neuraminidase; neurology; neuropathy; neutron number; newton; nicotinamide; nifedipine; nitrogen; nodule; normal [solution]; nucleoside; number; number in sample; number of molecules; number of neutrons in an atomic nucleus; population size; radiance; refractive index; spin density

0.02N fiftieth-normal [solution]

0.1N tenth-normal [solution]

0.5N half-normal [solution]

NI-NXII first to twelfth cranial nerves

2N double-normal [solution]

N/2 half-normal [solution]

N/10 tenth-normal [solution]

N/50 fiftieth-normal [solution]

n amount of substance expressed in moles; born [Lat. *natus*]; haploid chromosome number; index of refraction; nano; nerve; neuter; neutron; neutron number density; normal; nostril [Lat. *naris*]; number; number of density of molecule; principle quantum number; refractive index; rotational frequency; sample size

2n haploid chromosome; diploid

3n triploid

4n tetraploid

ν see *nu*

NA nalidixic acid; Narcotics Anonymous; network administrator; neuraminidase; neurologic age; neutralizing antibody; neutrophil antibody; nicotinic acid; Nomina Anatomica; nonadherent; noradrenalin; not admitted; not applicable; nuclear antibody; not available; nucleic acid; nucleus ambiguus; numerical aperture; nurse's aid; nursing assistant; nursing auxiliary

N/A not applicable

Na Avogadro's number; sodium [Lat. *natrium*]

nA nanoampere

NAA naphthaleneacetic acid; neutral amino acid; neutron activation analysis; neutrophil aggregation activity; nicotinic acid amide; no apparent abnormalities

NAACLS National Accrediting Agency for Clinical Laboratory Sciences

NAACOG Nurses Association of the American College of Obstetricians and Gynecologists

NAAP N-acetyl-4-amino-phenazone

NAB novarsenobenzene

NABP National Association of Boards of Pharmacy

NABPLEX National Association of Boards of Pharmacy Licensing Examination

NAC N-acetylcysteine; National Asthma Center; Noise Advisory Council

NACDS North American Clinical Dermatological Society

NACED National Advisory Council on the Employment of the Disabled

NAC-EDTA N-acetylcysteine EDTA

nAChR nicotinic acetylcholine receptor

NACOR National Advisory Committee on Radiation

NACSAP National Alliance Concerned with School-Age Parents

NAD new antigenic determinant; nicotinamide adenine dinucleotide; nicotinic acid dehydrogenase; no abnormal discovery; no active disease; no acute distress; no apparent distress; no appreciable disease; normal axis deviation; nothing abnormal detected

NAD$^+$ the oxidized form of NAD

NaD sodium dialysate

NADA New Animal Drug Application

NADABA N-adenoxyldiaminobutyric acid

NADG nicotinamide adenine dinucleotide glycohydrolase

NADH reduced nicotinamide adenine dinucleotide

NADL National Association of Dental Laboratories

NaDodSO₄ sodium dedecyl sulfate

NADP nicotinamide adenine dinucleotide phosphate

NADP⁺ oxidized form of nicotinamide adenine dinucleotide phosphate

NADPH reduced nicotinamide adenine dinucleotide phosphate

NAE net acid excretion

NaE, Naₑ exchangeable body sodium

NAEMT National Association of Emergency Medical Technicians

NaERC sodium efflux rate constant

NAF nafcillin; National Amputation Foundation; National Ataxia Foundation; net acid flux

NAG N-acetyl-D-glucosaminidase; narrow-angle glaucoma; nonagglutinable

NAGO neuraminidase and galactose oxidase

NAH 2-hydroxy-3-naphthoic acid hydrazide

NAHA National Association of Health Authorities

NAHCS National Association of Health Center Schools

NAHG National Association of Humanistic Gerontology

NAHI National Athletic Health Institute

NAHMOR National Association of Health Maintenance Organization Regulators

NAHPA National Association of Hospital Purchasing Agents

NAHSA National Association for Hearing and Speech Action

NAHSE National Association of Health Services Executives

NAHU National Association of Health Underwriters

NAHUC National Association of Health Unit Clerks-Coordinators

NAI net acid input; no accidental injury; no acute inflammation; nonadherence index

NAIC National Association of Insurance Commissioners

NAIR nonadrenergic inhibitory response

NAL nonadherent leukocyte

NALD neonatal adrenoleukodystrophy

NAM natural actomyosin

NAMCS National Ambulatory Medical Care Survey

NAME National Association of Medical Examiners; nevi, atrial myxoma, myxoid neurofibroma, ephelides [syndrome]

NAMH National Association for Mental Health

NAMN nicotinic acid mononucleotide

NAMRU Navy Medical Reserve Unit

NANA N-acetyl neuraminic acid

NANB non-A, non-B [hepatitis]

NANBH non-A, non-B hepatitis

NAND not-and

NAOO National Association of Optometrists and Opticians

NAOP National Alliance for Optional Parenthood

NAP nasion, point A, pogonion [convexity or concavity of the facial profile]; nerve action potential; neutrophil alkaline phosphatase; nodular adrenocortical pathology; nucleic acid phosphatase

NAPA N-acetyl-p-aminophenol; N-acetyl procainamide

NAPCA National Air Pollution Control Administration

NaPG sodium pregnanediol glucuronide

NAPH naphthyl; nicotinamide adenine dinucleotide phosphate

NAPHT National Association of Patients on Hemodialysis and Transplantation

NAPM National Association of Pharmaceutical Manufacturers

NAPN National Association of Physicians' Nurses

NAPNAP National Association of Pediatric Nurse Associates and Practitioners

NAPNES National Association for Practical Nursing Education and Services

NAPPH National Association of Private Psychiatric Hospitals

NAPT National Association for the Prevention of Tuberculosis

NAR nasal airway resistance; National Association for Retarded [Children, Citizens]; no action required

NARA Narcotics Addict Rehabilitation Act; National Association of Recovered Alcoholics

NARAL National Abortion Rights Action League

NARC narcotic; National Association for Retarded Children; nucleus arcuatus

narco narcotic, narcotic addict, drug enforcement agent

NARD National Association of Retail Druggists

NARES nonallergic rhinitis–eosinophilia syndrome

NARF National Association of Rehabilitation Facilities

NARMC Naval Aerospace and Regional Medical Center

NARMH National Association for Rural Mental Health

NARS National Acupuncture Research Society

NAS nasal; National Academy of Sciences; National Association of Sanitarians; neonatal airleak syndrome; neuroallergic syndrome; no added salt

NASA National Aeronautics and Space Administration

NASE National Association for the Study of Epilepsy

NASEAN National Association for State Enrolled Assistant Nurses

NASM Naval Aviation School of Medicine

NAS-NRC National Academy of Science-National Research Council

NASW National Association of Social Workers

NAT N-acetyltransferase; natal; neonatal alloimmune thrombocytopenia; no action taken; nonaccidental trauma

Nat native; natural

NaT sodium tartrate

NATCO North American Transplant Coordinator Organization

Natr sodium [Lat. *natrium*]

NB nail bed; neuro-Behçet [syndrome]; neuroblastoma; neurometric battery; newborn; nitrous oxide-barbiturate; normoblast; note well [Lat. *nota bene*]; nutrient broth

Nb niobium

nb newborn; note well [Lat. *nota bene*]

NBA neuron-binding activity

NBC non-battle casualty

NBCC nevoid basal cell carcinoma

NBCCS nevoid basal cell carcinoma syndrome

NBCIE nonbullous congential ichthyosiform erythroderma

NBD neurogenic bladder dysfunction; no brain damage

NBF no breast feeding

NBI neutrophil bactericidal index; no bone injury; non-battle injury

NBICU newborn intensive care unit

NBM no bowel movement; normal bone marrow; normal bowel movement; nothing by mouth

nbM newborn mouse

nbMb newborn mouse brain

NBME National Board of Medical Examiners; normal bone marrow extract

NBN newborn nursery

NBO non-bed occupancy

NBP needle biopsy of prostate; neoplastic brachial plexopathy

NBRT National Board for Respiratory Therapy

NBS N-bromosuccinimide; National Bureau of Standards; nevoid basal cell carcinoma syndrome; Nijmegen breakage syndrome; normal blood serum; normal bowel sounds; normal brain stem; nystagmus blockage syndrome

NBT nitroblue tetrazolium; non-tumor-bearing; normal breast tissue

NBTE nonbacterial thrombotic endocarditis

NBTNF newborn, term, normal, female

NBTNM newborn, term, normal, male

NBT PABA N-benzoyl-L-tyrosyl para-aminobenzoic acid

NBTS National Blood Transfusion Service

n-Bu n-butyl

NBW normal birth weight

NC nasal cannula; nasal clearance; neck complaint; neonatal cholestasis; neural crest; neurologic check; nevus comedonicus; night call; nitrocellulose; no casualty; no change; no charge; no complaints; noise criterion; noncirrhotic; noncontributory; normocephalic; nose cone; not completed; not cultured; nucleocapsid; nursing coordinator

N:C nuclear-cytoplasmic ratio

nC nanocoulomb

nc nanocurie; not counted

NCA National Certification Agency; National Council on Aging; National Council on Alcoholism; neurocirculatory asthenia; neutrophil chemotactic activity; nodulocystic acne; noncontractile area; nonspecific cross-reacting antigen; nuclear cerebral angiogram

n-CAD negative coronoradiographic documentation

NCAE National Council for Alcohol Education

NCAMI National Committee Against Mental Illness

NCAMLP National Certification Agency for Medical Laboratory Personnel

NcAMP nephrogenous cyclic adenosine monophosphate

NC/AT normal cephalic atraumatic

NCBI National Center for Biotechnology Information

NCC noncoronary cusp; nursing care continuity

NCCDC National Center for Chronic Disease Control

NCCEA Neurosensory Center Comprehensive Examination for Aphasia

NCCIP National Center for Clinical Infant Program

NCCLS National Committee for Clinical Laboratory Standards

NCCLVP National Coordinating Committee on Large Volume Parenterals

NCCMHC National Council for Community Mental Health Centers

NCCPA National Commission on Certification of Physician Assistants

NCCU newborn convalescent care unit

NCD National Commission on Diabetes; National Council on Drugs; neurocirculatory dystonia; nitrogen clearance delay; normal childhood disorder; not considered disabling

NCDA National Council on Drug Abuse

NCDV Nebraska calf diarrhea virus

NCE negative contrast echocardiography; new chemical entity; nonconvulsive epilepsy

NCEP National Cholesterol Education Program

NCF neutrophil chemotactic factor

NCFA Narcolepsy and Catalepsy Foundation of America

NCF(C) neutrophil chemotactic factor (complement)

NCHC National Council of Health Centers

NCHCA National Commission for Health Certifying Agencies

NCHCT National Center for Health Care Technology

NCHLS National Council of Health Laboratory Services

NCHPD National Council on Health Planning and Development

NCHS National Center for Health Statistics

NCHSR National Center for Health Services Research

NCI National Cancer Institute; noncriterion ischemic [animal]; nuclear contour index; nursing care integration

nCi nanocurie

NCIB National Collection of Industrial Bacteria

NCIH National Council for International Health

NCJ needle catheter jejunostomy

NCL neuronal ceroid lipofuscinosis

NCLEX-RN National Council Licensure Examination for Registered Nurses

N/cm² newtons per square centimeter

NCMC natural cell-mediated cytotoxicity

NCMH National Committee for Mental Health

NCMHI National Clearinghouse for Mental Health Information

NCMI National Committee Against Mental Illness

NCN National Council of Nurses

NCNR Natural Center for Nursing Research

NCP noncollagen protein

n-CPAP nasal continuous positive airway pressure

NCPE noncardiac pulmonary edema

NCPPB National Collection of Plant Pathogenic Bacteria

NCR National Research Council; nuclear/cytoplasmic ratio

NCRND National Committee for Research in Neurological Diseases

NCRP National Council on Radiation Protection [and Measurements]

NCRV National Committee for Radiation Victims

NCS National Collaborative Study; neocarcinostatin; nerve conduction study; newborn calf serum; no concentrated sweets; noncircumferential stenosis; nystagmus compensation syndrome

NCSN National Council for School Nurses

NCT neural crest tumor

NCTC National Cancer Tissue Culture; National Collection of Type Cultures

NCV nerve conduction velocity; noncholera vibrio

NCVS nerve conduction velocity study

NCYC National Collection of Yeast Cultures

ND Doctor of Naturopathy; nasal deformity; natural death; Naval Dispensary; neonatal death; neoplastic disease; neuropsychological deficit; neurotic depression; neutral density; new drug; New-

castle disease; no data; no disease; nondetectable; nondiabetic; nondisabling; normal delivery; normal development; Norrie disease; not detected, not determined; not diagnosed; not done; nurse's diagnosis; nutritionally deprived

N/D no defects; not done

N&D nodular and diffuse

N$_D$, n$_D$ refractive index

Nd neodymium

n$_D$ refractive index

NDA National Dental Association; New Drug Application; no data available; no detectable activity; no detectable antibody

NDC National Data Communications; National Drug Code; Naval Dental Clinic; nondifferentiated cell

NDCD National Drug Code Directory

NDD no dialysis days

NDDG National Diabetes Data Group

NDE near-death experience; nondiabetic extremity

NDF neutrophil diffraction factor; new dosage form

NDFDA nonadecafluoro-n-decanoic acid

NDGA nordihydroguaiaretic acid

NDI nephrogenic diabetes insipidus

NDIR nondispersive infrared analyzer

NDMA nitrosodimethylamine

nDNA native deoxyribonucleic acid

NDP net dietary protein; nucleoside diphosphate

NDR neonatal death rate; normal detrusor reflex

NDS Naval Dental School; new drug submission; normal dog serum

NDSB Narcotic Drugs Supervisory Board

NDT neurodevelopmental treatment; noise detection threshold; nondestructive test, nondestructive testing

NDTI National Disease and Therapeutic Index

NDV Newcastle disease virus

Nd/YAG neodymium/yttrium-aluminum-garnet [laser]

NE national emergency; necrotic enteritis; nephropathia epidemica; nerve ending; nerve excitation; neuroendocrinology; neuroepithelium; neurological examination; neutrophil elastase; no effect; no exposure; nocturnal exacerbation; nonelastic; nonendogenous; norepinephrine; noninvasive evaluation; not elevated; not enlarged; not equal; not evaluated; not examined; nutcracker esophagus

Ne neon

NEA neoplasm embryonic antigen; no evidence of abnormality

NEB neuroendocrine body

nebul spray [Lat. *nebula*]

NEC National Electrical Code; necrotizing enterocolitis; neuroendocrine cell; no essential changes; nonesterified cholesterol; not else classified or classifiable

NECHI Northeastern Consortium for Health Information

NED no evidence of disease; no expiration date; normal equivalent deviation

NEE needle electrode examination

NEEE Near East equine encephalomyelitis

NEEP negative end-expiratory pressure

NEF nephritic factor

NEFA nonesterified fatty acid

neg negative

NEHE Nurses for Environmental Health Education

NEI National Eye Institute

NEISS National Electronic Injury Surveillance System

NEJ neuroeffector junction

NEJM New England Journal of Medicine

NEM N-ethylmaleimide; no evidence of malignancy

nem nutritional milk unit [Ger. *Nahrungs Einheit Milch*]

NEMA National Eclectic Medical Association

nema nematode

NEMD nonspecific esophageal motor dysfunction

Neo neomycin

neo neoarsphenamine

NEP negative expiratory pressure; nephrology; neutral endopeptidase; no evidence of pathology

nep nephrectomy

NEPHGE nonequilibrated pH gradient electrophoresis

NERHL Northeastern Radiological Health Laboratory

NER no evidence of recurrence

NERD no evidence of recurrent disease

ner nervous

NERO noninvasive evaluation of radiation output

NES not elsewhere specified

NESO Northeastern Society of Orthodontists

NESP Nurse Education Support Program

NET nasoendotracheal tube; nerve excitability test

n et m night and day [Lat. *nocte et mane*]

Neu neuraminidase

neu neurilemma

neur, neuro, neurol neurology, neurological, neurologist

neuropath neuropathology

neut neuter, neutral; neutrophil

NEY neomycin egg yolk [agar]

NEYA neomycin egg yolk agar

NF nafcillin; National Formulary; nephritic factor; neurofibromatosis; neurofilament; neutral fraction; noise factor; normal flow; not filtered; not found

nF nanofarad

NFAIS National Federation of Abstracting and Indexing Services

NFB National Foundation for the Blind; nonfermenting bacteria

NFC National Fertility Center

NFD neurofibrillary degeneration

NFDR neurofaciodigitorenal [syndrome]

NFE nonferrous extract

NFH nonfamilial hematuria

NFIC National Foundation for Ileitis and Colitis

NFID National Foundation for Infectious Diseases

NFL nerve fiber layer

NFLD nerve fiber layer defect

NFLPN National Federation of Licensed Practical Nurses

NFMD National Foundation for Muscular Dystrophy

NFME National Fund for Medical Education

NFND National Foundation for Neuromuscular Diseases

NFNID National Foundation for Non-Invasive Diagnostics

NFPA National Fire Protection Association

NFS National Fertility Study

NFT neurofibrillary tangle

NFTD normal full term delivery

NFW nursed fairly well

NG nasogastric; new growth; nitroglycerin; nodose ganglion; no growth; not given

ng nanogram

NGA nutrient gelatin agar

NGC nucleus reticularis gigantocellularis

NGF nerve growth factor

NGGR nonglucogenic/glucogenic ratio

NGI nuclear globulin inclusions

NGL neutral glycolipid

NGR narrow gauze roll; nasogastric replacement

NGS normal goat serum

NGSA nerve growth stimulating activity

NGSF nongenital skin fibroblast

NGT normal glucose tolerance

NGU nongonococcal urethritis

NH natriuretic hormone; Naval Hospital; neonatal hepatitis; neurologically handicapped; nocturnal hypoventilation; nonhuman; nursing home

N(H) proton density

NHA National Health Association; National Hearing Association; National Hemophilia Association; nonspecific hepatocellular abnormality

NHANES National Health and Nutrition Examination Survey

NHBPCC National High Blood Pressure Coordinating Committee

NHC National Health Council; neighborhood health center; neonatal hypocalcemia; nonhistone chromosomal [protein]; nursing home care

NHCP nonhistone chromosomal protein

NHD normal hair distribution

NHDC National Hansen's Disease Center

NHDF normal human diploid fibroblast

NHDL non–high-density lipoprotein

NHDS National Hospital Discharge Survey

NHF National Health Federation; National Hemophilia Foundation; nonimmune hydrops fetalis

NHG normal human globulin

NHGJ normal human gastric juice

NHH neurohypophyseal hormone

NHI National Health Institute; National Health Insurance

NHIF National Head Injury Foundation

NHIS National Health Interview Survey

NHK normal human kidney

NHL nodular histiocytic lymphoma; non-Hodgkin's lymphoma

NHLBI National Heart, Lung, and Blood Institute

NHML non-Hodgkin's malignant lymphoma

NHMRC National Health and Medical Research Council

NHP nonhemoglobin protein; nonhistone protein; normal human pooled plasma; nursing home placement

NHPC National Health Planning Council

NHPF National Health Policy Forum

NHPIC National Health Planning Information Center

NHPPN National Health Professions Placement Network

NHR net histocompatibility ratio

NHRC National Health Research Center

NHS Nance-Horan syndrome; National Health Service; normal horse serum; normal human serum

NHSAS National Health Service Audit Staff
NHSC National Health Service Corps
NHSR National Hospital Service Reserve
NHT nonpenetrating head trauma
NI neuraminidase inhibition; neurological improvement; neutralization index; no information; noise index; not identified; not isolated; nucleus intercalatus
Ni nickel
NIA National Institute on Aging; nephelometric inhibition assay; niacin; no information available; Nutritional Institute of America
nia niacin
NIAAA National Institute of Alcohol Abuse and Alcoholism
NIADDK National Institute of Arthritis, Diabetes, Digestive and Kidney Diseases
NIAID National Institute of Allergy and Infectious Diseases
NIAMDD National Institute of Arthritis, Metabolism, and Digestive Diseases
NIB National Institute for the Blind
NIBP noninvasive blood pressure
NIBSC National Institute for Biological Standards and Control
NIC neurogenic intermittent claudication; nursing interim care
NICHD National Institute of Child Health and Development
NICU neonatal intensive care unit; neurological intensive care unit; neurosurgical intensive care unit; nonimmunologic contact urticaria
NID nonimmunological disease
NIDA National Institute of Drug Abuse
NIDD non-insulin-dependent diabetes
NIDDM non-insulin-dependent diabetes mellitus
NIDDY non-insulin-dependent diabetes in the young
NIDM National Institute for Disaster Mobilization
NIDR National Institute of Dental Research
NIDS nonionic detergent soluble

NIEHS National Institutes of Environmental Health Sciences
NIF negative inspiratory force; neutrophil immobilizing factor; nonintestinal fibroblast
Nig non-immunoglobulin
nig black [Lat. *niger*]
NIGMS National Institute of General Medical Sciences
NIH National Institutes of Health
NIHL noise-induced hearing loss
NIHR National Institute of Handicapped Research
NIHS National Institute of Hypertension Studies
NIIC National Injury Information Clearinghouse
NIIS National Institute of Infant Services
NIL noise interference level
NIMBY not in my backyard
NIMH National Institute of Mental Health
NIMP National Intern Matching Program
NIMR National Institute for Medical Research
NIMS National Infant Mortality Surveillance
NINCDS National Institute of Neurological and Communicative Disorders and Stroke
NINDB National Institute of Neurological Diseases and Blindness
NIOSH National Institute for Occupational Safety and Health
NIP nipple; no infection present; no inflammation present
NIPH National Institute of Public Health
NIPS neuroleptic-induced Parkinson syndrome
NIPTS noise-induced permanent threshold shift
NIR near infrared
nIR non-insulin-resistance
NIRA nitrite reductase
NIRD nonimmune renal disease
NIRMP National Intern and Resident Matching Program

NIRNS National Institute for Research in Nuclear Science

NIRS normal inactivated rabbit serum

NIS N-iodosuccinimide; no inflammatory signs

NIT National Intelligence Test

NITD noninsulin-treated disease

nit nitrous

nitro nitroglycerin

NIV nodule-inducing virus

NJ nasojejunal

NJPC National Joint Practice Commission

NK Commission on [Anatomical] Nomenclature [Ger. *Nomenklatur Kommission*]; natural killer [cell]; not known

n/k not known

NKA neurokinin A; no known allergies

nkat nanokatal

NKC nonketotic coma

NKCA natural killer cell activity

NKCF natural killer cytotoxic factor

NKDA no known drug allergies

NKFA no known food allergies

NKH nonketogenic hyperglycemia; nonketotic hyperosmotic

NKHA nonketotic hyperosmolar acidosis

NKHS nonketotic hyperosmolar syndrome; normal Krebs-Henseleit solution

NL neural lobe; neutral lipid; nodular lymphoma; normal; normal libido, normal limits

nl it is not clear [Lat. *non liquet*]; it is not permitted [Lat. *non licet*]; nanoliter; normal [value]

NLA National Leukemia Association; neuroleptoanesthesia; normal lactase activity

NLB needle liver biopsy

NLD nasolacrimal duct; necrobiosis lipoidica diabeticorum

NLDL normal low-density lipoprotein

NLE neonatal lupus erythematosus

Nle norleucine

NLF neonatal lung fibroblast; nonlactose fermentation

NLK neuroleukin

NLM National Library of Medicine; noise level monitor

NLMC nocturnal leg-muscle cramps

NLN National League for Nursing; no longer needed

NLNE National League for Nursing Education

NLP no light perception; nodular liquefying panniculitis; normal light perception; normal luteal phase

NLS Names Learning Test; nonlinear least squares; normal lymphocyte supernatant

NLT normal lymphocyte transfer; not less than; nucleus lateralis tuberis

NLX naloxone

NM near-miss; neomycin; neuromuscular; nictitating membrane; nitrogen mustard; nocturnal myoclonus; nodular melanoma; nonmotile; normetanephrine; not malignant; not measurable, not measured; not mentioned; not motile; nuclear medicine, technologist in nuclear medicine

N&M nerves and muslces; night and morning

Nm nutmeg [Lat. *nux moschata*]

N/m newtons per meter

N-m newton-meter

N/m² newtons per square meter

N x m newtons by meter

nM nanomolar

nm nanometer; night and morning [Lat. *nocte et mane*]

NMA National Malaria Association; National Medical Association; neurogenic muscular atrophy; *N*-nitroso-*N*-methylalanine

NMAC National Medical Audiovisual Center

NM(ASCP) Technologist in Nuclear Medicine certified by the American Society of Clinical Pathologists

NMC National Medical Care; Naval Medical Center; neuromuscular control; nonmotor condition; nucleus reticularis magnocellularis

NMCES National Medical Care Expenditure Survey

NMCUES National Medical Care Utilization and Expenditure Survey

NMD neuromyodysplasia

NMDA N-methyl-D-aspartate

NME National Medical Enterprises; neuromyeloencephalopathy

NMF N-methylformamide; National Medical Fellowship; National Migraine Foundation; nonmigrating fraction

NMFI National Master Facility Inventory

NMI no mental illness; normal male infant

NMJ neuromuscular junction

NML nodular mixed lymphoma

NMM nodular malignant melanoma

NMN nicotinamide mononucleotide; normetanephrine

NMNRU National Medical Neuropsychiatric Research Unit

nmol nanomole

NMOR N-nitrosomorpholine

NMOS N-type metal oxide semiconductor

NMP normal menstrual period; nucleoside monophosphate

NMPCA nonmetric principal component analysis

NMPTP N-methyl-4-phenyl-1,2,3,6-tetrahydropyridine

NMR neonatal mortality rate; nictitating membrane response; nuclear magnetic resonance

NMRDC Naval Medical Research and Development Command

NMRI Naval Medical Research Institute; nuclear magnetic resonance imaging

NMRL Naval Medical Research Laboratory

NMRU Naval Medical Research Unit

NMS Naval Medical School; neuroleptic malignant syndrome; neuromuscular spindle; normal mouse serum

N•m/s newton meters per second

NMSIDS near-miss sudden infant death syndrome

NMSS National Multiple Sclerosis Society

NMT neuromuscular tension; neuromuscular transmission; N-methyltransferase; no more than; nuclear medicine technology

NMTS neuromuscular tension state

NMTCB Nuclear Medicine Technology Certification Board

NMTD nonmetastatic trophoblastic disease

NMU neuromuscular unit; nitrosomethylurea

NN neonatal; nevocellular nevus; normally nourished; normal nutrition; nurse's notes

nn nerves; new name [Lat. *nomen novum*]

NNAS neonatal narcotic abstinence syndrome

NNC National Nutrition Consortium

NND neonatal death; New and Nonofficial Drugs; nonspecific nonerosive duodenitis

NNDC National Naval Dental Center

NNE neonatal necrotizing enterocolitis; nonneuronal enolase

NNEB National Nursery Examination Board

NNG nonspecific nonerosive gastritis

NNHS National Nursing Home Survey

NNI noise and number index

NNIS National Nosocomial Infections Study

NNM neonatal mortality

NNMC National Naval Medical Center

NNN Novy-MacNeal-Nicolle [medium]

NNNMU N-nitroso-N-methylurethane

NNO no new orders

n nov new name [Lat. *nomen novum*]

NNP nerve net pulse

NNR New and Nonofficial Remedies

NNS nonneoplastic syndrome

NNT nuclei nervi trigemini

NNWI Neonatal Narcotic Withdrawal Index

NO narcotics officer; nitric or nitrous oxide; none obtained; nonobese; nurse's office

No nobelium

No, no number [Lat. *numero*]

NOA National Optometric Association

NOAPP National Organization of Adolescent Pregnancy and Parenting

NOBT nonoperative biopsy technique

NOC not otherwise classified

noc, noct at night [Lat. *nocte*]

noct maneq at night and in the morning [Lat. *nocte maneque*]

NOD nodular melanoma; nonobese diabetic; notify of death

NOEL no observed effect level

NOF National Osteopathic Foundation

NOFT nonorganic failure-to-thrive

NOII nonocclusive intestinal ischemia

NOK next of kin

nom dub a doubtful name [Lat. *nomen dubium*]

NOMI nonocclusive mesenteric infarction

nom nov new name [Lat. *nomen novum*]

nom nud a name without designation [Lat. *nomen nudum*]

non-REM non-rapid eye movement [sleep]

non rep, non repetat do not repeat [Lat. *non repetatur*]

NOP not otherwise provided for

NOPHN National Organization for Public Health Nursing

NOR noradrenaline; normal; nortriptyline; nucleolar organizer region

NORC National Opinion Research Center

NOR-EPI norepinephrine

norleu norleucine

norm normal

NOS network operating system; non-organ-specific; not on staff; not otherwise specified

NOSAC nonsteroidal anti-inflammatory compound

NOSIE Nurses' Observation Scale for Inpatient Evaluation

NOSTA Naval Ophthalmic Support and Training Activity

NOT nocturnal oxygen therapy

NOTB National Ophthalmic Treatment Board

NOTT nocturnal oxygen therapy trial

nov n new name [Lat. *novum nomen*]

NOVS National Office of Vital Statistics

nov sp new species [Lat. *novum species*]

NP nasopharynx, nasopharyngeal; near point; neonatal-perinatal; neuritic plague; neuropathology; neurophysin; neuropsychiatry; new patient; newly presented; Niemann-Pick [disease]; nitrogen-phosphorus; nitrophenol; no pain; no pressure; nonpalpable; nonparalytic; nonpathogenic; nonphagocytic; normal plasma; normal pressure; nonpracticing; not perceptible; not performed; not pregnant; not present; nucleoplasmic; nucleoprotein; nucleoside phosphorylase; nurse practitioner; nursed poorly; nursing procedure; proper name [Lat. *nomen proprium*]

N-P need-persistence

Np neper; neptunium; neurophysin

np nucleotide pair

n p proper name [Lat. *nomen proprium*]

NPA National Pharmaceutical Association; National Pituitary Agency; near point accommodation

NPA-NIHHDP National Pituitary Agency–National Institutes of Health Hormone Distribution Program

NPB nodal premature beat; nonprotein bound

NPBF nonplacental blood flow

NPC nasopharyngeal carcinoma; near point of convergence; nodal premature contractions; nonparenchymal [liver] cell; nonproductive cough; nucleus of posterior commissure

NPCa nasopharyngeal carcinoma

NPCP National Prostatic Cancer Project; non-*Pneumocystis* pneumonia

NP cult nasopharyngeal culture

NPD narcissistic personality disorder; natriuretic plasma dialysate; negative pressure device; Niemann-Pick disease; nitrogen-phosphorus detector; nonpathologic diagnosis; normal protein diet

NPDL nodular poorly differentiated lymphocytic

NPDR nonproliferative diabetic retinopathy

NPE neurogenic pulmonary edema; neuropsychologic examination; no palpable enlargement; normal pelvic examination

NPF nasopharyngeal fiberscope; National Parkinson Foundation; National Pharmaceutical Foundation; National Psoriasis Foundation; no predisposing factor

NPFT Neurotic Personality Factor Test

NPH neutral protamine Hagedorn (insulin); normal pressure hydrocephalus

NPhx nasopharynx

NPI Narcissistic Personality Inventory; neuropsychiatric institution; no present illness; nucleoplasmic index

NPIC neurogenic peripheral intermittent claudication

NPII Neonatal Pulmonary Insufficiency Index

NPJT nonparoxysmal atrioventricular junctional tachycardia

NPK neuropeptide K

NPL National Physics Laboratory; neoproteolipid

NPM nothing per mouth

NPN nonprotein nitrogen

NPO nothing by mouth [Lat. *nulla per os*]; nucleus preopticus

NPO/HS nothing by mouth at bedtime [Lat. *nulla per os hora somni*]

NPP nitrophenylphosphate; normal pool plasma; nucleus tegmenti pedunculopontinus

NPPase nucleotide pyrophosphatase

NPPH nucleotide pyrophosphohydrolase

NPPNG nonpenicillinase-producing *Neisseria gonorrhoeae*

NP polio nonparalytic poliomyelitis

NPR net protein ratio; normal pulse rate; nucleoside phosphoribosyl

NPRL Navy Prosthetics Research Laboratory

NPS nail-patella syndrome

NPSA normal pilosebaceous appartus

NPSH nonprotein sulhydryl [group]

NPT neoprecipitin test; nocturnal penile tumescence; normal pressure and temperature

NPU net protein utilization

NPV negative pressure value; negative pressure ventilation; nuclear polyhidrosis virus; nucleus paraventricularis

NQA nursing quality assurance

4NQO 4-nitroquinoline 1-oxide

NQR nuclear quadruple resonance

NR do not repeat [Lat. *non repetatur*]; nerve root; neural retina; neutral red; noise reduction; nonreactive; nonrebreathing; no radiation; no reaction; no recurrence; no refill; no report; no respiration; no response; no result; nonresponder; nonretarded; normal range; normal reaction; normotensive rat; not readable; not recorded; not resolved; nurse; nutrition ratio; Reynold's number

N/R not remarkable

N$_R$ Reynold's number

nr near

NRA nitrate reductase; nucleus retroambigualis

NRB nonrejoining break

NRBC National Rare Blood Club; normal red blood cell; nucleated red blood cell

NRbc nucleated red blood cell

NRC National Research Council; normal retinal correspondence; not routine care; Nuclear Regulatory Commission

NRCC National Registry in Clinical Chemistry

NRCL nonrenal clearance

NRDL Naval Radiological Defense Laboratory

NREH normal renin essential hypertension

NREM nonrapid eye movement [sleep]

NRF Neurosciences Research Foundation; normal renal function

NRFC nonrosette-forming cell

NRFD not ready for data

NRGC nucleus reticularis gigantocellularis

NRH nodular regenerative hyperplasia

NRI nerve root involvement; nerve root irritation; nonrespiratory infection

NRK normal rat kidney

NRL nucleus reticularis lateralis

NRM National Registry of Microbiologists; normal range of motion; nucleus reticularis magnocellularis

NRMP National Resident Matching Progam

nRNA nuclear ribonucleic acid

nRNP nuclear ribonucleoprotein

NROM normal range of motion

NRP nucleus reticularis parvocellularis

NRPC nucleus reticularis pontis caudalis

NRPG nucleus reticularis paragigantocellularis

NRR net reproduction rate

NRRL Northern Regional Research Laboratory

NRS neurobehavioral rating scale; normal rabbit serum; normal reference serum; numerical rating scale

NRSCC National Reference System in Clinical Chemistry

NRSFPS National Reporting System for Family Planning Services

NRV nucleus reticularis ventralis

NS natural science; Neosporin; nephrosclerosis; nephrotic syndrome; nervous system; neurological surgery, neurosurgery; neurosecretion, neurosecretory; neurosyphilis; neurotic score; nodular sclerosis; nonsmoker; nonspecific; nonstimulation; nonstructural; nonsymptomatic; Noonan syndrome; normal saline; normal serum; normal sodium [diet]; Norwegian scabies; no sample; no sequelae; no specimen; not seen; not significant; not specified; not sufficient; not symptomatic; nuclear sclerosis; nursing services; Nursing Sister

N/S normal saline

Ns nasospinale; nerves

ns nanosecond; nonspecific; no sequelae; no specimen; not significant; nylon suture

NSA Neurological Society of America; normal serum albumin; no salt added; no significant abnormality; no significant anomaly

nsa no salt added

NSABP National Surgical Adjuvant Breast Project

NSAD no signs of acute disease

NSAE nonsupported arm exercise

NSAI nonsteroidal anti-inflammatory [drug]

NSAIA nonsteroidal anti-inflammatory agent

NSAID nonsteroidal anti-inflammatory drug

NSAM Naval School of Aviation Medicine

NSC neurosecretory cell; no significant change; nonservice connected; nonspecific suppressor cell; normal child with short stature

nsc nonservice connected; no significant change

NSCC National Society for Crippled Children

NSCD nonservice connected disability

NSCLC non-small-cell lung cancer

NSD Nairobi sheep disease; neonatal staphylococcal disease; neurosecretory dysfunction; night sleep deprivation; nominal single dose; nominal standard dose; normal standard dose; no significant defect; no significant deficiency; no significant deviation; no significant difference; no significant disease; normal spontaneous delivery

NSE neuron-specific enolase; nonspecific esterase; normal saline enema

nsec nanosecond

NSF National Science Foundation; nodular subepidermal fibrosis

NSFTD normal spontaneous full-term delivery

NSG neurosecretory granule

nsg nursing

NSGCT nonseminomatous germ cell tumor

NSG Hx nursing history

NSGI nonspecific genital infection

NSH National Society for Histotechnology

NSHD nodular sclerosing Hodgkin's disease

NSI negative self-image; no signs of infection/inflammation; non-syncytium-inducing

NSIDS near sudden infant death syndrome

NSILA nonsuppressible insulinlike activity

NSILP nonsuppressible insulinlike protein

NSJ nevus sebaceus of Jadassohn

NSM neurosecretory material; neurosecretory motor neuron; nonantigenic specific mediator; nutrient sporulation medium

N·s/m² newton seconds per square meter

NSMR National Society for Medical Research

NSN nephrotoxic serum nephritis; nicotine-stimulated neurophysin

NSNA National Student Nurse Association

NSND nonsymptomatic and nondisabling

NSO Neosporin ointment; nucleus supraopticus

NSP neuron specific protein

NSPB National Society for the Prevention of Blindness

NSPN neurosurgery progress note

NSQ Neuroticism Scale Questionnaire; not sufficient quantitiy

NSR nasal septal reconstruction; nonspecific reaction; normal sinus rhythm; not seen regularly

NSS normal saline solution; normal size and shape; not statistically significant; nutrition support services

NSSTT nonspecific ST and T [wave]

NST neospinothalamic [tract]; nonshivering thermogenesis; nonstress test; nutritional support team

NSTT nonseminomatous testicular tumor

NSU neurosurgical unit; nonspecific urethritis

NSurg neurosurgery, neurosurgeon

NSV nonspecific vaginitis/vaginosis

NSVD normal spontaneous vaginal delivery

NSVT nonsustained ventricular tachycardia

NSX neurosurgical examination

nsy nursery

NT nasotracheal; neotetrazolium; neurotensin; neutralization test; nicotine tartrate; nontender; nontumoral; normal temperature; normal tissue; normotensive; nortriptyline; not tested; N-terminal [fragment]; nucleotidase; nucleotide

5'NT 5'-nucleotidase

Nt amino terminal

nt nucleotide

N&T nose and throat

NTA natural thymocytotoxic autoantibody; nitrilotriacetic acid; Nurse Training Act

NTAB nephrotoxic antibody

NTBR not to be resuscitated

NTC neotetrazolium chloride

NTCC National Type Culture Collection

NTD neural tube defect; nitroblue tetrazolium dye; noise tone difference; 5'-nucleotidase

NTE neuropathy target esterase; neurotoxic esterase; not to exceed

NTF normal throat flora

NTG nitroglycerin; nitrosoguanidine; nontoxic goiter; normal triglyceridemia

NTGO nitroglycerin ointment

NTHH nontumorous, hypergastrinemic hyperchlorhydria

NTI nonthyroid illness

NTIG nontreated immunoglobulin

NTIS National Technical Information Service

NTLI neurotensin-like immunoreactivity

NTM nontuberculous mycobacteria

NTMI nontransmural myocardial infarction

NTN nephrotoxic nephritis

NTOS neurogenic thoracic outlet syndrome

NTP National Toxicology Program; nitroprusside; normal temperature and pressure; nucleoside triphosphate
NT&P normal temperature and pressure
NTR negative therapeutic reaction; normotensive rat; nutrition
ntr nutriton
NTRC National Toxins Research Center
NTS nasotracheal suction; nephrotoxic serum; nucleus tractus solitarius
NTT nearly total thyroidectomy
NTU Navy Toxicology Unit
NTV nerve tissue vaccine
nt wt net weight
NTX naltrexone
NTZ normal transformation zone
NU name unknown
nU nanounit
nu nude [mouse]
ν Greek letter *nu*; degrees of freedom; frequency; kinematic velocity; neutrino
NUC nonspecific ulcerative colitis; sodium urate crystal
Nuc nucleoside
nuc nucleated
nucl nucleus
NUD nonucler dyspepsia
NUG necrotizing ulcerative gingivitis
NUI number user identification
nullip nulliparous
numc number concentration
NURB Neville upper reservoir buffer
Nut nutrition
NUV near ultraviolet
NV negative variation; neovascularization; next visit; nonveteran; normal value; not vaccinated; not venereal; not verified; not volatile
Nv naked vision
N&V nausea and vomiting
NVA near visual acuity
NVB neurovascular bundle
NVD nausea, vomiting, and diarrhea; neck vein distention; nonvalvular disease; no venereal disease; Newcastle virus disease; number of vessels diseased
NVG neovascular glaucoma; nonventilated group
NVL no visible lesion
NVM neovascular membrane; nonvolatile matter
NVS neurologic vital signs
NVSS normal variant short stature
NW naked weight; nasal wash
NWB nonweightbearing
NWDA National Wholesale Druggists Association
NWR normotensive Wistar rat
NX naloxane
NXG necrobiotic xanthogranuloma
ny, nyst nystagmus
NYC New York City [medium]
NYD not yet diagnosed; not yet discovered
NYHAFC New York Heart Association Functional Class
NZ normal zone
NZB New Zealand black [mouse]
NZC New Zealand chocolate [mouse]
NZO New Zealand obese [mouse]
NZR New Zealand red [rabbit]
NZW New Zealand white [mouse]

O

O blood type in the ABO blood group; eye [Lat. *oculus*]; nonmotile strain of microorganisms [Ger. *ohne Hauch*]; objective findings; observed frequency in a contingency table; obstetrics; obvious; occipital electrode placement in electroencephalography; occiput; occlusal; oculus; [doctor's] office; often; ohm; old; opening; operator; operon; opium; oral, orally; orange [color]; orderly respirations [anesthesia chart]; ortho-; orthopedics; osteocyte; other; output; ovine; oxygen; pint [Lat. *octarius*]; respirations [anesthesia chart]; zero

O_2 both eyes; diatomic oxygen; molecular oxygen

O_3 ozone

o eye [Lat. *oculus*]; opening; ovary transplant; pint [Lat. *octarius*]; see *omicron*

ō negative; without

Ω see *ohm*

Ω see *omega*

ω see *omega*

OA obstructive apnea; occipital artery; occiput anterior; octanoic acid; ocular albinism; old age; oleic acid; opiate analgesia; opsonic activity; optic atrophy; oral alimentation; orotic acid; osteoarthritis; ovalbumin; overall assessment; Overeaters Anonymous; oxalic acid

O&A observation and assessment

O_2a oxygen availability

OAA Old Age Assistance; Opticians Association of America; oxaloacetic acid

OAAD ovarian ascorbic acid depletion

OAB ABO blood group; old age benefits

OABP organic anion binding protein

OAD obstructive airway disease; organic anionic dye

OADC oleate-albumin-dextrose-catalase [medium]

OAF open air factor; osteoclast activating factor

OAG open angle glaucoma

OAH ovarian androgenic hyperfunction

OAISO overaction of the ipsilateral superior oblique

OALF organic acid labile fluid

OALL ossification of anterior longitudinal ligament

OAM outer acrosomal membrane

OAP Office of Adolescent Pregnancy; old age pension, old age pensioner; ophthalmic artery pressure; osteoarthropathy; oxygen at atmospheric pressure

OAPP Office of Adolescent Pregnancy Programs

OAS old age security; oral allergy syndrome; osmotically active substance

OASD ocular albinism-sensorineural deafness [syndrome]

OASDHI Old-Age, Survivors, Disability and Health Insurance

OASDI Old-Age, Survivors, and Disability Insurance

OASI Old Age and Survivors Insurance

OASP organic acid soluble phosphorus

OAT ornithine aminotransferase

OAV oculoauriculovertebral [dysplasia]

OAVD oculoauriculovertebral dysplasia

OAW oral airways

OB obese, obesity; objective benefit; obliterative bronchiolitis; obstetrics, obstetrician; occult bleeding; olfactory bulb; oligoclonal band

O&B opium and belladonna

ob he (she) died [Lat. *obiit*]; obese [mouse]

OBB own bed bath

OBD organic brain disease

OBE Office of Biological Education

OBF organ blood flow

OBG, ObG obstetrics and gynecology, obstetrician-gynecologist

OBGS obstetrical and gynecological surgery

OB-GYN, ob-gyn obstetrics and gynecology, obstetrician-gynecologist

obj objective

obl oblique

ob/ob obese [mouse]

OBP ova, blood, parasites [in stool]

OBRA Omnibus Reconciliation Act

OBS obstetrical service; organic brain syndrome

Obs observation, observed; obstetrics, obstetrician

obs obsolete

Obst obstetrics, obstetrician

obst, obstr obstruction, obstructed

OC obstetrical conjugate; occlusocervical; office call; on call; only child; optic chiasma; oral contraceptive; original claim; organ culture; outer canthal [distance]; ovarian cancer; oxygen consumed

O&C onset and course

OCA oculocutaneous albinism; olivopontocerebellar atrophy; oral contraceptive agent

OCa ovarian carcinoma

OCAD occlusive carotid artery disease

O$_2$cap oxygen capacity

OCBF outer cortical blood flow

occ occasional; occiput, occipital; occlusion; occlusive; occupation; occurrence

occas occasional

occip occiput, occipital

occl occlusion, occlusive

OccTh occupational therapy, occupational therapist

occup occupation, occupational

occup Rx occupational therapy

OCD obsessive compulsive disorder; Office of Child Development; Office of Civil Defense; osteochondritis dissecans; ovarian cholesterol depletion

OCG omnicardiogram; oral cholecystogram

OCH oral contraceptive hormone

OCHS Office of Cooperative Health Statistics

OCIS Oncology Center Information System

OCM oral contraceptive medication

OCN oculomotor nucleus

OCP octacalcium phosphate; oral case presentation; oral contraceptive pill

OCR oculocardiac reflex; oculocerebrorenal [syndrome]; optical character recognition

oCRF ovine corticotropin-releasing factor

OCRG oxycardiorespirography

oCRH ovine corticotropin-releasing hormone

OCRL Lowe's oculocerebrorenal [syndrome]

OCRS oculocerebrorenal syndrome

OCS occipital condyle syndrome; Ondine's curse syndrome; open canalicular system; oral contraceptive steroid; outpatient clinic substation

OCSD oculocraniosomatic disease

OCT object classification test; optimal cutting temperature; oral contraceptive therapy; ornithine carbamoyltransferase; orthotopic cardiac transplantation; oxytocin challenge test

OCU observation care unit

OCV ordinary conversational voice

OD Doctor of Optometry; every day [Lat. *omni die*]; obtained absorbance; occipital dysplasia; occupational dermatitis; occupational disease; oculodynamic; Ollier disease; on duty; once a day; open drop [anesthesia]; optical density; optimal dose; originally derived; out-of-date; outside diameter; overdose, overdosage; right eye [Lat. *oculus dexter*]

O-D obstacle-dominance

od every day [Lat. *omni die*]; overdose

ODA right occipitoanterior [fetal position] [Lat. *occipito-dextra anterior*]

ODB opiate-directed behavior

ODC oritidine decarboxylase; ornithine decarboxylase; oxygen dissociation curve

ODD oculodentodigital [dysplasia]

OD'd overdosed [drug]

ODM ophthalmodynamometer, ophthalmodynamometry

ODOD oculo-dento-osseous dysplasia

Odont odontogenic
odorat odoriferous [Lat. *odoratus*]
ODP offspring of diabetic parents; right occipitoposterior [fetal position] [Lat. *occipito-dextra posterior*]
ODPHP Office of Disease Prevention and Health Promotion
ODS osmotic demyelination syndrome
ODSG ophthalmic Doppler sonogram
ODT oculodynamic tract; right occipitotransverse [fetal position] [Lat. *occipito-dextra transversa*]
ODTS organic dust toxic syndrome
ODU optical density unit
OE on examination; orthopedic examination; otitis externa
O/E observed/expected [ratio]
O&E observation and examination
Oe oersted
OEE osmotic erythrocyte enrichment; outer enamel epithelium
OEF oil immersion field; oxygen extraction fraction
OEIS omphalocele, exstrophy, imperforate anus, spinal defects [complex]
OEL occupational exposure limit
OEM opposite ear masked
OER osmotic erythrocyte [enrichment]; oxygen enhancement ratio
O₂ER oxygen extraction ratio
OERP Office of Education and Regional Programming
OES oral esophageal stethoscope; optical emission spectroscopy
oesoph esophagus [oesophagus]
OET oral endotracheal tube; oral esophageal tube
OF occipitofrontal; open field [test]; optical fundus; orbitofrontal; osmotic fragility; osteitis fibrosa; oxidation-fermentation
O/F oxidation-fermentation
OFA oncofetal antigen
OFAGE orthogonal field alternation gel electrophoresis
OFBM oxidation-fermentation basal medium

OFC occipitofrontal circumference; orbitofacial cleft; osteitis fibrosa cystica
OFCTAD occipito-facio-cervico-thoraco-abdomino-digital dysplasia
OFD object-film distance; occipital frontal diameter; oro-facial-digital [syndrome]
ofd object-film distance
Off official
OFHA occipitofrontal headache
OFM orofacial malformation
OG obstetrics and gynecology; occlusogingival; oligodendrocyte; optic ganglion; orange green; orogastric
O&G obstetrics and gynecology
OGF ovarian growth factor; oxygen gain factor
OGH ovine growth hormone
OGS oxygenic steroid
OGTT oral glucose tolerance test
OH every hour [Lat. *omni hora*]; hydroxycorticosteroid; obstructive hypopnea; occipital horn; occupational health; occupational history; open heart [surgery]; osteopathic hospital; out of hospital; outpatient hospital
17-OH 17-hydroxycorticosteroid
oh every hour [Lat. *omni hora*]
OHA oral hypoglycemic agents
OHAHA ophthalmoplegia-hypotonia-ataxia-hypacusis-athetosis [syndrome]
OHB₁₂ hydroxycobalamin
O₂Hb oxyhemoglobin
OHC occupational health center; outer hair cell
OH-Cbl hydroxycobalamin
OHCC hydroxycalciferol
OHCS hydroxycorticosteroid
OHD hydroxyvitamin D; Office of Human Development; organic heart disease
25-OH-D 25-hydroxyvitamin D
OHDA hydroxydopamine
16-OH-DHAS 16-alpha-hydroxydehydroepiandrosterone sulfate
8-OH-DPAT 8-hydroxy-2-(di-n-propylamino)tetralin

OHDS Office of Human Development Services
OHF Omsk hemorrhagic fever
OHFA hydroxy fatty acid
OHFT overhead frame trapeze
OHI Occupational Health Institute; operative hypertension indicator; oral hygiene index; Oral Hygiene Instruction
OHIAA hydroxyindoleacetic acid
OHI-S Oral Hygiene Instruction-Simplified
OHL oral hairy leukoplakia
OHN occupational health nurse
OHP hydroxyprogesterone; hydroxyproline; oxygen under high pressure
17-OHP 17-hydroxyprogesterone
OHR Office of Health Research
OHS obesity hypoventilation syndrome; ocular histoplasmosis syndrome; open heart surgery; ovarian hyperstimulation syndrome
OHSD hydroxysteroid dehydrogenase
OHSS ovarian hyperstimulation syndrome
OHT ocular hypertension
OI obturator internus; occasional insomnia; opportunistic infection; opsonic index; orgasmic impairment; orientation inventory; orthoiodohippurate; osteogenesis imperfecta; oubain insensitivity; oxygen intake
O-I outer and inner
OIC osteogenesis imperfecta congenita
OID optimal immunomodulating dose; Organism Identification Number
OIF observed intrinsic frequency; oil immersion field; Osteogenesis Imperfecta Foundation
OIH Office of International Health; orthoiodohippurate; ovulation-inducing hormone
OILD occupational immunologic lung disease
oint ointment
OIP organizing interstitial pneumonia
OIR Office of International Research
OIT organic integrity test
OJ orange juice

OKN optokinetic nystagmus
Ol oil [Lat. *oleum*]
ol left eye [Lat. *oculus laevus*]
OLA left occipitoanterior [fetal position] [Lat. *occipito-laeva anterior*]
OLB olfactory bulb; open liver biopsy
OLD obstructive lung disease; orthochromatic leukodystrophy
OLH ovine lactogenic hormone
oLH ovine luteinizing hormone
OLIDS open loop insulin delivery system
ol oliv olive oil [Lat. *oleum olivea*]
OLP left occipitoposterior [fetal position] [Lat. *occipito-laeva posterior*]
OLR otology, laryngology, and rhinology
ol res oleoresin
OLS oubain-like substance
OLT left occipitotransverse [fetal position] [Lat. *occipito-laeva transversa*]; orthotopic liver transplantation
OM occipitomental; occupational medicine; ocular movement; oculomotor; Osborne Mendel [rat]; osteomalacia; osteomyelitis; osteopathic manipulation; otitis media; outer membrane; ovulation method
om every morning [Lat. *omni mane*]
OMAC otitis media, acute catarrhal
OMAR Office of Medical Applications of Research
OMAS occupational maladjustment syndrome
OMB Office of Management and Budget
OMC Open Mutual Commissurotomy
OMCT Orientation-Memory-Concentration Test
OMD ocular muscle dystrophy; oculomandibulodyscephaly; organic mental disorder; oromandibular dystonia
OME office of medical examiner; otitis media with effusions
Ω Greek capital letter *omega*
Ω ohm
Ω⁻¹ Ω^{-1}, siemens
ω Greek lower case letter *omega*; angular velocity

OMH Office of Mental Health

OMI old myocardial infarction

o Greek letter *omicron*

OMM outer mitochondrial membrane

OMN oculomotor nerve

omn bih every two hours [Lat. *omni bihora*]

omn hor every hour [Lat. *omni hora*]

omn 2 hor every second hour [Lat. *omni secunda hora*]

omn man every morning [Lat. *omni mane*]

omn noct every night [Lat. *omni nocte*]

omn quad hor every quarter of an hour [Lat. *omni quadrante hora*]

omn sec hor every second hour [Lat. *omni secunda hora*]

OMP olfactory marker protein; ornithine monophosphate; outer membrane protein

OMPA octamethyl pyrophosphoramide; otitis media, purulent, acute

OMPC, OMPCh otitis media, purulent, chronic

om quar hor every quarter of an hour [Lat. *omni quadrante hora*]

OMS organic mental syndrome; otomandibular syndrome

OM&S osteopathic medicine and surgery

OMSA otitis media, suppurative, acute

OMSC otitis media secretory (or suppurative) chronic

OMT O-methyltransferase; osteopathic manipulative therapy

OMVC open mitral valve commissurotomy

ON every night [Lat. *omni nocte*]; occipitonuchal; office nurse; onlay; optic nerve; orthopedic nurse; osteonecrosis; overnight

ONC oncogene; oncology; Orthopaedic Nursing Certificate; over-the-needle catheter

OND Ophthalmic Nursing Diploma; orbitonasal dislocation; other neurological disorders

ONP operating nursing procedure; orthonitrophenyl

ONPG o-nitrophenyl-beta-D-galacto-pyranoside

ONS Oncology Nursing Society

ONTG oral nitroglycerin

ONTR orders not to resuscitate

OO oophorectomy

O&O on and off

OOA outer optic anlage

OOB out of bed

OOLR ophthalmology, otology, laryngology, and rhinology

OOM oogonial metaphase

OORR orbicularis oculi reflex response

OOW out of wedlock

OOWS objective opiate withdrawal scale

OP occipitoparietal; occiput posterior; octapeptide; olfactory peduncle; opening pressure; operation, operative; operative procedure; ophthalmology; opponens pollicis; organophosphorus; oropharynx; orthostatic proteinuria; osmotic pressure; osteoporosis; outpatient; ovine prolactin

O&P ova and parasites

Op ophthalmology; opisthocranion

op operation; operator

OPB outpatient basis

OPC oculopalatocerebral [syndrome]; outpatient clinic

OPCA olivopontocerebellar atrophy

OPCOS oligomenorrheic polycystic ovary syndrome

OPD obstetric prediabetic; optical path difference; otopalatodigital [syndrome]; outpatient department; outpatient dispensary

O'p-DDD mitotane

OpDent operative dentistry

OPDG ocular plethysmodynamography

OPG ocular pneumoplethysmography; oxypolygelatin

opg opening

OPH obliterative pulmonary hypertension; ophthalmia

OPH, Oph ophthalmology; ophthalmoscopy, ophthalmoscope

OphD Doctor of Ophthalmology

Ophth ophthalmology

OPI oculoparalytic illusion; Omnibus Personality Inventory

OPIDN organophosphorus-induced delayed neuropathy

OPK optokinetic

OPL outer plexiform layer; ovine placental lactogen

OPLL ossification of posterior longitudinal ligament

OPM occult primary malignancy; ophthalmoplegic migraine

OPN ophthalmic nurse

OPP osmotic pressure of plasma; oxygen partial pressure

opp opposite

OPPG oculopneumoplethysmography

OPRR Office of Protection from Research Risks

OPS operations; osteoporosis-pseudolipoma syndrome; outpatient service; outpatient surgery

OPSA ovarian papillary serous adenocarcinoma

OpScan optical scanning

OPSI overwhelming postsplenectomy infection

OPSR Office of Professional Standards Review

OPT outpatient; outpatient treatment

opt best [Lat. *optimus*]; optics, optician

OPTHD optimal hemodialysis

OPV oral polio vaccine

OPWL opiate withdrawal

OR a logical binary relation that is true if any argument is true, and false otherwise; [o]estrogen receptor; odds ratio; oil retention [enema]; open reduction; operating room; optic radiation; oral rehydration; orthopedic; orthopedic research

O-R oxidation-reduction

O$_R$ rate of outflow

Or orbitale

ORA opiate receptor agonist

ORANS Oak Ridge Analytical System

ORBC ox red blood cell

orch orchitis

ORD optical rotatory dispersion; oral radiation death

ORDS Office of Research, Demonstration, and Statistics

OREF Orthopedic Research and Education Foundation

ORF open reading frame

OR&F open reduction and fixation

orf open reading frame

Org, org organic

ORIF open reduction with internal fixation

OrJ orange juice

ORL otorhinolaryngology

ORM orosomucoid; other regulated material

ORN operating room nurse; orthopedic nurse

Orn ornithine

ORNL Oak Ridge National Laboratory

ORO oil red O

OROS oral osmotic

ORP oxidation-reduction potential

ORPM orthorhythmic pacemaker

ORS olfactory reference syndrome; oral rehydration solution; oral surgery, oral surgeon; Orthopaedic Research Society; orthopedic surgeon, orthopedic surgery; oxygen radical scavengers

ORT object relations technique; operating room technician; oral rehydration therapy

orth, ortho orthopedics, orthopedic

OS left eye [Lat. *oculus sinister*]; occipitosacral; occupational safety; office surgery; Omenn syndrome; opening snap; operating system; oral surgery; organ-specific; orthopedic surgeon, orthopedic surgery; Osgood-Schlatter [disease]; osteogenic sarcoma; osteosarcoma; osteosclerosis; oubain sensitivity; overall survival; oxygen saturation

Os osmium

os left eye [Lat. *oculus sinister*]

OSA obstructive sleep apnea; Office of Services to the Aging; Optical Society of America; ovarian sectional area

OSAS obstructive sleep apnea syndrome

osc oscillation

OSCE Objective Structured Clinical Exam

OSF organ system failure; outer spiral fiber; overgrowth stimulating factor

OSHA Occupational Safety and Health Adminstration

OSH Act Occupational Safety and Health Act of 1970

OSM ovine submaxillary mucin; oxygen saturation meter

osm osmole; osmosis, osmotic

Osm/kg osmoles per kilogram

Osm/l osmoles per liter

osmol osmole

OSRD Office of Scientific Research and Development

OSS over-the-shoulder strap

oss osseous

OST object sorting test

osteo osteoarthritis; osteomyelitis; osteopathy

OSUK Ophthalmological Society of the United Kingdom

OT objective test; oblique talus; occlusion time; occupational therapist, occupational therapy; ocular tension; office therapy; old term (in anatomy); old tuberculin; olfactory threshold; optic tract; orientation test ; original tuberculin; ornithine transcarbamylase; orotracheal; orthopedic treatment; otolaryngology; otology; oxytocin; oxytryptamine

Ot otolaryngology

OTA ornithine transaminase; orthotoluidine arsenite

OTC ornithine transcarbamylase; oval target cell; over-the-counter; oxytetracycline

OTD oral temperature device; organ tolerance dose

OTE optically transparent electrode

OTF oral transfer factor

OTI ovomucoid trypsin inhibitor

OTM orthotoluidine manganese sulfate

OTO otology; otorhinolaryngology

Otol otology, otologist

OTR Ovarian Tumor Registry; Occupational Therapist, Registered

OTReg Occupational Therapist, Registered

OTS occipital temporal sulcus; orotracheal suction

OTT orotracheal tube

OTU olfactory tubercle; operational taxonomic unit

OU observation unit; Oppenheimer-Urbach [syndrome]

ou both eyes together [Lat. *oculi unitas*]; each eye [Lat. *oculus uterque*]

OULQ outer upper left quadrant

OURQ outer upper right quadrant

OUS overuse syndrome

OV oculovestibular; office visit; osteoid volume; outflow volume; ovalbumin; ovary; overventilation; ovulation

Ov ovary

ov ovum

OVA ovalbumin

ova ovariectomy

OVC ovarian cancer

OVD occlusal vertical dimension

OvDF ovarian dysfunction

OVX ovariectomized

OW once weekly; open wedge; outer wall; oval window

O/W oil in water

OWR Osler-Weber-Rendu [syndrome]; ovarian wedge resection

OWS outerwear syndrome

OX optic chiasma; oxacillin; oxalate; oxide; orthopedic examination; oxytocin

Ox oxygen

OXA oxaprotiline

OXP oxypressin

OXT oxytocin

OXY, oxy oxygen

OYE old yellow enzyme

oz ounce

oz ap apothecaries' ounce (U.S.)

oz apoth apothecaries' ounce (U.K.)

oz t ounce troy (U.S.)

oz tr ounce troy (U.K.)

P

P an electrocardiographic wave corresponding to a wave of depolarization crossing the atria; by weight [Lat. *pondere*]; father [Lat. *pater*]; handful [Lat. *pugilus*]; near [Lat. *proximum*]; near point [Lat. *punctum proximum*]; pain; parietal electrode placement in electroencephalography; parity; part; partial pressure; *Pasteurella*; paternal; patient; penicillin; percent; percussion; perforation; permeability; peta-; pharmacopeia; phenophthalein; phenylalanine; phosphate group; phosphorus; physiology; pig; pint; placebo; plan; plasma; *Plasmodium; Pneumocystis;* point; poise; poison, poisoning; polarity; polarization; pole; polymyxin; pons; population; porcelain; porcine; porphyrin; position; positive; posterior; postpartum; power; precipitin; precursor; prednisone; premolar; presbyopia; pressure; primary; primipara; probability; product; progesterone; prolactin; proline; properdin; propionate; protein; *Proteus*; proximal; *Pseudomonas*; psychiatry; pulmonary; pulse; pupil; radiant power; significance probability [value]; sound power; weight [Lat. *pondus*]

P₁, P-one first parental generation
P₂ pulmonic second sound
P₃ proximal third
³²P radioactive phosphorus

P-50 oxygen half-saturation pressure
p atomic orbital with angular momentum quantum number 1; freeze preservation; the frequency of the more common allele of a pair; momentum; papilla; phosphate; pico-; pint; pond; pressure; probability; proton; pupil; short arm of chromosome; sound pressure

p after
p- para
5p- cri-du-chat syndrome
Π see *pi*
π see *pi*
ψ see *psi*
φ see *phi*

PA panic attack; pantothenic acid; paralysis agitans; paranoia; passive aggressive; pathology; periarteritis; peridural artery; periodic acid; periodontal abscess; pernicious anemia; phakic-aphakic; phenylalkylamine; phosphatidic acid; phenylalanine; phosphoarginine; photoallergy; phthalic anhydride; physician assistant; pituitary-adrenal; plasma adsorption; plasma aldosterone; plasminogen activator; platelet adhesiveness; platelet aggregation; platelet-associated; polyamine; polyarteritis; polyarthritis; post-aural; posteroanterior; prealbumin; predictive accuracy; pregnancy-associated; presents again; primary aldosteronism; primary amenorrhea; primary anemia; prior to admission; proactivator; proanthocyanidin; procainamide; prolonged action; propionic acid; prostate antigen; protective antigen; proteolytic action; prothrombin activity; protrusio acetabuli; *Pseudomonas aeruginosa;* psychoanalysis; psychogenic aspermia; pulmonary artery; pulmonary atresia; pulpoaxial; puromycin aminonucleoside; pyruvic acid; pyrrolizidine alkaloid; yearly [Lat. *per annum*]

P_A alveolar pressure
P-A posteroanterior
P&A percussion and auscultation
Pa pascal; pathologist, pathology; protactinium; *Pseudomonas aeruginosa;* pulmonary arterial [pressure]
P_A partial pressure of arterial fluid
pA picoampere
pa through the anus [Lat. *per anum*]; yearly [Lat. *per annum*]
PAA partial agonist activity; phenylacetic acid; phosphonoacetic acid; physical abilities analysis; plasma angioten-

sinase activity; polyacrylamide; polyamino acid; pyridine acetic acid

PAB para-aminobenzoate; performance assessment battery; pharmacologic autonomic block; premature atrial beat; purple agar base

PABA para-aminobenzoic acid

PABD predeposit autologous blood donation

PABP pulmonary artery balloon pump

PAC papular acrodermatitis of childhood; parent-adult-child; phenacetin, aspirin, and caffeine; plasma aldosterone concentration; platelet-associated complement; Policy Advisory Committee; premature atrial contraction

pac pachytene

PACE Pacing and Clinical Electrophysiology; personalized aerobics for cardiovascular enhancement; pulmonary angiotensin I converting enzyme

PA$_{CO}$ mean alveolar gas volume

P$_{ACO_2}$ partial pressure of carbon dioxide in alveolar gas

P$_{aCO2}$ partial pressure of carbon dioxide in arterial blood

PACP pulmonary alveolar-capillary permeability; pulmonary artery counterpulsation

PACS picture archiving and communication system

PACT papillary carcinoma of thyroid; precordial acceleration tracing

PACU postanesthetic care unit

PAD percutaneous abscess drainage; percutaneous automated discectomy; peripheral artery disease; phenacetin, aspirin, and desoxyephedrine; photon absorption densitometry; primary affective disorder; psychoaffective disorder; pulmonary artery diastolic; pulsatile assist device

PADP pulmonary artery diastolic pressure

PADUA progressive augmentation by dilating the urethra anterior

PAE progressive assistive exercise

p ae equal parts [Lat. *partes aequales*]

paed pediatrics, pediatric [*paediatrics, paediatric*]

PAEDP pulmonary artery end-diastolic pressure

PAES popliteal artery entrapment syndrome

PAF paroxysmal atrial fibrillation; phosphodiesterase-activating factor; platelet-activating factor; platelet-aggregating factor; pollen adherence factor; premenstrual assessment form; pulmonary arteriovenous fistula

PA&F percussion, auscultation, and fremitus

PAF-A platelet-activating factor of anaphylaxis

PAFD percutaneous abscess and fluid drainage; pulmonary artery filling defect

PAFI platelet-aggregation factor inhibitor

PAFIB paroxysmal atrial fibrillation

PAFP pre-Achilles fat pad

PAG periaqueductal gray [matter]; polyacrylamide gel; pregnancy-associated globulin

pAg protein A-gold [technique]

PAGE polyacrylamide gel electrophoresis

PAGIF polyacrylamide gel isoelectric focusing

PAGMK primary African green monkey kidney

PAH para-aminohippurate; polycyclic aromatic hydrocarbon; pulmonary artery hypertension; pulmonary artery hypotension

PAHA para-aminohippuric acid; procainamide-hydroxylamine

PAHO Pan-American Health Office

PAHVC pulmonary alveolar hypoxic vasoconstrictor

PAI plasminogen activator inhibitor

PAIC procedures, alternatives, indications, and complications

PAIDS paralyzed academic investigator's disease syndrome; pediatric acquired immunodeficiency syndrome

PAIgG platelet-associated immunoglobulin G

PAIRS Pain and Impairment Relationship Scale

PAIS partial androgen insensitivity syndrome; phosphoribosylaminoimidazole synthetase

PAJ paralysis agitans juvenilis

PAL pathology laboratory; posterior axillary line; product of activated lymphocytes; pyogenic abscess of the liver

pal palate

PALP placental alkaline phosphatase

palp palpation, palpate

palpi palpitation

PALS parietolateral lymphocyte sheath; prison-acquired lymphoproliferative syndrome

PAM pancreatic acinar mass; penicillin aluminum monostearate; phenylalaline mustard; p-methoxyamphetamine; postauricular myogenic; pralidoxime; pregnancy-associated α-macroglobulin; primary amebic meningoencephalitis; pulmonary alveolar macrophage; pulmonary alveolar microlithiasis; pulse amplitude modulation; pyridine aldoxime methiodide

PAMC pterygoarthromyodysplasia congenital

PAMD primary adrenocortical micronodular dysplasia

PAME primary amebic meningoencephalitis

PAMP pulmonary artery mean pressure

PAN periarteritis nodosa; periodic alternating nystagmus; peroxyacylnitrate; polyarteritis nodosa; positional alcohol nystagmus; puromycin aminonucleoside

pan pancreas, pancreatic, pancreatectomy

PAND primary adrenocortical nodular dysplasia

PANS puromycin aminonucleoside

PANSS Positive and Negative Syndrome Scale

PAO peak acid output; peripheral airway obstruction; plasma amine oxidase; polyamine oxidase; pustulotic arthroosteitis

PAo airway opening pressure; ascending aortic pressure; pulmonary artery occlusion pressure

P$_{AO2}$ partial pressure of oxygen in alveolar gas

PaO$_2$ partial pressure of oxygen in arterial blood

PAOD peripheral arterial occlusive disease; peripheral arteriosclerotic occlusive disease

PAOP pulmonary artery occlusion pressure

PAP Papanicolaou [test]; papaverine; passive-aggressive personality; patient assessment program; peak airway pressure; phosphoadenosine phosphate; peroxidase antibody to peroxidase; peroxidase-antiperoxidase [method]; placental acid/alkaline phosphatase; positive airway pressure; primary atypical pneumonia; prostatic acid phosphatase; pseudoallergic reaction; pulmonary alveolar proteinosis; pulmonary artery pressure; purified alternate pathway

Pap Papanicolaou test

pap papilla

PAPF platelet adhesiveness plasma factor

papova papilloma-polyoma-vacuolating agent [virus]

PAPP para-aminopropiophenone; pregnancy-associated plasma protein

PAPPC pregnancy-associated plasma protein C

PAPS 3'-phosphoadenosine-5'-phosphosulfate

Paps papillomas

Pap sm Papanicolaon smear

PAPUFA physiologically active polyunsaturated fatty acid

parv small [Lat. *parvus*]

pa-pv pulmonary arterial pressure–pulmonary venous pressure

PAPVC partial anomalous pulmonary venous connection

PAPVR partial anomalous pulmonary venous return

PAQ Personal Attitudes Questionnaire

PAR passive avoidance reaction; perennial allergic rhinitis; photosynthetically active radiation; physiological aging rate; platelet aggregate ratio; postanesthesia recovery; postanesthesia room; Program for Alcohol Recovery; proximal alveolar region; pulmonary arteriolar resistance

par paraffin; paralysis

PARA, Para, para number of pregnancies producing viable offspring

para paraplegic; parathyroid, parathyroidectomy

para 0 nullipara

para I primipara

para II secundipara

para III tripara

para IV quadripara

par aff the part affected [Lat. *pars affecta*]

parasit parasitology; parasite, parasitic

parasym parasympathetic

parent parenteral

parox paroxysm, paroxysmal

PARR postanesthesia recovery room

PARS Personal Adjustment and Role Skills Scale

part aeq equal parts [Lat. *partes aequales*]

part dolent painful parts [Lat. *partes dolentes*]

part vic in divided doses [Lat. *partitis vicibus*]

PARU postanesthetic recovery unit

PAS para aminosalicylate; Parent Attitude Scale; patient appointments and scheduling; periodic acid–Schiff [reaction]; peripheral anterior synechia; persistent atrial standstill; Personality Assessment Scale; photoacoustic spectroscopy; phosphatase acid serum; posterior airway space; pregnancy advisory service; premature atrial stimulus; Professional Activity Study; progressive accumulated stress; pulmonary arterial stenosis; pulmonary artery systolic

Pas pascal-second

Pa x s pascals per second

PASA para-aminosalicylic acid; primary acquired sideroblastic anemia; proximal articular set angle

PASAT Paced Auditory Serial Addition Task

PAS-C para-aminosalicylic acid crystallized with ascorbic acid

PASD after diastase digestion

PASG pneumatic antishock garment

PASH periodic acid–Schiff hematoxylin

PASM periodic acid–silver methenamine

pass passive

PAST periodic acid–Schiff technique

Past Pasteurella

PASVR pulmonary anomalous superior venous return

PAT Pain Apperception Test; paroxysmal atrial tachycardia; patient; phenylaminotetrazole; physical abilities test; picric acid turbidity; platelet aggregation test; polyamine acetyltransferase; preadmission assessment team/test; preadmission testing; predictive ability test; pregnancy at term; psychoacoustic test

pat patella; patent; paternal origin; patient

PATE psychodynamic and therapeutic education; pulmonary artery thromboembolism

PATH pathology, pathological; pituitary adrenotropic hormone

path pathogenesis, pathogenic; pathology, pathological

PAT-SED pseudoachondroplastic dysplasia

PA-T-SP periodic acid–thiocarbohydrazide–silver proteinate

PAV percutaneous aortic valvuloplasty; poikiloderma atrophicans vasculare; posterior arch vein

pavex passive vascular exercise

PAVF pulmonary arteriovenous fistula

PAVNRT paroxysmal atrioventricular nodal reciprocal tachycardia

PAW peripheral airways; pulmonary artery wedge

Paw mean airway pressure

PAWP pulmonary arterial wedge pressure

PAWS primary withdrawal syndrome

PB British pharmacopeia [*Pharmacopoeia Britannica*]; paraffin bath; Paul-Bunnell [antibody]; periodic breathing; peripheral blood; peroneus brevis; phenobarbital; phenoxybenzamine phonetically balanced; pinealoblastoma; polymyxin B; premature beat; pressure breathing; protein binding; punch biopsy

Pb lead [Lat. *plumbum*]; phenobarbital; presbyopia

P&B pain & burning; phenobarbital and belladonna

PBA polyclonal B-cell activity; pressure breathing assist; prolactin-binding assay; prune belly anomaly; pulpobuccoaxial

PBB polybrominated biphenyl

Pb-B lead in blood

PBBs polybrominated biphenyls

PBC peripheral blood cell; point of basal convergence; pre-bed care; primary biliary cirrhosis; progestin-binding complement

PBD postburn day

PBE tuberculin from *Mycobacterium tuberculosis bovis* [Ger. *Perlsucht Bacillen-emulsion*]

PBF peripheral blod flow; placental blood flow; pulmonary blood flow

PBFe protein-bound iron

PBG porphobilinogen

PBG-S porphobilinogen synthase

PBH pulling boat hands

PBHB poly-beta-hydroxybutyrate

PBI parental bonding instrument; penile pressure/brachial pressure index; protein-bound iodine

PbI lead intoxication

PBIgG platelet surface bound immunoglobulin G

PBK phosphorylase B kinase

PBL peripheral blood leukocyte; peripheral blood lymphocyte

PBLC peripheral blood lymphocyte count

PBLT peripheral blood lymphocyte transformation

PBM peripheral basement membrane; peripheral blood mononuclear [cell]; placental basement membrane

PBMC peripheral blood mononuclear cell

PBMV pulmonary blood mixing volume

PBN paralytic brachial neuritis; peripheral benign neoplasm; polymyxin B sulfate, bacitracin, and neomycin

PBNA partial body neutron activation

PBO penicillin in beeswax and oil; placebo

PBP penicillin-binding protein; porphyrin biosynthesis pathway; prostate-binding protein; pseudobulbar palsy; pulsatile bypass pump

PBPI penile–brachial pulse index

PBS perfusion-pressure breakthrough syndrome; phenobarbital sodium; phosphate-buffered saline; planar bone scan; primer binding site; prune belly syndrome; pulmonary branch stenosis

PBSP prognostically bad signs during pregnancy

PBT Paul-Bunnell test; phenacetin breath test; profile-based therapy

PBT$_4$ protein-bound thyroxine

PBV predicted blood volume; pulmonary blood volume

PBW posterior bite wing

PBZ personal breathing zone; phenylbutazone; phenoxybenzamine; pyribenzamine

PC avoirdupois weight [Lat. *pondus civile*]; packed cells; paper chromatography; paracortex; parent cell; particulate component; partition coefficient; penicillin; pentose cycle; peritoneal cell; pharmacology; pheochromocytoma; phosphate cycle; phosphatidylcholine; phosphocreatine; phosphorylcholine; photoconduction; physicians' corporation; pill counter; piriform cortex; plasma concentration; plasma cortisol; plasmacytoma; plasmin complex; platelet concentrate; platelet count; pneumotaxic center; polycentric; polyposis coli; poor condition; poor coordination; portacaval; portal cirrhosis; postcoital; posterior cervical; posterior chamber; posterior commissure; posterior cortex; precordial; prenatal care; present complaint; primary closure; printed circuit; procollagen; productive cough; professional corporation; prostatic carcinoma; protein C; proximal colon; pseudocyst; pubococcygeus [muscle]; pulmonary capillary; pulmonary circulation; pulmonic closure; Purkinje cell; pyloric canal; pyruvate carboxylase

pc after meals [Lat. *post cibum*]; parsec; percent; picocurie

PCA para-chloramphetamine; parietal cell antibody; passive cutaneous anaphylaxis; patient care assistant/aide; patient-controlled analgesia; perchloric acid; percutaneous carotid angiography; polyclonal antibody; porous coated anatomic [prosthesis]; portacaval anastomosis; posterior cerebral artery; posterior communicating aneurysm/artery; precoronary care area; President's Council on Aging; principal components analysis; procoagulant activity; prostatic carcinoma; pyrrolidine carboxylic acid

PCB paracervical block; polychlorinated biphenyl; portacaval bypass; procarbazine

PcB near point of convergence to the intercentral base line [*punctum convergens basalis*]

PC-BMP phosphorylcholine—binding myeloma protein

PCC Pasteur Culture Collection; percutaneous cecostomy; pheochromocytoma; phosphate carrier compound; plasma catecholamine concentration; pneumatosis cystoides coli; Poison Control Center; precoronary care; premature chromosome condensation; primary care clinic; prothrombin complex concentration

PCc periscopic concave

pcc premature chromosome condensation

PCCU post-coronary care unit

PCD papillary collecting duct; paraneoplastic cerebellar degeneration; paroxysmal cerebral dysrhythmia; phosphate-citrate-dextrose; plasma cell dyscrasia; polycystic disease; posterior corneal deposits; premature centromere division; primary ciliary dyskinesia; prolonged contractile duration; pulmonary clearance delay

PCDC plasma clot diffusion chamber

PCDF polychorinated dibenzofuran

PCE physical capacity evaluation; pseudocholinesterase

PCF peripheral circulatory failure; pharyngoconjunctival fever; platelet complement fixation; posterior cranial fossa; prothrombin conversion factor

pcf pounds per cubic feet

PCFT platelet complement fixation test

PCG paracervical ganglion; phonocardiogram; primate chorionic gonadotropin; pubococcygeus [muscle]

PCH paroxysmal cold hemoglobinuria; polycyclic hydrocarbon

PCHE pseudocholinesterase

PCI prophylactic cranial irradiation

pCi picocurie

PCI pneumatosis cystoides intestinales

PCIC Poison Control Information Center

PC-IRV pressure-controlled inverted ratio ventilation

PCIS Patient-Care Information System; postcardiac injury syndrome

PCK polycystic kidney

PCKD polycystic kidney disease

PCL pacing cycle length; persistent corpus luteum; plasma cell leukemia; posterior chamber lens; posterior cruciate ligament

PCM primary cutaneous melanoma; process control monitor; protein-calorie malnutrition; protein carboxymethylase

PCMO Principal Clinical Medical Officer

PCMT pacemaker circus movement tachycardia

PCN penicillin; primary care nursing

PCNA proliferating cell nuclear antigen

PCNB pentachloronitrobenzene

PCNL percutaneous nephrostolithotomy

PCNV postchemotherapy nausea and vomiting; Provisional Committee on Nomenclature of Viruses

PCO patient complains of; polycystic ovary; predicted cardiac output

P_{CO} partial pressure of carbon monoxide

P_{CO_2}, pCO_2 partial pressure of carbon dioxide

PCOD polycystic ovarian disease

PCOS polycystic ovary syndrome

PCP parachlorophenate; patient care plan; pentachlorophenol; 1-(1-phenylcyclohexyl)piperidine; peripheral coronary pressure; persistent cough and phlegm; phencyclidine; *Pneumocystis carinii* pneumonia; postoperative constrictive pericarditis; primary care physician; prochlorperazine; procollagen peptide; pulmonary capillary pressure; pulse cytophotometry

PCPA para-chlorophenylalanine

PCPL pulmonary capillary protein leakage

pcpn precipitation

PCQ polychloroquaterphenyl

PCR patient contact record; phosphocreatinine; plasma clearance rate; polymerase chain reaction; protein catabolism rate

PCr phosphocreatine

PCS palliative care service; Patient Care System; patterns of care study; pelvic congestion syndrome; pharmacogenic confusional syndrome; portacaval shunt; post–cardiac surgery; postcardiotomy syndrome; postcholecystectomy syndrome; postconcussion syndrome; premature centromere separation; primary cancer site; prolonged crush syndrome; proportional counter spectrometry; proximal coronary sinus; pseudotumor cerebri syndrome

pcs preconscious

PCSM percutaneous stone manipulation

PCT peripheral carcinoid tumor; plasma clotting time; plasmacrit test; plasmacytoma; polychlorinated triphenyl; polychlorinated triphenyl; porphyria cutanea tarda; portacaval transposition; positron computed tomography; progesterone challenge test; prothrombin consumption time; proximal convoluted tubule

pct percent

PCU pain control unit; primary care unit; pulmonary care unit

PCV packed cell volume; polycythemia vera; postcapillary venule

PCV-M polycythemia vera with myeloid metaplasia

PCW pericanalicular web; primary capillary wedge; purified cell walls

PCWP pulmonary capillary wedge pressure

PCx periscopic convex

PCZ procarbazine; prochlorperazine

PD Doctor of Pharmacy; Dublin Pharmacopoeia; interpupillary distance; Paget disease; pancreatic duct; papilla diameter; paralyzing dose; Parkinson disease; parkinsonian dementia; paroxysmal discharge; pars distalis; patent ductus; pediatric, pediatrics; percentage difference; percutaneous drain; peritoneal dialysis; personality disorder; phenyldichlorarsine; phosphate dehydrogenase; phosphate dextrose; photosensitivity dermatitis; Pick disease; plasma defect; poorly differentiated; posterior division; postnasal drainage; postural drainage; potential difference; pregnanediol; present disease; pressor dose; prism diopter; problem drinker; progression of disease; protein degradation; problem degradation; protein diet; psychotic depression; pulmonary disease; pulpodistal; pulse duration; pupillary distance; pyloric dilator

2-PD two-point discrimination

Pd palladium; pediatrics

pd for the day [Lat. *pro die*]; prism diopter

PDA patent ductus arteriosus; posterior descending artery; pulmonary disease anemia

PdA pediatric allergy

PDAB para-dimethylaminobenzaldehyde

PD/AR photosensitivity dermatitis and actinic reticuloid syndrome

PDB Paget disease of bone; paradichlorobenzene; phosphorus-dissolving bacteria; preventive dental [health] behavior

PDC parkinsonism dementia complex; pediatric cardiology; penta-decylcatechol; physical dependence capacity; plasma dioxin concentration; preliminary diagnostic clinic; private diagnostic clinic

PdC pediatric cardiology

PDCD primary degenerative cerebral disease

PD-CSE pulsed Doppler cross-sectional echocardiography

PDD pervasive developmental disorder; platinum diamminodichloride [cisplatin]; primary degenerative dementia; pyridoxine-deficient diet

PDE paroxysmal dyspnea on exertion; phosphodiesterase; progressive dialysis encephalopathy; pulsed Doppler echocardiography

PdE pediatric endocrinology

PDF Parkinson's Disease Foundation; peritoneal dialysis fluid; pyruvate dehydrogenase

PDG parkinsonism-dementia complex of Guam; phosphogluconate dehydrogenase

PDGA pteroyldiglutamic acid

PDGF platelet-derived growth factor

PDGS partial form of DiGeorge's syndrome

PDH past dental history; phosphate dehydrogenase; progressive disseminated histoplasmosis; pyruvate dehydrogenase

PDHa pyruvate dehydrogenase in active form

PDHC pyruvate dehydrogenase complex

PdHO pediatric hematology-oncology

PDI periodontal disease index; plan-do integration; psychomotor development index

Pdi transdiaphragmatic pressure

PDIE phosphodiesterase

P-diol pregnanediol

PDL pancreatic duct ligation; periodontal ligament; poorly differentiated lymphocyte; population doubling level; progressive diffuse leukoencephalopathy

pdl poundal; pudendal

PDLC poorly differentiated lung cancer

PDLD poorly differentiated lymphocytic–diffuse

PDLL poorly differentiated lymphocytic lymphoma

PDLN poorly differentiated lymphocytic–nodular

PDMS patient data management system; pharmacokinetic drug monitoring service

PDN prednisone

PdNEO pediatric neonatology

PdNEP pediatric nephrology

PDP pattern disruption point; piperidinopyrimidine; platelet-derived plasma; primer-dependent deoxynucleic acid polymerase; Product Development Protocol

PDPD prolonged-dwell peritoneal dialysis

PDPI primer-dependent deoxynucleic acid polymerase index

PDQ Personality Diagnostic Questionnaire; Physician's Data Query; Premenstrual Distress Questionnaire; protocol data query

PDR pediatric radiology; peripheral diabetic retinopathy; *Physicians' Desk Reference*; postdelivery room; primary drug resistance; proliferative diabetic retinopathy

PdR pediatric radiology

pdr powder

PDRB Permanent Diability Rating Board

PDRT Portland Digit Recognition

PDS pain-dysfunction syndrome; paroxysmal depolarizing shift; patient data system; pediatric surgery; peritoneal dialysis system; plasma-derived serum; polydioxanone sutures; predialyzed serum

PdS pediatric surgery

PDSG pigment dispersion syndrome glaucoma

PDT photodynamic therapy; population doubling time

PDUF pulsed Doppler ultrasonic flowmeter

PDUR Predischarge Utilization Review

PDV peak disatolic velocity

PDW platelet distribution width

PE Edinburgh Pharmacopoeia; pancreatic extract; paper electrophoresis; partial epilepsy; pelvic examination; penile erection; pericardial effusion; peritoneal exudate; pharyngoesophageal; phenylethylamine; phenylephrine; phosphatidyl ethanolamine; photographic effect; phycoerythrin; physical education; physical examination; physical exercise; physiological ecology; pigmented epithelium; pilocarpine-epinephrine; placental extract; plasma exchange; pleural effusion; point of entry; polyethylene; potential energy; powdered extract; preeclampsia; preexcitation; present evaluation; pressure equalization; prior to exposure; probable error; professional engineer; pseudoexfoliation; pulmonary edema; pulmonary embolism; pyrogenic exotoxin

Pe pressure on expiration

PEA pelvic examination under anesthesia; phenylethyl alcohol; phenylethylamine; polysaccharide egg antigen

PEAP positive end-airway pressure

PEBG phenethylbiguanide

PEC pelvic cramps; peritoneal exudate cell; pyrogenic exotoxin C

PED, ped pediatrics

PeDS Pediatric Drug Surveillance

PEEP positive end-expiratory pressure, peak end-expiratory pressure

PEEPi intrinsic peak end-expiratory pressure

PEF peak expiratory flow; Psychiatric Evaluation Form; pulmonary edema fluid

PEFR peak expiratory flow rate

PEFV partial expiratory flow volume

PEG Patient Evaluation Grid; percutaneous endoscopic gastrostomy; pneumoencephalogram, pneumoencephalography; polyethylene glycol

PEI phosphate excretion index; physical efficiency index; polyethyleneimine

PEL peritoneal exudate lymphocyte; permissible exposure limit

pelidisi weight ten line divided sitting height [Lat. *pondus decies linearis divisus sidentis (altitudo)*]

PEM peritoneal exudate macrophage; prescription event monitoring; primary enrichment medium; probable error of measurement; protein energy malnutrition

PEMA phenylethylmalonamide

Pen penicillin

Pent pentothal

PEO progressive external ophthalmoplegia

PEP peptidase; phospho(enol)pyruvate; pigmentation, edema, and plasma cell dyscrasia [syndrome]; polyestradiol phosphate; postencephalitic parkinsonism; pre-ejection period; protein electrophoresis

Pep peptidase

PEPA peptidase A

PEPB peptidase B

PEPC peptidase C

PEPc corrected pre-ejection period

PEPCK phosphoenolpyruvate carboxykinase

PEPD peptidase D

PEPE peptidase E

PEPI pre-ejection period index

PEPP positive expiratory pressure plateau

PEPS peptidase S

PER peak ejection rate; protein efficiency ratio

per perineal; periodicity, periodic

percus percussion

perf perforation

PERG pattern electroretinogram

PERI Psychiatric Epidemiology Research Interview

periap periapical

Perio periodontics

PERK prospective evaluation of radial keratotomy [protocol]

PERLA pupils equal, react to light and accommodation

per op emet when the action of emetic is over [Lat. *peracta operatione emetici*]

perp perpendicular

PERRLA pupils equal, round, react to light and accommodation

PERS Patient Evaluation Rating Scale

PERT program evaluation and review technique

PES photoelectron spectroscopy; physicians' equity services; polyethylene sulfonate; postextrasystolic; preepiglottic space; preexcitation syndrome; primary empty sella [syndrome]; pseudoexfoliative syndrome

PESP postextrasystolic potentiation

Pess pessary

PET peak ejection time; poor exercise tolerance; positron emission tomography; preeclamptic toxemia; progressive exercise test; psychiatric emergency team

PET$_{CO2}$ end-tidal pressure of carbon dioxide

PETH pink-eyed, tan-hooded [rat]

PETN pentaerythritol tetranitrate

petr petroleum

PETT pendular eye-tracking test; positron emission transverse tomography

PEU plasma equivalent unit

PEV peak expiratory velocity

pev peak electron volts

PEW pulmonary extravascular water

PEWV pulmonary extravascular water volume

PEx physical examination

PF pair feeding; peak flow; perfusion fluid; pericardial fluid; peritoneal fluid; permeability factor; personality factor; picture-frustration [study]; plantar flexion; plasma factor; platelet factor; pleural fluid; power factor; primary fibrinolysin; prostatic fluid; pulmonary factor; pulmonary function; Purkinje fiber; purpura fulminans; push fluids

P-F picture-frustration [test]

P$_f$ final pressure

PF$_{1-4}$ platelet factors 1 to 4

Pf *Plasmodium falciparum*

pF picofarad

PFA p-fluorophenylalanine; phosphonoformate

PFAS performic acid–Schiff [reaction]

PFC pair-fed control [mice]; pelvic flexion contracture; perfluorocarbon; pericardial fluid culture; persistent fetal circulation; plaque-forming cell

pFc noncovalently bonded dimer of the C-terminal immunoglobulin of the Fc fragment

PFD polyostotic fibrous dysplasia

PFDA perfluoro-n-decanoic acid

PFFD proximal focal femoral deficiency

PFG peak flow gauge

PFGE pulsed field gel electrophoresis

PFIB perfluoroisobutylene

PFK phosphofructokinase

PFKL phosphofructokinase, liver type

PFKM phosphofructokinase, muscle type

PFKP phosphofructokinase, platelet type

PFL profibrinolysin

PFM peak flow meter

PFN partially functional neutrophil

PFO patent foramen ovale

PFP peripheral facial paralysis; platelet-free plasma

PFPS patellofemoral pain syndrome

PFQ personality factor questionnaire

PFR parotid flow rate; peak flow rate

PFRC predicted functional residual capacity

PFS primary fibromyalgia syndrome; protein-free supernatant; pulmonary function score

PFT pancreatic function test; parafascicular thalamotomy; posterior fossa tumor; prednisone, fluorouracil, and tax-omifen; pulmonary function test

PFTBE progressive form of tick-borne encephalitis

PFU plaque-forming unit; pock-forming unit

PFUO prolonged fever of unknown origin

PFV physiologic full value

PG paregoric; parotid gland; pentagastrin; pepsinogen; peptidoglycan; Pharmacopoeia Germanica; phosphate glutamate; phosphatidylglycerol; phosphogluconate; pigment granule; pituitary gonadotropin; plasma glucose; plasma triglyceride; polyfalacturonate; postgraduate; pregnanediol glucuronide; pregnant; progesterone; prolyl hydrolase; propylene glycol; Prospect Hill [virus]; prostaglandin; proteoglycan; pyoderma gangrenosum

Pg nasopharyngeal electrode placement in electroencephalography; gastric pressure; pogonion; pregnancy, pregnant

pg picogram; pregnant

PGA pepsinogen A; phosphoglyceric acid; polyglandular autoimmune [syndrome]; prostaglandin A; pteroylglutamic acid

PGA$_{1-3}$ prostaglandins A$_1$ to A$_3$

PGAM phosphoglycerate mutase

PGAS persisting galactorrhea-amenorrhea syndrome; polyglandular autoimmune syndrome

PGB prostaglandin B

PGC primordial germ cell

PGD phosphogluconate dehydrogenase; phosphoglyceraldehyde dehydrogenase; prostaglandin D

PGD$_2$ prostaglandin D$_2$

6-PGD 6-phosphogluconate dehydrogenase

PGDH phosphogluconate dehydrogenase

PGDR plasma glucose disappearance rate

PGE platelet granule exract; posterior gastroenterostomy

PGE, PGE$_1$, PGE$_2$ prostaglandins E, E$_1$, E$_2$

PGF, PGF$_1$, PGF$_2$ prostaglandins F, F$_1$, F$_2$

PGFT phosphoribosylglycinamide formyltransferase

PG prostaglandin G

PGG polyclonal gamma globulin

PGG$_2$ prostaglandin G$_2$

PGH pituitary growth hormone; porcine growth hormone; prostaglandin H

PGH$_2$ prostaglandin H$_2$

PGI phosphoglucose isomerase; potassium, glucose, and insulin; prostaglandin I

PGI$_2$ prostaglandin I$_2$

PGK phosphoglycerate kinase

PGL persistent generalized lymphadenopathy; phosphoglycolipid

PGlyM phosphoglyceromutase

PGM phosphoglucomutase

PGN proliferative glomerulonephritis

PGO ponto-geniculo-occipital [spike]

PGP phosphoglyceroyl phosphatase; postgamma proteinuria; prepaid group practice; progressive general paralysis

PGR progesterone receptor; psychogalvanic response

PgR progesterone receptor

PGS peristent gross splenomegaly; plant growth substance; postsurgical gastroparesis syndrome; prostaglandin synthetase

PGSI prostaglandin synthetase inhibitor

PGSR phosphogalvanic skin response

PGTR plasma glucose tolerance rate

PGTT prednisolone glucose tolerance test

PGU peripheral glucose uptake; postgonococcal urethritis

PGUT phosphogalactose uridyl transferase

PGV proximal gastric vagotomy

PGX prostacyclin

PGY postgraduate year

PGYE peptone, glucose yeast extract

PH parathyroid hormone; partial hepatectomy; partial hysterectomy; passive hemagglutination; past history; patient's history; persistent hepatitis; personal history; pharmacopeia; physical history; porphyria hepatica; posterior hypothalamus; previous history; primary hyperparathyroidism; prostatic hypertrophy; pseudohermaphroditism; public health; pulmonary hypertension; pulmonary hypoplasia

Ph pharmacopeia; phenyl; Philadelphia [chromosome]; phosphate

Ph¹ Philadelphia chromosome

pH hydrogen ion concentration

pH₁ isoelectric point

ph phial; phot

PHA passive hemagglutination-inhibition assay; peripheral hyperalimentation; phenylalanine; phytohemagglutinin; phytohemagglutinin antigen; pseudohypoaldosteronism; pulse-height analyzer

pH_A arterial blood hydrogen tension

PHAL phytohemagglutinin-stimulated lymphocyte

phal phalangeal

PHA-LCM phytohemagglutinin-stimulated leukocyte conditioned medium

PHAP phytohemagglutinin protein

phar pharmaceutical; pharmacy; pharynx

Phar B Bachelor of Pharmacy [Lat. *Pharmaciae Baccalaureus*]

Phar C pharmaceutical chemist

Phar D Doctor of Pharmacy [Lat. *Pharmaciae Doctor*]

PHARM pharmacy

Phar M Master of Pharmacy [Lat. *Pharmaciae Magister*]

pharm pharmacist; pharmacology; pharmacopeia; pharmacy

PHB polyhydroxybutyrate; preventive health behavior

PhB, Phb Pharmacopoeia Britannica

PHBB propylhydroxybenzyl benzimidazole

PHC personal health costs; posthospital care; premolar hypodontia, hyperhidrosis, [premature] canities [syndrome]; primary health care; primary hepatic carcinoma; proliferative helper cell

PhC pharmaceutical chemist

Ph¹ c Philadelphia chromosome

PHCC primary hepatocellular carcinoma

PHD pathological habit disorder; postheparin plasma diamine oxidase; potentially harmful drug

PhD Doctor of Pharmacy [Lat. *Pharmaciae Doctor*]; Doctor of Philosophy [Lat. *Philosophiae Doctor*]

PHE periodic health examination

Phe phenylalanine

PhEEM photoemission electron microscopy

Pheo pheochromocytoma

PHF paired helical filament; personal hygiene facility

PHFG primary human fetal glia

PhG Graduate in Pharmacy; Pharmacopoeia Germanica

phgly phenylglycine

PHI passive hemagglutination inhibition; past history of illness; phosphohexose isomerase; physiological hyaluronidase inhibitor

PhI Pharmacopoeia Internationalis

φ Greek letter *phi*; magnetic flux; osmotic coefficient

PHIM posthypoxic intention myoclonus

PHK platelet phosphohexokinase; postmortem human kidney

PHLA postheparin lipolytic activity

PHLS Public Health Laboratory Service

PHM peptide histidine methionine; posterior hyaloid membrane; pulmonary hyaline membrane

PhM Master of Pharmacy [Lat. *Pharmaciae Magister*]; pharyngeal muscle

PhmG Graduate in Pharmacy

PHN paroxysmal noctural hemoglobinuria; passive Heymann nephritis; postherpetic neuralgia; public health nursing, public health nurse

PH₂O partial pressure of water vapor

phos phosphate

PHP postheparin phospholipase; prehospital program; prepaid health plan; primary hyperparathyroidism; pseudohypoparathyroidism

p-HPPO p-hydroxyphenyl pyruvate oxidase

PHPT primary hyperparathyroidism; pseudohypoparathyroidism

pHPT primary hyperparathyroidism

PHPV persistent hyperplastic primary vitreous

PHR peak heart rate; photoreactivity

PHS Physician's Health Study; pooled human serum; posthypnotic suggestion; Public Health Service

PHSC pleuripotent hemopoietic stem cell

pH-stat apparatus for maintaining the pH of a solution

PHT phenytoin; portal hypertension; primary hyperthyroidism; pulmonary hypertension

PhTD Doctor of Physical Therapy

PHV peak height velocity; Prospect Hill virus

PHX pulmonary histiocytosis X

Phx past history; pharynx

PHY pharyngitis; physical; physiology

PHYS physiology

PhyS physiologic saline [solution]

phys physical; physician

Phys Ed physical education

physio physiology; physiotherapy

Phys Med physical medicine

Phys Ther physical therapy

PI first meiotic prophase; isoelectric point; pacing impulse; package insert; pancreatic insufficiency; parainfluenza; pars intermedia; patient's interest; performance intensity; perinatal injury; periodontal index; permeability index; personal injury; personality inventory; Pharmacopoeia Internationalis; phosphatidylinositol; physically impaired; pineal body; plaque index; plasmin inhibitor; pneumatosis intestinalis; poison ivy; ponderal index; postictal immobility; postinfection; postinfluenza; postinjury; postinoculation; preinduction [examination]; premature infant; prematurity index; preparatory interval; present illness; primary infarction; primary infection; principal investigator; product information; proinsulin; prolactin inhibitor; protamine insulin; protease inhibitor; proximal intestine; pulmonary incompetence; pulmonary infarction; pulsatility index

P$_I$ inspiratory pressure

Pi, P$_i$ inorganic phosphate

Pi parental generation; pressure in inspiration; protease inhibitor

pI isoelectric point

Π Greek capital letter *pi*

π Greek lower case letter *pi;* the ratio of circumference to diameter, 3.1415926536

PIA photoelectric intravenous angiography; plasma insulin activity; preinfarction angina; Psychiatric Institute of America

PIAT Peabody Individual Achievement Test

PIAVA polydactyly–imperforate anus–vertebral anomalies [syndrome]

PIBC percutaneous intraaortic balloon counterpulsation [catheter]

PIC Personality Inventory for Children; polymorphism information content

PICA percutaneous transluminal coronary angioplasty; Porch Index of Communicative Abilities; posterior inferior cerebellar artery; posterior inferior communicating artery

PICC peripherally inserted central catheter

PICD primary irritant contact dermatitis

PICFS postinfective chronic fatigue syndrome

PICSO pressure-controlled intermittent coronary sinus occlusion

PICU pediatric intensive care unit; pulmonary intensive care unit

PID pain intensity difference [score]; pelvic inflammatory disease; photoionization detector; plasma iron disappearance; postinertia dyskinesia; prolapsed/protruded intervertebral disk

PIDRA portable insulin dosage regulating apparatus

PIDS primary immunodeficiency syndrome

PIDT plasma iron disappearance time

PIE postinfectious encephalomyelitis preimplantation embryo; prosthetic infectious endocarditis; pulmonary infiltration with eosinophilia; pulmonary interstitial emphysema

PIF paratoid isoelectric focusing variant protein; peak inspiratory flow; proinsulin-free; prolactin-inhibiting factor; proliferation-inhibiting factor; prostatic interstitial fluid

PIFG poor intrauterine fetal growth

PIFR peak inspiratory flow rate

PIFT platelet immunofluorescence test

pigm pigment, pigmented

PIH periventricular-intraventricular hemorrhage; phenyl isopropylhydrazine; pregnancy-induced hypertension; prolactin-inhibiting hormone

PII plasma inorganic iodine; primary irritation index

PIIP portable insulin infusion pump

PIIS posterior inferior iliac spine

PIL patient information leaflet

pil pill [Lat. *pilula*]

πm pi meson

PILBD paucity of interlobular bile ducts

PIM penicillamine-induced myasthenia

PIN product identification number

PINN proposed international nonproprietary name

PINV postimperative negative variation

PIO$_2$ partial pressure of inspired oxygen

PION posterior ischemic optic neuropathy

PIP paralytic infantile paralysis; peak inflation pressure, peak inspiratory pressure; piperacillin; pressure inversion point; proximal interphalangeal; Psychotic Inpatient Profile; psychosis, intermittent hyponatremia, polydipsia [syndrome];

posterior interphalangeal; probable intrauterine pregnancy

PIPE persistent interstitial pulmonary emphysema

PIPJ proximal interphalangeal joint

PIQ Performance Intelligence Quotient

PIR postinhibition rebound

PIRI plasma immunoreactive insulin

PIRS plasma immunoreactive secretion

PIS preinfarction syndrome; primary immunodeficiency syndrome; Provisional International Standard

pIs isoelectric point

PISCES percutaneously inserted spinal cord electrical stimulation

PIT pacing-induced tachycardia; patella inhibition test; picture identification test; pitocin; pitressin; plasma iron turnover

pit pituitary

PITC phenylisothiocyanate

PITR plasma iron turnover rate

PIU polymerase-inducing unit

PIV parainfluenza virus; polydactyly–imperforate anus–vertebral anomalies [syndrome]

PIVD protruded intervertebral disk

PIVH peripheral intravenous hyperalimentation; periventricular-intraventricular hemorrhage

PIVKA protein induced by vitamin K absence or antagonism

PIXE particle-induced x-ray emission; proton-induced x-ray emission

PJ pancreatic juice; Peutz-Jeghers [syndrome]

PJB premature junctional beat

PJC premature junctional contractions

PJP pancreatic juice protein

PJS peritoneojugular shunt; Peutz-Jeghers syndrome

PJT paroxysmal junctional tachycardia

PK penetrating keratoplasty; pericardial knock; pharmacokinetics; pig kidney; Prausnitz-Küstner [reaction]; protein kinase; psychokinesis; pyruvate kinase

pK negative logarithm of the dissociation constant

pK' apparent value of a pK; negative

logarithm of the dissociation constant of an acid

pk peck

PkA prekallikrein activator

pK$_a$ negative logarithm of the acid ionization constant

PKAR protein kinase activation ratio

PKase protein kinase

PKD polycystic kidney disease; proliferative kidney disease

PKI potato kallikrein inhibitor

PKK plasma prekallikrein

PKN parkinsonism

PKP penetrating keratoplasty

PKR phased knee rehabilitation; Prausnitz-Küstner reaction

PKT Prausnitz-Küstner test

PKU phenylketonuria

PKV killed poliomyelitis vaccine

pkV peak kilovoltage

PL palmaris longus; pancreatic lipase; perception of light; peroneus longus; phospholipid; photoluminescence; placebo; placental lactogen; plantar; plasma lemma; plastic surgery; platelet lactogen; polarized light; preleukemia; prolymphocytic leukemia; pulpolingual; Purkinje's layer

Pl poiseuille

P$_L$ transpulmonary pressure

pl picoliter; placenta; plasma; platelet

PL/I programming language I (one)

PLA peripheral laser angioplasty; phenyl lactate; phospholipase A; phospholipid antibody; placebo therapy; plasminogen activator; platelet antigen; polylactic acid; potentially lethal arrhythmia; procaine/lactic acid; pulp linguoaxial

P$_{LA}$ left atrial pressure

PLa pulpolabial

Pla left atrial pressure

PLA2 phospholipase A2

PLAP placental alkaline phosphatase

PLB parietal lobe battery; phospholipase B; porous layer bead

PLC phospholipase C; primary liver cancer; proinsulin-like component; pro-

tein-lipid complex; pseudolymphocytic choriomeningitis

PLCC primary liver cell cancer

PLCO postoperative low cardiac output

PLD peripheral light detection; phospholipase D; platelet defect; polycystic liver disease; posterior latissimus dorsi [muscle]; potentially lethal damage

PLDH plasma lactic dehydrogenase

PLDR potentially lethal damage repair

PLE paraneoplastic limbic encephalopathy; protein-losing enteropathy; pseudolupus erythematosus

PLED periodic lateral epileptiform discharge

PLES parallel-line equal space

PLET polymyxin, lysozyme, EDTA, and thallous acetate [in heart infusion agar]

PLEVA pityriasis lichenoides et varioliformis acuta

PLF perilymphatic fistula; posterior lung fiber

PLFS perilymphatic fistula syndrome

PLG plasminogen; L-propyl-L-leucyl-glucinamide

P-LGV psittacosis-lymphogranuloma venereum

PLH placental lactogenic hormone

PLI professional liability insurance

PLL peripheral light loss; poly-L-lysine; pressure length loop; prolymphocytic leukemia

PLM percent labeled mitoses; periodic leg movement; plasma level monitoring; polarized light microscopy

PLMV posterior leaf mitral valve

PLN peripheral lymph node

PLND pelvic lymph node dissection

PLO polycystic lipomembranous osteodysplasia

PLP phospholipid; plasma leukapheresis; polypeptide; polystyrene latex particles; pyridoxal phosphate

PLR pupillary light reflex

PLS Papillon-Lefèvre syndrome; polydactyly-luxation syndrome; preleukemic syndrome; primary lateral sclerosis;

prostaglandin-like substance; pulmonary leukostasis syndrome

PLT pancreatic lymphocytic infiltration; platelet; primed lymphocyte test; primed lymphocyte typing; psittacosis–lymphogranuloma venereum–trachoma [group]

plumb lead [Lat. *plumbum*]

PLUT Plutchnik [geriatric rating scale]

PLV poliomyelitis live vaccine; panleukopenia virus; phenylalanine, lysine, and vasopressin; posterior light ventricle

PLWS Prader-Labhart-Willi syndrome

plx plexus

PLZ phenelzine

PM after noon [Lat. *post meridiem*]; mean pressure; pacemaker; papillary muscle; papular mucinosis; partial meniscectomy; perinatal mortality; peritoneal macrophage; petit mal epilepsy [Fr. *petit mal*]; photomultiplier; physical medicine; plasma membrane; platelet membrane; platelet microsome; pneumomediastinum; poliomyelitis; polymorph, polymorphonuclear; polymyositis; porokeratosis of Mibelli; posterior mitral; postmenstrual; postmortem; premarketing [approval]; premenstrual; premolar; presystolic murmur; pretibial myxedema; preventive medicine; primary motivation; prostatic massage; protein methylesterase; protocol management; pterygoid muscle; pubertal macromastia; pulmonary macrophage; pulpomesial

Pm paratid midle [band protein]; promethium

pM picomolar

pm picometer

PMA index of prevalence and severity of gingivitis, where P = papillary gingiva, M = marginal gingiva, and A = attached gingiva; papillary, marginal, attached [gingiva]; para-methoxyamphetamine; Pharmaceutical Manufacturers Association; phenylmercuric acetate; phorbol myristate acetate; phosphomolybdic acid; premarket approval; primary mental abilities; progressive muscular atrophy; pyridylmercuric acetate

PMB papillomacular bundle; parahydroxymercuribenzoate; polychrome methylene blue; polymorphonuclear basophil; polymyxin B; postmenopausal bleeding

PMC phenylmercuric chloride; physical medicine clinic; pleural mesothelial click; premature mitral closure; pseudomembranous colitis

PMD posterior mandibular depth; primary myocardial disease; programmed multiple development; progressive muscular dystrophy

PM/DM polymyositis/dermatomyositis

PMDS peristent müllerian duct syndrome; primary myelodysplastic syndrome

PME polymorphonuclear eosinophil; progressive myoclonus epilepsy

PMEA 9-(2-phosphomethoxyethyl) adenine

PMF progressive massive fibrosis; proton motive force; pterygomaxillary fossa

pmf proton motive force

PMGCT primary mediastinal germ-cell tumor

PMH past medical history; posteromedial hypothalamus

PMHR predicted maximum heart rate

PMI past medical illness; patient medication instruction; perioperative myocardial infarction; point of maximal impulse; point of maximal intensity; posterior myocardial infarction; postmyocardial infarction; present medical illness; previous medical illness

PMIS postmyocardial infarction syndrome; PSRO (see p. 251) Management Information System

PML polymorphonuclear leukocyte; posterior mitral leaflet; progressive multifocal leukodystrophy; progressive multifocal leukoencephalopathy; prolapsing mitral leaflet; pulmonary microlithiasis

PMLE polymorphous light eruption

PMM pentamethylmelamine; protoplast maintenance medium

PMMA polymethylmethacrylate

PMN polymorphonuclear; polymorphonuclear neutrophil; polymorphonucleotide

PMNC percentage of multinucleated cells; peripheral blood mononuclear cell

PMNG polymorphonuclear granulocyte

PMNL peripheral blood monocytes and polymorphonuclear leukocytes; polymorphonuclear leukocyte

PMNN polymorphonuclear neutrophil

PMNR periadenitis mucosa necrotica recurrens

PMO postmenopausal osteoporosis; Principal Medical Officer

pmol picomole

PMP pain management program; patient management program; patient medication profile; persistent mentoposterior [fetal position]; previous menstrual period

PMPS postmastectomy pain syndrome

PMQ phytylmenaquinone

PMR perinatal mortality rate; periodic medical review; physical medicine and rehabilitation; polymyalgia rheumatica; prior medical record; proportionate morbidity/mortality ratio; proton magnetic resonance

PM&R physical medicine and rehabilitation

PMRAFNS Princess Mary's Royal Air Force Nursing Service

PMRS physical medicine and rehabilitation service

PMS patient management system; perimenstrual syndrome; periodic movements during sleep; phenazine methosulfate; postmarketing surveillance; postmenstrual stress; postmitochondrial supernatant; pregnant mare serum; premenstrual syndrome, premenstrual symptoms; psychotic motor syndrome

PMSC pluripotent myeloid stem cell

PMSF phenylmethylsulfonyl fluoride

PMSG pregnant mare serum gonadotropin

PMT phenol O-methyltransferase; photomultiplier tube; Porteus maze test; premenstrual tension; pyridoxyl-methyl-tryptophan

PMTS premenstrual tension syndrome

PMTT pulmonary mean transit time

PMV paramyxovirus; percutaneous mitral balloon valvotomy; prolapse of mitral valve

PMVL posterior mitral valve leaflet

PMW pacemaker wires

PN papillary necrosis; parenteral nutrition; penicillin; perceived noise; percussion note; periarteritis nodosa; peripheral nerve; peripheral neuropathy; phrenic nerve; plaque neutralization; pneumonia; polyarteritis nodosa; polyneuritis; polyneuropathy; polynuclear; positional nystagmus; posterior nares; postnatal; practical nurse; predicted normal; primary nurse; progress note; protease nexin; psychiatry and neurology; psychoneurotic; pyelonephritis; pyridine nucleotide

P/N positive/negative

P&N psychiatry and neurology

P$_{N_2}$ partial pressure of nitrogen

Pn pneumatic; pneumonia

pn pain

PNA Paris Nomina Anatomica; peanut agglutinin; pentosenucleic acid

P$_{Na}$ plasma sodium

PNAvQ positive-negative ambivalent quotient

PNB p-nitrobiphenyl; perineal needle biopsy; premature nodal beat

PNBT p-nitroblue tetrazolium

PNC penicillin; peripheral nucleated cell; pneumotaxic center; premature nodal contracture

PND paroxysmal nocturnal dyspnea; partial neck dissection; postnasal drainage; postnasal drip; postnatal death; principal neutralizing determinant; purulent nasal drainage

PNdb perceived noise decibel

PNE plasma norepinephrine; pneumoencephalography; pseudomembranous necrotizing enterocolitis

PNET peripheral neuroepithelioma; primitive neuroectodermal tumor
pneu pneumonia
PNF proprioceptive neuromuscular facilitation
PNG penicillin G
PNH paroxysmal nocturnal hemoglobinuria; polynuclear hydrocarbon
PNHA Physicians National Housestaff Association
PNI peripheral nerve injury; postnatal infection
PNID Peer Nomination Inventory for Depression
PNK polynucleotide kinase
PNL peripheral nerve lesion; polymorphonuclear neutrophilic leukocyte
PNLA percutaneous needle lung aspiration
PNM perinatal mortality; peripheral dysostosis, nasal hypoplasia, and mental retardation [syndrome]; peripheral nerve myelin
PNMR postnatal mortality risk
PNMT phenyl-ethanolamine-N-methyltransferase
PNO Principal Nursing Officer
PNP pancreatic polypeptide; para-nitrophenol; pediatric nurse practitioner; peripheral neuropathy; pneumoperitoneum; polyneuropathy; psychogenic nocturnal polydipsia; purine nucleoside phosphorylase
P-NP para-nitrophenol
PNPase polynucleotide phosphorylase
PNPB positive-negative pressure breathing
PNPP para-nitrophenylphosphate
PNPR positive-negative pressure respiration
PNS paraneoplastic syndrome; parasympathetic nervous system; partial nonprogressive stroke; peripheral nerve stimulation; peripheral nervous system; posterior nasal spine; practical nursing student
PNT partial nodular transformation; patient

Pnt patient
PNU protein nitrogen unit
Pnx pneumothorax
PNZ posterior necrotic zone
PO by mouth, orally [Lat. *per os*]; parieto-occipital; parietal operculum; period of onset; perioperative; posterior; postoperative; predominant organism
P$_o$ opening pressure
PO$_2$, P$_{O_2}$, pO2 partial pressure of oxygen
Po polonium; porion
po by mouth [Lat. *per os*]
POA pancreatic oncofetal antigen; phalangeal osteoarthritis; preoptic area; primary optic atrophy
POAG primary open-angle glaucoma
POA-HA preoptic anterior hypothalamic area
POB penicillin, oil, beeswax; phenoxybenzamine; place of birth
POC particulate organic carbon; postoperative care; probability of chance
pocill small cup [Lat. *pocillum*]
pocul cup [Lat. *poculum*]
POD peroxidase; place of death; podiatry; polycystic ovary disease; postoperative day
PODx preoperative diagnosis
POE pediatric orthopedic examination; point of entry; polyoxyethylene; postoperative endophthalmitis; proof of eligibility
POEMS polyneuropathy, organomegaly, endocrinopathy, M protein, skin changes [syndrome]
POF position of function; premature ovarian failure; primary ovarian failure; pyruvate oxidation factor
PofE portal of entry
POG polymyositis ossificans generalisata
Pog pogonion
pOH hydroxide ion concentration in a solution
POHI physically or otherwise health-impaired

POHS presumed ocular histoplasmosis syndrome

POI Personal Orientation Inventory

poik poikilocyte, poikilocytosis

POIS Parkland On-Line Information Systems

pois poison, poisoning, poisoned

pol polish, polishing

polio poliomyelitis

Poly polymorphonuclear

poly-A, poly(A) polyadenylic acid

poly-C, poly(C) polycytidylic acid

poly-G, poly(G) polyguanylic acid

poly-I, poly(I) polyinosinic acid

poly-IC, poly-I:C copolymer of polyinosinic and polycytidylic acids; synthetic RNA polymer

polys polymorphonuclear leukocytes

poly-T, poly(T) polythymidylic acid

poly-U, poly(U) polyuridylic acid

POM pain on motion; prescription only medicine

POMC propiomelanocortin

POMP principal outer material protein

POMR problem-oriented medical record

POMS Profile of Mood States

PON paraoxonase; particulate organic nitrogen

pond by weight [Lat. *pondere*]; heavy [Lat. *ponderosus*]

POP diphosphate group; pain on palpation; paroxypropione; persistent occipitoposterior [fetal position]; pituitary opioid peptide; plasma osmotic pressure; plaster of Paris; polymyositis ossificans progressiva

Pop popliteal; population

POPOP 1,4-bis-(5-phenoxazol-2-yl) benzene

POR physician of record; postocclusive oscillatory response; prevalence odds ratio; problem-oriented record

PORH postoperative reactive hyperemia

PORP partial ossicular replacement prosthesis

PORT Patient Outcome Research Team; postoperative respiratory therapy

POS periosteal osteosarcoma; polycystic ovary syndrome; psychoorganic syndrome

pos positive

POSC problem-oriented system of charting

POSM patient-operated selector mechanism

POSS proximal over-shoulder strap

POSSUM Pictures of Standard Syndromes and Undiagnosed Malformations

post posterior

post cib after a meal [Lat. *post cibrum*]

postgangl postganglionic

postop, post-op postoperative

post sing sed liq after very loose stool [Lat. *post singulas sedes liquidas*]

POT periostitis ossificans toxica; postoperative treatment

pot potassium; potential

potass potassium

POU placenta, ovary, and uterus

PoV portal vein

POW Powassan [encephalitis]

powd powder

POX point of exit

PP diphosphate group; emphysema [pink puffers]; near point of accommodation [Lat. *punctum proximum*]; pacesetter potential; palmoplantar; pancreatic polypeptide; paradoxical pulse; parietal pulse; partial pressure; perfusion pressure; peritoneal pseudomyxoma; persisting proteinuria; Peyer patches; pinprick; placental protein; planned parenthood; placenta previa; plasma pepsinogen; plasmapheresis; plasma protein; plaster of Paris; polypropylene; polystyrene agglutination plate; population planning; posterior papillary; posterior pituitary; postpartum; postprandial; precocious puberty; preferred provider; primapara; private practice; proactivator plasminogen; protoporphyria; protoporphyrin; proximal phalanx; pseudomyxoma peritonei; pterygoid process; pulmonary pressure; pulse pressure; pulsus paradoxus; purulent pericarditis; pyrophosphate

P-P prothrombin proconvertin

P-5'-P pyridoxal-5'-phosphate

PP₁ free pyrophosphate

pp near point of accommodation [Lat. *punctum proximum*]; postprandial; postpartum

PPA first shake well [Lat. *phiala prius agitata*]; palpation, percussion, auscultation; pepsin A; phenylpropanolamine; phenylpyruvic acid; Pittsburgh pneumonia agent; polyphosphoric acid; postpartum amenorrhea; postpill amenorrhea; pure pulmonary atresia

PP&A palpation, percussion, and auscultation

Ppa pulmonary artery pressure

PPAS peripheral pulmonary artery stenosis

Ppaw pulmonary artery wedge pressure

PPB platelet-poor blood; pneumococcal pneumonia and bacteremia; positive pressure breathing

PPb postparotid basic protein

ppb parts per billion

PPBS postprandial blood sugar

PPC pentose phosphate cycle; peripheral posterior curve; plasma prothrombin conversion; pneumopericardium; progressive patient care; proximal palmar crease

PPCA plasma prothrombin conversion accelerator; proserum prothrombin conversion accelerator

PPCD polymorphous posterior corneal dystropy

PPCE postproline cleaving enzyme

PPCF peripartum cardiac failure; plasma prothrombin conversion factor

PPCM postpartum cardiomyopathy

PPD paraphenylenediamine; percussion and postural drainage; permanent partial disability; phenyldiphenyloxadiazole; postpartum day; primary physical dependence; progressive perceptive deafness; purified protein derivative;

Siebert purified protein derivative of tuberculin

PPDS phonologic programming deficit syndrome

PPD-S purified protein derivative–standard

PPE palmoplantar erythrodysesthesia; personal protective equipment; polyphosphoric ester; porcine pancreatic elastase; pulmonary permeability edema

PPES palmar-plantar erythrodysesthesia syndrome

PPF pellagra preventive factor; phagocytosis promoting factor; phosphonoformate; plasma protein fraction

PPFA Planned Parenthood Federation of America

PPG photoplethysmography

ppg picopicogram

PPGA postpill galactorrhea-amenorrhea

PPGF polypeptide growth factor

PPGP prepaid group practice

ppGpp 3'-pyrophosphoryl-guanosine-5'-diphosphate

PPH past pertinent history; persistent pulmonary hypertension; postpartum hemorrhage; primary pulmonary hypertension; protocollagen proline hydroxylase

pphm parts per hundred million

PPHN persistent pulmonary hypertension of the newborn

PPHP pseudopseudohypoparathyroidism

ppht parts per hundred thousand

PPI partial permanent impairment; patient package insert; present pain intensity; purified porcine insulin

PPi, PP₁ inorganic pyrophosphate

PPID peak pain intensity difference [score]

PPIE prolonged postictal encephalopathy

PPK palmoplantar keratosis

PPL penicilloyl polylysine

Ppl intrapleural pressure

PPLO pleuropneumonia-like organism

PPM permanent pacemaker; phosphopentomutase; pigmented pupillary membrane; posterior papillary muscle

ppm parts per million; pulses per minute

PPMA progressive postmyelitis muscular atrophy

PPN partial parenteral nutrition; pedunculopontine nucleus

PPNA peak phrenic nerve activity

PPNAD primary pigmented nodular adrenocortical disease

PPNG penicillinase-producing *Neisseria gonorrhoeae*

PPO platelet peroxidase; preferred provider organization

PPP palatopharyngoplasty; palmoplantar pustulosis; pentose phosphate pathway; Pickford projective pictures; platelet-poor plasma; polyphoretic phosphate; porcine pancreatic polypeptide; portal perfusion pressure; purified placental protein

PPPBL peripheral pulses palpable both legs

PPPI primary private practice insurance

PPR physician-patient relation; posterior primary ramus; Price precipitation reaction

PPr paraprosthetic

PPRC Physician Payment Review Commission

PPRF paramedian pontine reticular formation; postpartum renal failure

PPRWP poor precordial R-wave progression

PPS Personal Preference Scale; polyvalent pneumococcal polysaccharide; popliteal pterygium syndrome; postpartum sterilization; postperfusion syndrome; postpericardiotomy syndrome; postpolio syndrome; postpump syndrome; primary acquired preleukemic syndrome; prospective payment system; protein plasma substitute; pulse per second

PPSH pseudovaginal perineoscrotal hypospadias

PPT parietal pleural tissue; partial prothrombin time; peak-to-peak threshold;

plant protease test; polypurine tract; postpartum thyroiditis; pulmonary platelet trapping

ppt parts per trillion; precipitation, precipitate; prepared

pptd precipitated

PPTL postpartum tubul ligation

PPV pneumococcal polysaccharide vaccine; porcine parvovirus; positive predictive value; positive pressure ventilation; progressive pneumonia virus; pulmonary plasma volume

PPVr regional pulmonary plasma volume

PPVT Peabody Picture Vocabulary Test

PPVT-R Peabody Picture Vocabulary Test, Revised

Ppw pulmonary wedge pressure

PPY pancreatic polypeptide

PQ paraquat; permeability quotient; physician's questionnaire; plastoquinone; pronator quadratus; pyrimethamine-quinine

PR by way of the rectum [Lat. *per rectum*]; far point [of accommodation] [Lat. *punctum remotum*]; palindromic rheumatism; parallax and refraction; partial reinforcement; partial remission; partial response; peer review; perfusion rate; peripheral resistance; per rectum; phenol red; photoreaction; physical rehabilitation; pityriasis rosea; posterior root; postmyalgia rheumatica; postural reflex; potency ratio; preference record; pregnancy; pregnancy rate; preretinal; pressoreceptor; pressure; prevention; Preyer's reflex; proctology; production rate; profile; progesterone receptor; progressive relaxation; progressive resistance; progress report; prolactin; prolonged remission; propranolol; prosthion; protein; public relations; pulmonary rehabilitation; pulse rate; pulse repetition; pyramidal response

P-R the time between the P wave and the beginning of the QRS complex in electrocardiography [interval]

P&R pelvic and rectal [examination]; pulse and respiration

Pr praseodymium; prednisolone; presbyopia; primary; prism; production rate [of steroid hormones]; prolactin; propyl

pr far point of accommodation [Lat. *punctum remotum*]; pair; per rectum; prism

PRA phosphoribosylamine; physician recognition award; plasma renin activity; progesterone receptor assay

prac, pract practice, practitioner

PrA-HPA protein A hemolytic plaque assay

PRAS pre-reduced anaerobically sterilized [medium]; pseudo-renal artery syndrome

p rat aetat in proportion to age [Lat. *pro ratione aetatis*]

PRB Prosthetics Research Board

PRBC packed red blood cells; placental residual blood volume

PRBV placental residual blood volume

PRC packed red cells; peer review committee; phase response curve; plasma renin concentration; professional review committee

PRCA pure red cell aplasia

PRD partial reaction of degeneration; postradiation dysplasia

PRE photoreacting enzyme; pigmented retinal epithelium; progressive resistive exercise

pre preliminary

pre-AIDS pre–acquired immune deficiency syndrome

precip precipitate, precipitated, precipitation

PRED prednisone

prefd preferred

preg, pregn pregnancy, pregnant

prelim preliminary

prem premature, prematurity

preop, pre-op preoperative

prep, prepd prepare, prepared

preserv preserve, preserved, preservation

press pressure

prev prevention, preventive; previous

PREVMEDU preventive medicine unit

PRF partial reinforcement; patient report form; plasma recognition factor; pontine reticular formation; progressive renal failure; prolactin releasing factor

pRF polyclonal rheumatoid factor

PRFM premature rupture of fetal membranes

PRG phleborheography; purge

PRGS phosphoribosylglycineamide synthetase

PRH past relevant history; prolactin releasing hormone

PRI Pain Rating Index; phosphate reabsorption index; phosphoribose isomerase

PRIAS Packard's radioimmunoassay system

PRICES protection, rest, ice, compression, elevation, support [first aid]

PRIH prolactin release-inhibiting hormone

PRIME Prematriculation Program in Medical Education

PRIMEX primary care extender

primip primipara

prim luc first thing in the morning [Lat. *prima luc*]

prim m first thing in the morning [Lat. *primo mane*]

PRIND prolonged reversible ischemic neurologic deficit

PRIST paper radioimmunosorbent test

PRK photorefractive keratectomy; primary rabbit kidney

PRL, Prl prolactin

PRM phosphoribomutase; photoreceptor membrane; premature rupture of membranes; Primary Reference Material

PrM preventive medicine

PRN polyradiculoneuropathy

prn as required [Lat. *pro re nata*]

PRNT plaque reduction neutralization test

PRO Professional Review Organization; pronation

Pro proline; prophylactic; prothrombin

pro protein

prob probable
proc proceedings, procedure; process
proct, procto proctology, proctologist, proctoscopy
prod production, product
prog progress, progressive
progn prognosis
prolong prolongation, prolonged
PROM passive range of motion; premature rupture of fetal membranes; prolonged rupture of fetal membranes; programmable read only memory
PROMIS Problem-Oriented Medical Information System
pron pronator, pronation
PROP propranolol
ProPac Prospective Payment Assessment Commission
proph prophylactic, prophylaxis
pro rect recatal [Lat. *pro recto*]
pros prostate, prostatic
prosth prosthesis, prosthetic
PROTO protoporphyrin
prov provisional
prox proximal
PRP physiologic rest position; pityriasis rubra pilaris; platelet-rich plasma; polyribosyl ribitol phosphate; postural rest position; pressure rate product; primary Raynaud's phenomenon; progressive rubella panencephalitis; proliferative retinopathy photocoagulation; Psychotic Reaction Profile
PRPP phosphoribosyl pyrophosphate
PRR proton relaxation rate; pulse repetition rate
PrR progesterone receptor
PRRE pupils round, regular, and equal
PR-RSV Prague Rous sarcoma virus
PRS Personality Rating Scale; Pierre Robin syndrome; plasma renin substrate
PRSIS Prospective Rate Setting Information System
PRT *Penicillium roqueforti* toxin; pharmaceutical research and testing; phosphoribosyl transferase; postoperative respiratory therapy; prospective randomized trial

PRTH-C prothrombin time control
PRU peripheral resistance unit
PRV polycythemia rubra vera; pseudorabies virus
PRVEP pattern reversal visual evoked potential
PRW polymerized ragweed
PRX pseudoexfoliation
Prx prognosis
PRZF pyrazofurin
PS pacemaker syndrome; paired stimulation; paradoxical sleep; paraspinal; parasympathetic; parotid sialography; partial seizure; pathological stage; patient's serum; pediatric surgery; performing scale [I.Q.]; periodic syndrome; pferdestärke; phosphate saline [buffer]; phosphatidyl serine; photosensitivity, photosensitization; photosynthesis; phrenic stimulation; physical status; physiologic saline; plastic surgery; polysaccharide; polystyrene; population sample; Porter-Silber [chromogen]; prescription; presenting symptom; prostatic secretion; protein synthesis; protamine sulfate; protein S; Proteus syndrome; psychiatric; pulmonary stenosis; pyloric stenosis
P/S polisher-stimulator; polyunsaturated/saturated [fatty acid ratio]
P&S paracentesis and suction
Ps prescription; *Pseudomonas;* psoriasis
ps per second; picosecond
PSA polyethylene sulfonic acid; progressive spinal ataxia; prolonged sleep apnea; prostate specific antigen; psoriatic arthritis
Psa systemic blood pressure
PSAC President's Science Advisory Committee
PSAGN poststreptococcal acute glomerulonephritis
PSAn psychoanalysis
PSAP pulmonary surfactant apoprotein
PSB protected specimen brush
PSbetaG pregnancy-specific beta-1-glycoprotein
PSC patient services coordination; Por-

ter-Silber chromogen; posterior subcapsular cataract; primary sclerosing cholangitis; pulse synchronized contractions

PsChE pseudocholinesterase

PSCI Primary Self Concept Inventory

Psci pressure at slow component intercept

PSD particle size distribution; peptone, starch, and dextrose; periodic synchronous discharge; poststenosis dilation; postsynaptic density

PSDA psychoactive substance abuse and dependence

PSDES primary symptomatic diffuse esophageal spasm

PSE paradoxical systolic expansion; penicillin-sensitive enzyme; portal systemic encephalopathy; Present State Examination; purified spleen extract

psec picosecond

PSF peak scatter factor; pseudosarcomatous fasciitis

PSG peak systolic gradient; phosphate, saline, and glucose; polysomnogram; presystolic gallop

PSGN poststreptococcal glomerulonephritis

PSH postspinal headache

PsHD pseudoheart disease

PSI posterior sagittal index; problem solving information; prostaglandin synthetic inhibitor; psychosomatic inventory

psi pounds per square inch

ψ Greek letter *psi*; wave function

psia pounds per square inch absolute

pSIDS partially unexplained sudden infant death syndrome

PSIFT platelet suspension immunofluorescence test

PSIL preferred frequency speech interference level

PSIS posterior sacroiliac spine

PSL parasternal line; potassium, sodium chloride, and sodium lactate [solution]; prednisolone

PSM postmitochondrial supernatant; presystolic murmur

PSMA proximal spinal muscular atrophy

PSMed psychosomatic medicine

PSMF protein-sparing modified fast

PSMT psychiatric services management team

PSO proximal subungual onychomycosis

PSP pancreatic spasmolytic peptide; paralytic shellfish poisoning; parathyroid secretory protein; periodic short pulse; phenolsulfonphthalein; phosphoserine phosphatase; positive spike pattern; posterior spinal process; postsynaptic potential; prednisone sodium phosphate; progressive supranuclear palsy; pseudopregnancy

PSQ Parent Symptom Questionnaire; Patient Satisfaction Questionnaire

PSR pain sensitivity range; portal systemic resistance; proliferative sickle retinopathy; pulmonary stretch receptor

PSRC Plastic Surgery Research Council

PSRO Professional Standards Review Organization

PSS painful shoulder syndrome; physiologic saline solution; porcine stress syndrome; primary Sjögren syndrome; progressive systemic scleroderma; progressive systemic sclerosis; psoriasis severity scale; Psychiatric Status Schedule; pure sensory stroke

pSS primary Sjögren syndrome

PST pancreatic suppression test; paroxysmal supraventricular tachycardia; penicillin, streptomycin, and tetracycline; peristimulus time; phenolsulfotransferase; platelet survival time; poststenotic; poststimulus time; prefrontal sonic treatment; protein-sparing therapy; proximal straight tubule

PSTI pancreatic secretory trypsin inhibitor

PSU photosynthetic unit; primary sampling unit

PSurg plastic surgery

PSVER pattern shift visual evoked response

PSVT paroxysmal supraventricular tachycardia
PSW primary surgical ward; psychiatric social worker
PSWT psychiatric social work training
PSX pseudoexfoliation
Psy psychiatry; psychology
psych psychology, psychological
psychiat psychiatry, psychiatric
psychoan psychoanalysis, psychoanalytical
psychol psychology, psychological
psychopath psychopathology, psychopathological
psychosom psychosomatic
psychother psychotherapy
psy-path psychopathic
Ps-ZES pseudo-Zollinger-Ellison syndrome
PT parathormone; parathyroid; paroxysmal tachycardia; part time; patient; pericardial tamponade; permanent and total; pharmacy and therapeutics; phenytoin; photophobia; phototoxicity; physical therapy, physical therapist; physical training; physiotherapy; pine tar; plasma thromboplastin; pneumothorax; polyvalent tolerance; posterior tibial [artery pulse]; posttetanic; posttransfusion; posttransplantation; posttraumatic; premature termination [of pregnancy]; preterm; propylthiouracil; prothrombin time; pulmonary tuberculosis; psychotherapy; pulmonary thrombosis; pyramidal tract; temporal plane
P&T permanent and total [disability]; pharmacy and therapeutics
Pt patient; platinum
pt let it be continued [Lat. *perstetur*]; part; patient; pint; point
PTA parallel tubular arrays; parathyroid adenoma; percutaneous transluminal angioplasty; peroxidase-labeled antibody; persistent truncus arteriosus; phosphotungstic acid; physical therapy assistant; plasma thromboplastin antecedent; posttraumatic amnesia; pretreatment

anxiety; prior to admission; prior to arrival; prothrombin activity
PTAH phosphotungstic acid hematoxylin
PTAP purified diphtheria toxoid precipitated by aluminum phosphate
PTAT pure tone average threshold
PTB patellar tendon bearing; prior to birth
PTb pulmonary tuberculosis
PTBA percutaneous transluminal balloon angioplasty
PTBD percutaneous transhepatic biliary drainage; percutaneous transluminal balloon dilatation
PTBE pyretic tick-borne encephalitis
PTBNA protected transbronchial needle aspirate
PTBPD posttraumatic borderline personality disorder
PTBS posttraumatic brain syndrome
PTC percutaneous transhepatic cholangiography; phase transfer catalyst; phenothiocarbazine; phenylthiocarbamide; phenylthiocarbamoyl; plasma thromboplastin component; premature tricuspid closure; prior to conception; prothrombin complex; pseudotumor cerebri
PTCA percutaneous transluminal coronary angioplasty
PtcCO$_2$ transcutaneous partial pressure of carbon dioxide
PTCER pulmonary transcapillary escape rate
PtcO$_2$ transcutaneous oxygen tension
PTCR percutaneous transluminal coronary recanalization
PTD percutaneous transluminal dilatation; permanent total disability; personality trait disorder; prior to delivery
PTE parathyroid extract; posttraumatic epilepsy; pretibial edema; proximal tibial epiphysis; pulmonary thromboembolism
PTED pulmonary thromboembolic disease
PteGlu pteroylglutamic acid
PTEN pentaerythritol tetranitrate
pter end of short arm of chromosome

PTF patient treatment file; plasma thromboplastin factor

PTFA prothrombin time fixing agent

PTFE polytetrafluoroethylene

PTFS posttraumatic fibromyalgia syndrome

PTG parathyroid gland

PTH parathormone; parathyroid; parathyroid hormone; percutaneous transhepatic drainage; phenylthiohydantoin; plasma thromboplastin component; posttransfusion hepatitis

PTHLP parathyroid-hormone-like protein

PTHrP parathyroid-hormone-related protein

PTHS parathyroid hormone secretion [rate]

PTI pancreatic trypsin inhibitor; persistent tolerant infection; Pictorial Test of Intelligence; pulsatility transmission index

PTL peritoneal telencephalic leukoencephalomyopathy; pharyngotracheal lumen; plasma thyroxine level posterior tricuspid leaflet

PTLC precipitation thin-layer chromatography

PTLD posttransplanatation lymphoproliferative disorder; prescribed tumor lethal dose

PTM posterior trabecular meshwork; posttransfusion mononucleosis; posttraumatic meningitis; pulse time modulation

Ptm pterygomaxillary [fissure]

PTMA phenyltrimethylammonium

PTMDF pupils, tension, media, disc, fundus

PTN pain transmission neuron; posterior tibial nerve

pTNM TNM (see p. 305) staging of tumors as determined by correlation of clinical, pathologic, and residual findings

PTO Klemperer's tuberculin [Ger. *Perlsucht Tuberculin Original*]

PTP pancreatic thread protein; percuta-neous transhepatic portography; posterior tibial pulse; posttetanic potential; posttransfusion purpura; proximal tubular pressure

Ptp transpulmonary pressure

PTPI posttraumatic pulmonary insufficiency

PTPS postthrombophlebitis syndrome

PTR patellar tendon reflex; patient termination record; patient to return; peripheral total resistance; plasma transfusion reaction; psychotic trigger reaction; tuberculin *Mycobacterium tuberculosis bovis* [Ger. *Perlsucht Tuberculin Rest*]

PTr porcine trypsin

PTRA percutaneous transluminal renal angioplasty

PTRIA polystyrene-tube radioimmunoassay

Ptrx pelvic traction

PTS para-toluenesulfonic acid; postthrombotic syndrome; posttraumatic syndrome; prior to surgery

Pts, pts patients

PTSD posttraumatic stress disorder

PTSH poststimulus time histogram

PTSS posttraumatic stress syndrome

PTT partial thromboplastin time; particle transport time; posterior tibial tendon (transfer); pulmonary transit time; pulse transmission time

ptt partial thromboplastin time

PTU propylthiouracil

PTX pentoxifylline; picrotoxinin; pneumothorax

PTx parathyroidectomy; pelvic traction

PTZ pentylenetetrazol

PU by way of the urethra [Lat. *per urethra*]; palindromic unit; passed urine; pepsin unit; peptic ulcer; pregnancy urine; 6-propyluracil; prostatic urethra

Pu plutonium; purine; purple

pub public

PUBS purple urine bag syndrome

PUC pediatric urine collector

PUD peptic ulcer disease; pudendal

PuD pulmonary disease

PUF pure ultrafiltration
PUFA polyunsaturated fatty acid
PUH pregnancy urine hormones
PUI platelet uptake index
PUL, pul, pulm pulmonary
pulv powder [Lat. *pulvis*]
pulv gros coarse powder [Lat. *pulvis grossus*]
pulv subtil smooth powder [Lat. *pulvis subtilis*]
pulv tenu very fine powder [Lat. *pulvis tenuis*]
PUM peanut-reactive urinary mucin
PUMS permanently unfit for military service
PUN plasma urea nitrogen
PUO pyrexia of unknown origin
PUPPP pruritic urticarial papules and plaques of pregnancy
PUR polyurethrane
Pur purple
pur purulent
purg purgative
PUT provocative use test; putamen
PUU puumala [virus]
PUVA psoralen ultraviolet A-range
PV by way of the vagina [Lat. *per vaginam*]; pancreatic vein; papillomavirus; paraventricular; paravertebral; pemphigus vulgaris; peripheral vascular; peripheral vein; peripheral vessel; pityriasis versicolor; plasma viscosity; plasma volume; polio vaccine; polycythemia vera; polyoma virus; polyvinyl; portal vein; postvasectomy; postvoiding; pressure velocity; process variable; pulmonary vein
P-V pressure-volume [curve]
P&V pyloroplasty and vagotomy
Pv *Proteus vulgaris*; venous pressure
PVA polyvinyl acetate; polyvinyl alcohol
PVAc polyvinyl acetate
PVB cis-platinum, vinblastine, bleomycin; paravertebral block; premature ventricular beat
PVC persistent vaginal cornification; polyvinyl chloride; postvoiding cystogram; predicted vital capacity; premature

ventricular contraction; primary visual cortex; pulmonary venous congestion
PVCM paradoxical vocal cord motion
PV$_{CO2}$ partial pressure of carbon dioxide in mixed venous blood
PVD patient very disturbed; peripheral vascular disease; portal vein dilation; postural vertical dimension; premature ventricular depolarization; pulmonary vascular disease
PVE premature ventricular extrasystole
P-VEP pattern visual evoked potential
PVF peripheral visual field; portal venous flow; primary ventricular fibrillation
PVFS postviral fatigue syndrome
PVG pulmonary valve gradient
PVH periventricular hemorrhage
PVI peripheral vascular insufficiency; perivascular infiltration
PVK penicillin V potassium
PVL perivalvular leakage; permanent vision loss
PVM pneumonia virus of mice; proteins, vitamins, and minerals
PVMed preventive medicine
PVN paraventricular nucleus; predictive value negative
PVNPS post-Viet Nam psychiatric syndrome
PVO pulmonary venous obstruction
PV$_{O2}$ partial oxygen pressure in mixed venous blood
PVOD pulmonary vascular obstructive disease; pulmonary veno-occlusive disease
PVP penicillin V potassium; peripheral vein plasma; peripheral venous pressure; polyvinylpyrrolidone; portal venous pressure; pulmonary venous pressure
PVP-I polyvinylpyrrolidone-iodine
PVR peripheral vascular resistance; postvoiding residual; pulmonary vascular resistance; pulse volume recording
PVRI pulmonary vascular resistance index
PVS percussion, vibration, suction; persistent vegetative state; persistent viral

syndrome; Plummer-Vinson syndrome; poliovirus susceptibility; polyvinyl sponge; premature ventricular systole; programmed ventricular stimulation; pulmonary valvular stenosis

PVT paroxysmal ventricular tachycardia; portal vein thrombosis; pressure, volume, and temperature; private patient

PVW posterior vaginal wall

PVY potato virus Y

pvz pulverization

PW peristaltic wave; plantar wart; posterior wall [of the heart]; pressure wave; psychological warfare; pulmonary wedge [pressure]; pulsed wave

Pw progesterone withdrawal

PWA person(s) with AIDS

PWB partial weight bearing

PWBC peripheral white blood cell

PWBRT prophylactic whole brain radiation therapy

PWC peak work capacity; physical work capacity

PWCA pure white cell aplasia

PWCR Prader-Willi chromosome region

pwd powder

PWDS postweaning diarrhea syndrome

PWE posterior wall excursion

PWI posterior wall infarct

PWLV posterior wall of left ventricle

PWM pokeweed mitogen

PWP pulmonary wedge pressure

PWS port wine stain; Prader-Willi syndrome

pwt pennyweight

PX pancreatectomized; peroxidase; physical examination

Px past history; physical examination; pneumothorax; prognosis

PXE pseudoxanthoma elasticum

PXM projection x-ray microscopy; pseudoexfoliation material

PXS pseudoexfoliation syndrome

Py phosphopyridoxal; polyoma [virus]; pyridine; pyridoxal

PYA psychoanalysis

PyC pyogenic culture

PYE peptone yeast extract

PYG peptone-yeast extract-glucose [broth]

PYGM peptone-yeast-glucose-maltose [broth]

PYLL potential years of life lost

PYM psychosomatic

PYP pyrophosphate

Pyr pyridine; pyruvate

PyrP pyridoxal phosphate

PZ pancreozymin; pregnancy zone; proliferative zone

Pz 4-phenylazobenzylycarbonyl; parietal midline electrode placement in electroencephalography

pz pièze

PZE piezoelectric

PZA pyrazinamide

PZ-CCK pancreozymin-cholecystokinin

PZI protamine zinc insulin

PZP pregnancy zone protein

PZQ praziquantel

PZT lead zirconate titanate

Q

Q cardiac output; coulomb [electric quantity]; electric charge; 1,4-glucan branching enzyme; glutamine; heat; qualitative; quantity; quart; quartile; Queensland [fever]; query [fever]; question; quinacrine; quinidine; quinone; quotient; radiant energy; reactive power; reaction energy; temperature coefficient; see QRS [wave]

Q_{10} temperature coefficient

q each, every [Lat. *quaque*]; electric charge; long arm of chromosome; quart; quintal

QA quality assurance

QAC quaternary ammonium compound

QAF quality adjustment factor

QALE quality-adjusted life expectancy

QALY quality-adjusted life years

QAM quality assurance monitoring

qam every morning [Lat. *quaque ante meridiem*]

QAP quality assurance program; quinine, atabrine, and pamaquine

QAR quantitative autoradiography

QARANC Queen Alexandra's Royal Army Nursing Corps

QARNNS Queen Alexandra's Royal Naval Nursing Service

QAS quality assurance standard

QAUR quality assurance and utilization review

QB whole blood

Q_B total body clearance

QBV whole blood volume

QC quality control; quinine colchicine

Qc pulmonary capillary blood flow

QCIM Quarterly Cumulative Index Medicus

Q_{CO_2} carbon dioxide evolution by a tissue

QCT quantitative computed tomography

QD Qi deficiency

qd every day [Lat. *quaque die*]

qds to be taken four times a day [Lat. *quater die sumendum*]

QED quantum electrodynamics

QEE quadriceps extension exercise

QEEG quantitative electroencephalography

QEF quail embryo fibroblasts

QENF quantifying examination of neurologic function

QEONS Queen Elizabeth's Overseas Nursery Service

QEW quick early warning

QF quality factor; query fever; quick freeze; relative biological effectiveness

Q fever query fever

qh every hour [Lat. *quaque hora*]

q2h every two hours [Lat. *quaque secunda hora*]

q3h every three hours [Lat. *quaque tertia hora*]

q4h every four hours [Lat. *quaque quarta hora*]

QHDS Queen's Honorary Dental Surgeon

QHNS Queen's Honorary Nursing Sister

QHP Queen's Honorary Physician

QHS Queen's Honorary Surgeon

qhs every hour of sleep [Lat. *quaque hora somni*]

qid four times daily [Lat. *quater in die*]

QIDN Queen's Institute of District Nursing

QJ quadriceps jerk

ql as much as desired [Lat. *quantum libet*]

QLS Quality of Life Scale

QM quinacrine mustard

qm every morning [Lat. *quaque mane*]

QMI Q-wave myocardial infarction

QMT quantitative muscle test

QMWS quasi-morphine withdrawal syndrome

qn every night [Lat. *quaque nocte*]

QNB quinuclidinyl benzilate

QNS quantity not sufficient; Queen's Nursing Sister

qns quantity not sufficient
Qo oxygen consumption
Qo₂ oxygen quotient; oxygen utilization
qod every other day [Lat. *quaque altera die*]
qoh every other hour [Lat. *quaque altera hora*]
qon every other night [Lat. *quaque altera nocte*]
QP quanti-Pirquet [reaction]
Qp pulmonary blood flow
qp as much as desired [Lat. *quantum placeat*]
QPC quality of patient care
Qpc pulmonary capillary blood flow
QPEEG quantitative pharmaco-electro-encephalography
qPM every night
qq each, every [Lat. *quoque*]
qqd every day [Lat. *quoque die*]
qqh every four hours [Lat. *quaque quarta hora*]
qq hor every hour [Lat. *quaque hora*]
QR quality review; quantity is correct [Lat. *quantum rectum*]; quieting response; quinaldine red
qr quadriradial; quantity is correct [Lat. *quantum rectum*]; quarter
QRB Quality Review Bulletin
QRS in electrocardiography, the complex consisting of Q, R, and S waves, corresponding to depolarization of ventricles [complex]; in electrocardiography, the loop traced by QRS vectors, representing ventricular depolarization [interval]
QRS-ST the junction between the QRS complex and the ST segment in the electrocardiogram [junction]
QRS-T the angle between the QRS and T vectors in vectorcardiography [angle]
QRZ wheal reaction time [Ger. *Qaddel Reaktion Zeit*]

QS quiet sleep
Qs systemic blood flow
qs as much as will suffice [Lat. *quantum sufficit*]; sufficient quantity [Lat. *quantum satis*]
QSAR quantitative structure-activity relationship
q sat to a sufficient quantity [Lat. *quantum satis*]
QSPV quasistatic pressure volume
QSS quantitative sacroiliac scintigraphy
QST quantitative sensory test
q suff as much as suffices [Lat. *quantum sufficit*]
QT cardiac output; Quick test
Q-T in electrocardiography, the time from the beginning of the QRS complex to the end of the T wave [interval]
qt quantity; quart; quiet
QTc Q-T interval corrected for heart rate
Q-Tc corrected Q-T [interval]
qter end of long arm of chromosome
quad quadrant; quadriceps; quadriplegic
quadrupl four times as much [Lat. *quadruplicato*]
qual quality, qualitative
quant quantity, quantitative
quar quarintine
QUART quadrantectomy, axillary dissection, radiotherapy
Quat, quat four [Lat. *quattuor*]
QUEST Quality, Utilization, Effectiveness, Statistically Tabulated
QUICHA quantitative inhalation challenge apparatus
quinq five [Lat. *quinque*]
quint fifth, quintan [Lat. *quintus*]
quot quotient
quotid daily, quotidian [Lat. *quotidie*]
quot op sit as often as necessary [Lat. *quoties opus sit*]
qv as much as you desire [Lat. *quantum vis*]; which see [Lat. *quod vide*]
QYD Qi and Yin deficiency

R

R arginine; Behnken's unit; Broadbent registration point; a conjugative plasmid responsible for resistance to various elements; any chemical group (particularly an alfyl group); electrical resistance; far point [Lat. *remotum*]; in electrocardiography, the first positive deflection during the QRS complex [wave]; gas constant; organic radical; race; racemic; radioactive; radiology; radius; ramus; Rankine [scale]; rate; ratio; reaction; Réaumur [scale]; rectal; rectified; red; registered trademark; regression coefficient; regular; regular insulin; regulator [gene]; rejection factor; relapse; relaxation; release [factor]; remission; remote; repressor; residue; resistance; respiration; respiratory exchange ratio; response; responder; rest; restricted; reverse [banding]; rhythm; ribose; *Rickettsia*; right; Rinne [test]; roentgen; rough [colony]; rub; take [Lat. *recipe*]

R′ in electrocardiography, the second positive deflection during the QRS complex

+R Rinne's test positive

-R Rinne's test negative

°R degree on the Rankine scale; degree on the Réaumur scale

R1, R2, R3, etc. years of resident study

r correlation coefficient; radius; ratio; recombinant; regional; ribose; ribosomal; ring chromosome; roentgen; sample correlation coefficient

r² coefficient of determination

ρ see *rho*

RA radioactive; ragocyte; ragweed antigen; rapidly adapting [receptors]; reciprocal asymmetrical; refractory anemia; refractory ascites; renal artery; renin-angiotensin; repeat action; residual air; retinoic acid; rheumatoid arthritis; right angle; right arm; right atrium; right auricle

R$_A$ airway resistance

Ra radial; radium; radius

rA riboadenylate

RAA renin-angiotensin-aldosterone [system]

RAAMC Royal Australian Army Medical Corps

RAAS renin-angiotensin-aldosterone system

RAB remote afterloading brachytherapy

RABA rabbit antibladder antibody

Rab rabbit

rac racemate, racemic

RAD radial artery catheter; radiation absorbed dose; radical; reactive airways disease; right atrium diameter; right axis deviation; roentgen administered dose

Rad radiology; radiotherapy; radium

rad radiation absorbed dose; radial; radian; radical; radius; root [Lat. *radix*]

RADA rosin amine-D-acetate

RADC Royal Army Dental Corps

RADIO radiotherapy

radiol radiology

RadLV radiation leukemia virus

RADP right acromiodorsoposterior

RADS reactive airways dysfunction syndrome; retrospective assessment of drug safety

rad/s rad per second; radian per second

rad ther radiation therapy

RADTS rabbit antidog thymus serum

RAE right atrial enlargement

RAEB refractory anemia with excess blasts

RAEBiT, RAEB-T refractory anemia with excess blasts in transformation

RAEM refractory anemia with excess myeloblasts

RAF repetitive atrial firing; rheumatoid arthritis factor

RAFMS Royal Air Force Medical Services

RAG ragweed

258

Ragg rheumatoid agglutinin

RAH regressing atypical histiocytosis; right atrial hypertrophy

RAHO rabbit antibody to human ovary

RAHTG rabbit antihuman thymocyte globulin

RAI radioactive iodine; resting ankle index; right atrial involvement

RAID radioimmunodetection

RAIS reflection-absorption infrared spectroscopy

RAIU radioactive iodine uptake

RALPH renal-anal-lung-polydactyly-hamartoblastoma [syndrome]

RALT routine admission laboratory tests

RAM random-access memory; rapid alternating movements; rectus abdominis muscle; rectus abdominis myocutaneous [flap]; research aviation medicine; right anterior measurement

RAMC Royal Army Medical Corps

RAMP radioactive antigen microprecipitin; right atrial mean pressure

RAMT rabbit antimouse thymocyte

RANA rheumatoid arthritis nuclear antigen

RAN resident's admission notes

rANP rat atrial natriuretic peptide

RAO right anterior oblique

RaONC radiation oncology

RAP recurrent abdominal pain; regression-associated protein; renal artery pressure; rheumatoid arthritis precipitin; right atrial pressure

RAPD relative afferent pupillary defect

RAPK reticulate acropigmentation of Kitamura

RAPM refractory anemia with partial myeloblastosis

RAPO rabbit antibody to pig ovary

RAR rat insulin receptor; right arm reclining; right arm recumbent

RARLS rabbit anti-rat lymphocyte serum

RARS refractory anemia with ring sideroblasts

RARTS rabbit anti-rat thymocyte serum

RAS rapid atrial stimulation; recurrent aphthous stomatitis; reflex activating stimulus; renal artery stenosis; renin-angiotensin system; reticular activating system; rheumatoid arthritis serum

RA-S refractory anemia with ringed sideroblasts

ras retrovirus-associated DNA sequence; scrapings or filings [Lat. *rasurae*]

RASS rheumatoid arthritis and Sjögren syndrome

RAST radioallergosorbent test

RAT repeat action tablet; rheumatoid arthritis test

RATG rabbit antithymocyte globulin

RATHAS rat thymus antiserum

rAT-P recombinant antitrypsin Pittsburgh

RATx radiation therapy

RAU radioactive uptake

RAV Rous-associated virus

RAVC retrograde atrioventricular conduction; Royal Army Veterinary Corps

RAVLT Rey Auditory Verbal Learning Test

R$_{AW}$ airway resistance

RAZ razoxane

RB radiation burn; rating board; rebreathing; reticulate body; retinoblastoma; right bundle

Rb retinoblastoma; rubidium

RBA relative binding affinity; rescue breathing apparatus; right basilar artery; right brachial artery; rose bengal antigen

RBAP repetitive bursts of action potential

RBAS rostral basilar artery syndrome

RBB right bundle branch

RBBB right bundle-branch block

RBBsB right bundle-branch system block

RBBx right breast biopsy

RBC red blood cell; red blood corpuscle; red blood count

rbc red blood cell

RBCD right border cardiac dullness

RBCM red blood cell mass

RBCV red blood cell volume

RBD recurrent brief depression; relative biological dose; right border of dullness

RBE relative biological effectiveness

RBF regional blood flow; regional bone mass; renal blood flow

Rb Imp rubber base impression

RBL rat basophilic leukemia; Reid's baseline

RBN retrobulbar neuritis

RBNA Royal British Nurses Association

RBOW rupture of the bag of waters

RBP retinol-binding protein; riboflavin-binding protein

RBRVS resource-based relative value scale

RBS random blood sugar; Rutherford backscattering

RbSA rabbit serum albumin

RBV right brachial vein

RBW relative body weight

RBZ rubidazone

RC an electronic circuit containing a resistor and capacitor in series; radiocarpal; reaction center; recrystallization; red cell; red cell casts; red corpuscle; Red Cross; referred care; regenerated cellulose; respiration ceases; respiratory care; respiratory center; rest cure; retention catheter; retrograde cystogram; rib cage; root canal; routine cholecystography

R&C resistance and capacitance

Rc conditioned response; receptor

RCA red cell agglutination; relative chemotactic activity; renal cell carcinoma; right carotid artery; right coronary artery

RCAMC Royal Canadian Army Medical Corps

rCBF regional cerebral blood flow

RCBV regional cerebral blood volume

RCC radiological control center; rape crisis center; ratio of cost to charges; receptor-chemoeffector complex; red cell cast; red cell count; renal cell carcinoma; right common carotid

RCCM Regional Committee for Community Medicine

RCCT random controlled clinical trial

RCD relative cardiac dullness

RCDA recurrent chronic dissecting aneurysm

RCDP rhizomelic chondrodysplasia punctata

RCDR relative corrected death rate

RCE reasonable compensation equivalent

RCF red cell ferritin; red cell folate; relative centrifugal field/force; ristocetin cofactor

RCG radioelectrocardiography

RCGP Royal College of General Practitioners

RCH rectocolic hemorrhage

RCHF right congestive heart failure

RCHMS Regional Committee for Hospital Medical Services

RCI respiratory control index

RCIA red cell immune adherence

RCIRF radiologic contrast-induced renal failure

RCIT red cell iron turnover

RCITR red cell iron turnover rate

RCL renal clearance

RCM radiographic contrast medium; red cell mass; reinforced clostridial medium; replacement culture medium; right costal margin; Royal College of Midwives

rCMRGlc regional cerebral metabolic rate for glucose

rCMRO$_2$ regional cerebral metabolic rate for oxygen

RCN right caudate nucleus; Royal College of Nursing

RCoF ristocetin cofactor

RCOG Royal College of Obstetricians and Gynaecologists

RCP red cell protoporphyrin; retrocorneal pigmentation; riboflavin carrier protein; Royal College of Physicians

rCP regional cerebral perfusion

rcp reciprocal translocation

RCPath Royal College of Pathologists

RCPH red cell peroxide hemolysis

RCPSGlas Royal College of Physicians and Surgeons, Glasgow

RCR relative consumption rate; respiratory control ratio

RCRA Resource Conservation and Recovery Act

RCS rabbit aorta-contracting substance; red cell suspension; reticulum cell sarcoma; right coronary sinus; Royal College of Science; Royal College of Surgeons

RCSE Royal College of Surgeons, Edinburgh

RCT random controlled trial; retrograde conduction time; root canal therapy; Rorschach content test

rct a marker showing the ability of virulent strains to replicate at 40°C, while vaccine strain shows no replication

RCU respiratory care unit

RCV red cell volume

RCVS Royal College of Veterinary Surgeons

RD radial deviation; rate difference; Raynaud's disease; reaction of degeneration; registered dietitian; Reiter's disease; related donor; renal disease; resistance determinant; respiratory disease; retinal detachment; Reye's disease; rheumatoid disease; right deltoid; Riley-Day [syndrome]; Rolland-Desbuquois [syndrome]; rubber dam; ruminal drinking; ruptured disk

Rd rate of disappearance

rd rutherford

R&D research and develpment

RDA recommended daily allowance; recommended dietary allowance; Registered Dental Assistant; right dorsoanterior [fetal position]

RDB random double-blind [trial]

RDC research diagnostic criteria

RDDA recommended daily dietary allowance

RDDP ribonucleic acid–dependent deoxynucleic acid polymerase

RDE receptor-destroying enzyme

RDES remote data entry system

RDFC recurring digital fibroma of childhood

RDH Registered Dental Hygienist

RDHBF regional distribution of hepatic blood flow

RDI recommended daily intake; respiratory disturbance index; rupture-delivery interval

RDLBBB rate-dependent left bundle-branch block

RDM readmission

rDNA recombinant (or ribosomal) deoxyribonucleic acid

RDP right dorsoposterior [fetal position]

RDQ respiratory disease questionnaire

RDS respiratory distress syndrome; reticuloendothelial depressing substance; rhodanese

RDT retinal damage threshold; routine dialysis therapy

RDV rice dwarf virus

RDW red blood cell distribution width index

RE radium emanation; readmission; rectal examination; reflux esophagitis; regional enteritis; renal and electrolyte; resistive exercise; resting energy; restriction endonuclease; reticuloendothelial; retinol equivalent; right ear; right eye

R_E respiratory exchange ratio

R&E research and education

Re rhenium

R_e Reynold's number

REA radiation emergency area; radioenzymatic assay; renal anastomosis; right ear advantage

REAB refractory anemia with excess of blasts

readm readmission

REAS reasonably expected as safe; retained, excluded antrum syndrome

REAT radiological emergency assistance team

REB roentgen-equivalent biological

REC receptor

rec fresh [Lat. *recens*]; recessive; recombinant chromosome; record; recovery; recurrence, recurrent

recen fresh [Lat. *recens*]

RECG radioelectrocardiography

recip recipient; reciprocal

recon the smallest unit of DNA capable of recombination [recombination + Gr. *on* quantum]

recond reconditioned, reconditioning
recumb recumbent
recryst recrystallization
rect rectal; rectification, rectified; rectum; rectus [muscle]
recur recurrence, recurrent
RED radiation experience data; rapid erythrocyte degeneration
red reduction
redig in pulv let it be reduced to powder [Lat. *redigatur in pulverem*]
red in pulv reduced to powder [Lat. *reductus in pulverem*]
redox oxidation-reduction
REE rapid extinction effect; rare earth element; resting energy expenditure
REEDS retention of tears, ectrodactyly, ectodermal dysplasia, and strange hair, skin and teeth [syndrome]
REEG radioelectroencephalography
R-EEG resting electroencephalography
ReEND reproductive endocrinology
REEP right end-expiratory pressure
reev re-evaluate
reex re-examine
REF ejection fraction at rest; referred; refused; renal erythropoietic factor
ref reference; reflex
Ref Doc referring doctor
REFI regional ejection fraction image
ref ind refractive index
refl reflex
REFMS Recreation and Education for Multiple Sclerosis [Victims]
Ref Phys referring physician
REFRAD released from active duty
REG radiation exposure guide; radioencephalogram, radioencephalography
Reg registered
reg region
regen regenerated, regenerating, regeneration
reg rhy regular rhythm
reg umb umbilical region [Lat. *regio umbilici*]
regurg regurgitation
REH renin essential hypertension
rehab rehabilitation, rehabilitated

REL rate of energy loss; recommended exposure limit; resting expiratory level
rel relative
RELE resistive exercise of lower extremities
REM rapid eye movement; recent-event memory; reticular erythematous mucinosis; return electrode monitor; roentgen–equivalent–man
rem removal
REMA repetitive excess mixed anhydride
REMAB radiation-equivalent-manikin absorption
REMCAL radiation-equivalent-manikin calibration
remit remittent
REMP roentgen-equivalent-man period
REMS rapid eye movement sleep
REN renal
ren renew [Lat. *renovetur*]
ren sem renew only once [Lat. *renovetum semel*]
REO respiratory enteric orphan [virus]
REP rest-exercise program; retrograde pyelogram; roentgen equivalent–physical
rep let it be repeated [Lat. *repetatur*]; replication; roentgen equivalent–physical
repol repolarization
REPS reactive extensor postural synergy
rept let it be repeated
RER renal excretion rate; respiratory exchange ratio; rough endoplasmic reticulum
RERF Radiation Effects Research Foundation
RES radionuclide esophageal scintigraphy; reticuloendothelial system
res research; resection; resident; residue; resistance
RESNA Rehabilitation Engineering Society of North America
resp respiration, respiratory; response
REST Raynaud's phenomenon, esophageal motor dysfunction, sclerodactyly,

and telangiectasia [syndrome]; regressive electroshock therapy

resusc resuscitation

RET reticular; reticulocyte; retina; retention; retained; right esotropia

ret rad equivalent therapeutic

retard retardation, retarded

ret cath retention catheter

retic reticulocyte

REV reticuloendotheliosis virus

ReV regulator of virion

rev reverse; review; revolution

re-x reexamination

Rex regulator x

RF radial fiber; radiofrequency; receptive field; Reitland-Franklin [unit]; relative flow; relative fluorescence; release factor; renal failure; replicative form; resistance factor; respiratory failure; reticular formation; retroperitoneal fibromatosis; rheumatic fever; rheumatoid factor; riboflavin; risk factor; root canal filling; rosette formation

R^F rate of flow

Rf respiratory frequency; rutherfordium

R$_f$ in paper or thin-layer chromatography, the distance that a spot of a substance has moved from the point of application

rf radiofrequency

RFA right femoral artery; right frontoanterior [fetal position]

RFB retained foreign body

RFC retrograde femoral catheter; rosette-forming cell

RFE relative fluorescence efficiency

RFFIT rapid fluorescent focus inhibition test

RFI recurrence-free interval; renal failure index

RFL right frontolateral [fetal position]

RFLA rheumatoid-factor-like activity

RFLP restriction fragment length polymorphism

RFLS rheumatoid-factor-like substance

Rfm rifampin

RFP recurrent facial paralysis; request for proposal; right frontoposterior [fetal position]

RFPS (Glasgow) Royal Faculty of Physicians and Surgeons of Glasgow

RFR refraction

RFS renal function study

RFT rod-and-frame test; right frontotransverse [fetal position]

RFV right femoral vein

RFW rapid filling wave

RG right gluteal

rG regular gene

RGBMT renal glomerular basement membrane thickness

RGC radio-gas chromatography; remnant gastric cancer; retinal ganglion cell; right giant cell

RGD range-gated Doppler

RGE relative gas expansion

RGH rat growth hormone

RGM right gluteus medius

rGM-CSF recombinant granulocyte-macrophage colony-stimulating factor

RGN Registered General Nurse

RGP retrograde pyelography

RGR relative growth rate

RGU regional glucose utilization

RH radiant heat; radiological health; reactive hyperemia; recurrent herpes; regulatory hormone; relative humidity; releasing hormone; renal hemolysis; retinal hemorrhage; right hand; right heart; right hemisphere; right hyperphoria; room humidifier

Rh rhesus [factor]; rhinion; rhodium

Rh+ rhesus positive

Rh− rhesus negative

rh rheumatic

r/h roentgens per hour

RHA Regional Health Authority; right hepatic artery

RhA rheumatoid arthritis

RHB right heart bypass

RHBF reactive hyperemia blood flow

RHBs Regional Hospital Boards

RHC resin hemoperfusion column; respiration has ceased; right heart catheterization; right hypochondrium

RHCSA Regional Hospitals Consultants' and Specialists' Association

RHD radiological health data; relative hepatic dullness; renal hypertensive disease; rheumatic heart disease

RHE retinohepatoendocrinologic [syndrome]

RHEED reflection high-energy electron diffraction

rheo rheology

rheu, rheum rheumatic, rheumatoid

RHF right heart failure

RHG right hand grip

rhG-CSF recombinant human granulocyte colony-stimulating factor

rhGM-CSF recombinant human granulocyte macrophage colony-stimulating factor

RHI Rural Health Initiative

Rhin rhinology

rhino rhinoplasty

RHJSC Regional Hospital Junior Staff Committee

RHL recurrent herpes labialis; right hepatic lobe

RHLN right hilar lymph node

rhm roentgens per hour at 1 meter

RhMK rhesus monkey kidney

RhMk rhesus monkey

RhMkK rhesus monkey kidney

RHMV right heart mixing volume

RHN Rockwell hardness number

RHO right heeloff

ρ Greek letter *rho*; correlation coefficient; electric charge density; electrical resistivity; mass density; reactivity

RHR renal hypertensive rat; resting heart rate

r/hr roentgens per hour

RHS Ramsay Hunt syndrome; reciprocal hindlimb-scratching [syndrome]; right hand side; right heelstrike

RHT renal homotransplantation

rH-TNF recombinant human tumor necrosis factor

RHU registered health underwriter; rheumatology

rHuEpo recombinant human erythropoietin

rHuTNF recombinant human tumor-necrosing factor

RI radiation intensity; radioactive isotope; radioimmunology; recession index; recombinant inbred [strain]; refractive index; regenerative index; regional ileitis; regular insulin; relative intensity; release inhibition; remission induction; renal insufficiency; replicative intermediate; respiratory illness; respiratory index; retroactive inhibition; retroactive interference; ribosome; rosette index (or inhibition)

RIA radioimmunoassay

RIA-DA radioimmunoassay double antibody [test]

RIAS Roter International Analysis Scheme

Rib riboflavin; ribose

RIBS Rutherford ion backscattering

RIC right internal carotid [artery]; Royal Institute of Chemistry

RICE rest, ice, compression, and elevation

RICM right intercostal margin

RiCoF ristocetin cofactor

RICU respiratory intensive care unit

RID radial immunodiffusion; remission-inducing drug; ruptured intervertebral disc

RIF release-inhibiting factor; rifampin; right iliac fossa; rosette-inhibiting factor

RIFA radioiodinated fatty acid

RIFC rat intrinsic factor concentrate

rIFN recombinant interferon

RIG rabies immune globulin

RIGH rabies immune globulin, human

RIH right inguinal hernia

RIHSA radioactive iodinated human serum albumin

rIL recombinant interleukin

RILT rabbit ileal loop test

RIM radioisotope medicine; recurrent induced malaria; relative-intensity measure

RIMR Rockefeller Institute for Medical Research

RIMS resonance ionization mass spectrometry

RIN rat insulinoma

RINB Reitan-Indiana Neuropsychological Battery

RIND reversible ischemic neurologic deficit

RINN recommended international nonproprietary name

RIO right inferior oblique

RIP radioimmunoprecipitation; reflex inhibiting pattern

RIPA radioimmunoprecipitation assay

RIPH Royal Institute of Public Health

RIPHH Royal Institute of Public Health and Hygiene

RIPP resistive-intermittent positive pressure

RIR relative incidence rates; right interior rectus [muscle]

RIRB radioiodinated rose bengal

RIS rapid immunofluorescence staining; resonance ionization spectroscopy

RISA radioactive iodinated serum albumin; radioimmunosorbent assay

RIST radioimmunosorbent test

RIT radioimmune trypsin; radioiodinated triolein; radioiodine treatment; rosette inhibition titer

RITC rhodamine isothiocyanate

RIU radioactive iodine uptake

RIVC right inferior vena cava

RIVD ruptured intervertebral disc

RK rabbit kidney; radial keratotomy; right kidney

RKG radiocardiogram

RKH Rokitansky-Küster-Hauser [syndrome]

RKM rokitamycin

RKV rabbit kidney vacuolating [virus]

RKY roentgen kymography

RL radiation laboratory; reduction level; resistive load; reticular lamina; right lateral; right leg; right lung; Ringer's lactate [solution]

R&L right and left

RLC residual lung capacity

RLD related living donor; ruptured lumbar disc

RLE right lower extremity

RLF retrolental fibroplasia; right lateral femoral

RLL right lower limb; right lower lobe

RLM right lower medial

RLN recurrent laryngeal nerve; regional lymph node

RLNC regional lymph node cell

RLND regional lymph node dissection

RLO residual lymphatic output

RLP radiation leukemia protection; ribosome-like particle

RLQ right lower quadrant

RLR right lateral rectus [muscle]

RLS restless leg syndrome; Ringer's lactate solution; Roussy-Levy syndrome

RLSB right lower scapular border

R-Lsh right-left shunt

RLV Rauscher leukemia virus

RLWD routine laboratory work done

RM radical mastectomy; random migration; range of movement; red marrow; reference material; relative mobility; rehabilitation medicine; Riehl's melanosis; reinforced maneuver; resistive movement; respiratory movement; routine management; ruptured membranes

Rm relative mobility; remission

rm remission; room

RMA Registered Medical Assistant; relative medullary area; right mentoanterior [fetal position]

RMB right mainstem bronchus

RMBF regional myocardial blood flow

RMC reticular magnocellular [nucleus]; right middle cerebral [artery]

RMCA right middle cerebral artery

RMCL right midclavicular line

RMD retromanubrial dullness

RME rapid maxillary expansion; resting metabolic expenditure; right mediolateral episiotomy

RMEC regional medical education center

RMF right middle finger

RMK rhesus monkey kidney

RML radiation myeloid leukemia; regional medical library; right mediolateral; right middle lobe

RMLB right middle lobe bronchus

RMLS right middle lobe syndrome

RMLV Rauscher murine leukemia virus

RMM rapid micromedia method

RMN Registered Mental Nurse

RMO Regional Medical Officer; Resident Medical Officer

RMP rapidly miscible pool; regional medical program; resting membrane potential; ribulose monophosphate pathway; rifampin; right mentoposterior [fetal position]

RMPA Royal Medico-Psychological Association

RMR relative maximum respone; resting metabolic rate; right medial rectus [muscle]

RMS rectal morphine sulfate [suppository]; red man syndrome; repetitive motion syndrome; respiratory muscle strength; rheumatic mitral stenosis; rhodomyosarcoma; rigid man syndrome; root-mean-square

rms root-mean-square

RMSD root-mean-square deviation

RMSF Rocky Mountain spotted fever

RMT Registered Music Therapist; relative medullary thickness; retromolar trigone; right mentotransverse [fetal position]

RMUI relief medication unit index

RMuLV Rauscher murine leukemia virus

RMV respiratory minute volume

RN radionuclide; red nucleus; Registered Nurse; residual nitrogen; reticular nucleus

Rn radon

RNA radionuclide angiography; Registered Nurse Anesthetist; ribonucleic acid; rough, noncapsulated, avirulent [bacterial culture]

RNAA radiochemical neutron activation analysis

RNAse, RNase ribonuclease

RND radical neck dissection; radionu-

clide dacryography; reactive neurotic depression

RNFP Registered Nurse Fellowship Program

RNIB Royal National Institute for the Blind

RNICU regional neonatal intensive care unit

RNID Royal National Institute for the Deaf

RNP ribonucleoprotein

RNR ribonucleotide reductase

RNS reference normal serum; repetitive nerve stimulation

RNSC radionuclide superior cavography

Rnt roentgenology

RNV radionuclide venography

rNTP ribonuclease-5′-triphosphate

RNVG radionuclide ventriculography

RO radiation output; ratio of; relative odds; reverse osmosis; Ritter-Oleson [technique]; routine order; rule out

R/O rule out

ROA right occipitoanterior [fetal position]

ROAD reversible obstructive airways disease

ROAT repeat open application test

ROATS rabbit ovarian antitumor serum

rob robertsonian translocation

ROC receiver operating characteristic; receptor-operated channels; relative operating characteristic; resident on call; residual organic carbon

ROCF Rey-Osterrieth Complex Figure

rOEF regional oxygen extraction fraction

roent roentgenology

ROH rat ovarian hyperemia [test]

ROI reactive oxygen intermediate; region of interest; right occipitolateral [fetal position]

ROIH right oblique inguinal hernia

ROM range of motion; read only memory; rupture of membranes

Rom Romberg [sign]

rom reciprocal ohm meter

ROM CP range of motion complete and painfree

ROP retinopathy of prematurity; right occipitoposterior [fetal position]

ROPS rollover protective structure

Ror Rorschach [test]

ROS reactive oxygen species; review of systems; rod outer segment

RoS rostral sulcus

ROSS review of subjective symptoms

ROT real oxygen transport; remedial occupational therapy; right occipito-transverse [fetal position]

rot rotating, rotation

ROU recurrent oral ulcer

ROW Rendu-Osler-Weber [syndrome]

RP radial pulse; radiopharmaceutical; rapid processing [of film]; Raynaud's phenomenon; reactive protein; readiness potential; rectal prolapse; refractory period; regulatory protein; relapsing polychondritis; respiratory rate; rest pain; resting potential; resting pressure; retinitis pigmentosa; retrograde pyelogram; retroperitoneal; reverse phase; rheumatoid polyarthritis; ribose phosphate

R/P respiratory pulse [rate]

R$_p$ pulmonary resistance

RPA radial photon apsorptiometry; resultant physiologic acceleration; reverse passive anaphylaxis; right pulmonary artery

RPase ribonucleic acid polymerase

RPC relapsing polychondritis; relative proliferative capacity

RPCF, RPCFT Reiter protein complement fixation [test]

RPCGN rapidly progressive crescenting glomerulonephritis

RPD removable partial denture

RPE rate of perceived exertion; recurrent pulmonary embolism; retinal pigment epithelium

RPF relaxed pelvic floor; renal plasma flow; retroperitoneal fibrosis

RPG radiation protection guide; retrograde pyelogram; rheoplethysmography

RPGMEC Regional Postgraduate Medical Education Committee

RPGN rapidly progressive glomerulonephritis

RPh Registered Pharmacist

RPHA reversed passive hemagglutination

RPHAMFCA reversed passive hemagglutination by miniature centrifugal fast analysis

RP-HPLC reverse phase-high performance liquid chromatography

RPI relative percentage index; reticulocyte production index, ribose 5-phosphate isomerase

RPIPP reverse phase ion-pair partition

RPLAD retroperitoneal lymphadenectomy

RPLC reverse phase liquid chromatography

RPLD repair of potentially lethal damage

RPM, rpm rapid processing mode; revolutions per minute

RPMD rheumatic pain modulation disorder

RPMI Roswell Park Memorial Institute [medium]

RPO right posterior oblique

RPP heart rate–systolic blood pressure product; retropubic prostatectomy

RPPI role perception picture inventory

RPPR red cell precursor production rate

RPR rapid plasmin reagin [test]

RPr retinitis proliferans

RPRCT rapid plasma reagin cord test

RPS renal pressor substance; revolutions per second

rps revolutions per second

RPT rapid pull-through; refractory period of transmission; Registered Physical Therapist

RPTA renal percutaneous transluminal angioplasty

RPTC regional poisoning treatment center

Rptd ruptured

RPV right portal vein; right pulmonary vein

RPVP right posterior ventricular pre-excitation

RQ recovery quotient; reportable quantity; respiratory quotient

RR radiation reaction; radiation response; rate ratio; recovery room; relative response; relative risk; renin release; respiratory rate; respiratory reserve; response rate; retinal reflex; rheumatoid rosette; risk ratio; Riva-Rocci [sphygmomanometer]

R&R rate and rhythm; rest and recuperation

RRA radioreceptor assay; registered record administrator

RRC residency review committee; risk reduction component; routine respiratory care; Royal Red Cross

RRE radiation-related eosinophilia

RRE, RR&E round, regular, and equal [pupils]

RRF residual renal function

RR-HPO rapid recompression–high pressure oxygen

RRI recurrent respiratory infection; reflex relaxation index; relative response index

RRIS recurrent respiratory infection syndrome

RRL Registered Record Librarian

rRNA ribosomal ribonucleic acid

rRNP ribosomal ribonucleoprotein

RRP relative refractory period

RRpm respiratory rate per minute

RRR regular rhythm and rate; renin release rate (or ratio)

RR&R regular rate and rhythm

RRS retrorectal space; Richards-Rundle syndrome

RRT random response technique; Registered Respiratory Therapist; relative retention time

RRU respiratory resistance unit

RS random sample; rating schedule; Raynaud syndrome; recipient's serum; rectal sinus; rectal suppository; rectosigmoid; Reed-Steinberg [cell]; reinforcing stimulus; Reiter syndrome; relative stimulus; renal specialist; respiratory syncytial [virus]; response to stimulus; resting subject; reticulated siderocyte; Rett syndrome; review of symptoms; Reye syndrome; right sacrum; right septum; right side; right stellate [ganglion]; Ringer solution; Roberts syndrome; Rous sarcoma

Rs *Rauwolfia serpentina;* systemic resistance

R/s roentgens per second

r$_s$ rank correlation coefficient

RSA rabbit serum albumin; regular spiking activity; relative specific activity; relative standard accuracy; reticulum cell sarcoma; right sacroanterior [fetal position]; right subclavian artery

Rsa systemic arterial resistance

RSB reticulocyte standard buffer; right sternal border

RSC rat spleen cell; rested state contraction; reversible sickle-cell

RScA right scapuloanterior [fetal position]

RSCN Registered Sick Children's Nurse

RScP right scapuloposterior [fetal position]

RSD reflex sympathetic dystrophy; relative standard deviation

RSDS reflex sympathetic dystrophy syndrome

RSEP right somatosensory evoked potential

RSES Rosenberg Self-Esteem Scale

RSH Royal Society of Health

RSI repetition strain injury

RSIC Radiation Shielding Information Center

R-SIRS Revised, Seriousness of Illness Rating Scale

RSIVP rapid-sequence intravenous pyelography

RSL right sacrolateral [fetal position]

RSLD repair of sublethal damage

RSM risk screening model; Royal Society of Medicine

RSMR relative standard mortality rate

RSN right substantia nigra

RSNA Radiological Society of North America

RSO Resident Surgical Officer; right superior oblique [muscle]

RSP removable silicone plug; right sacroposterior [fetal position]

RSPCA Royal Society for the Prevention of Cruelty to Animals

RSPH Royal Society for the Promotion of Health

RSPK recurrent spontaneous psychokinesis

RSR regular sinus rhythm; relative survival rate; right superior rectus [muscle]

rSr an electrocardiographic complex

RSS rat stomach strip; rectosigmoidoscopy; Russell-Silver syndrome

RSSE Russian spring-summer encephalitis

RSSR relative slow sinus rate

RST radiosensitivity test; reagin screen test; right sacrotransverse [fetal position]; rubrospinal tract

R$_{st}$ in paper or thin layer chromatography, the distance that a spot of a substance has moved, relative to a reference standard spot

RSTI Radiological Service Training Institute

RSTL relaxed skin tension lines

RSTMH Royal Society of Tropical Medicine and Hygiene

RSTS retropharyngeal soft tissue space

RSV respiratory syncytial virus; right subclavian vein; Rous sarcoma virus

RSVC right superior vena cava

RT radiologic technologist; radiotelemetry; radiotherapy; radium therapy; rapid tranquilization; reaction time; reading test; reciprocating tachycardia; recreational therapy; rectal temperature; reduction time; Registered Technician; renal transplantation; resistance transfer; respiratory therapist/therapy; response time; rest tremor; retransformation; reverse transcriptase; right; right thigh; room temperature; Rubinstein-Taybi [syndrome]

RT3, rT$_3$ reverse triiodothyronine

Rt right; total resistance

rT ribothymidine

rt right

RTA renal tubular acidosis; reverse transcriptase assay; road traffic accident

RTAD renal tubular acidification defect

RT(ARRT) Radiologic Technologist certified by the American Registry of Radiologic Technologists

RTC random control trial; rape treatment center; renal tubular cell; residential treatment center; return to clinic

RTD routine test dilution

Rtd retarded

RTECS Registry of Toxic Effects of Chemical Substances

RTF resistance transfer factor; respiratory tract fluid

RTG-2 rainbow trout gonadal tissue cells

rTHF recombinant tumor necrosis factor

RTI respiratory tract infection; reverse transcriptase inhibition

rtl rectal

rt lat right lateral

RTM registered trademark

RTN renal tubular necrosis

RT(N)(ARRT) Radiologic Technologist (Nuclear Medicine) certified by the American Registry of Radiologic Technologists

RTO return to office; right toeoff

RTOG radiation therapy oncology group

RTP renal transplantation patient; reverse transcriptase-producing [agent]

RTR Recreational Therapist, Registered; red blood cell turnover rate; retention time ratio

RT(R)(ARRT) Registered Technologist, Radiography certified by the American Registry of Radiologic Technologists)

RTS real time scan; right toestrike; Rubinstein-Taybi syndrome

RT(T)(ARRT) Radiologic Technologist (Radiation Therapy) certified by the American Registry of Radiologic Technologists

RTRR return to recovery room

RTU relative time unit

RTW return to work

RTV room temperature vulcanization

RU radioulnar; rat unit; reading unit; residual urine; resin uptake; resistance unit; retrograde urogram; right upper; roentgen unit

Ru ruthenium

ru radiation unit

RU-1 human embryonic lung fibroblasts

rub red [Lat. *ruber*]

RUD recurrent ulcer of the duodenal bulb

RUE right upper extremity

RUL right upper eyelid; right upper lateral; right upper limb; right upper lobe

RuMP ribulose monophosphate pathway

RUOQ right upper outer quadrant

rupt ruptured

RUP right upper pole

RUQ right upper quadrant

RUR resin-uptake ratio

RURTI recurrent upper respiratory tract infection

RUS radioulnar synostosis

RUSB right upper sternal border

RUV residual urine volume

RUX right upper extremity

RV random variable; rat virus; Rauscher virus; rectovaginal; reinforcement value; renal vein; residual volume; respiratory volume; retroversion; return visit; rheumatoid vasculitis; rhinovirus; right ventricle, right ventricular; rubella vaccine; rubella virus; Russell viper

R$_V$ radius of view

RVA re-entrant ventricular arrhythmia; right ventricle activation; right vertebral artery

RVAD right ventricular assist device

RVAW right ventricle anterior wall

RVB red venous blood

RVC rectovaginal constriction

RVD relative vertebral density; right ventricular dysplasia

RVDO right ventricular diastolic overload

RVDV right ventricular diastolic volume

RVE right ventricular enlargement

RVECP right ventricular endocardial potential

RVEDD right ventricular end-diastolic diameter

RVEDP right ventricular end-diastolic pressure

RVEDVI right ventricular end-diastolic volume index

RVEF right ventricular ejection fraction; right ventricular end-flow

RVET right ventricular ejection time

RVF renal vascular failure; Rift Valley fever; right ventricular failure; right visual field

RVFP right ventricular filling pressure

RVG right ventral glutens [muscle]; right visceral ganglion

RVH renovascular hypertension; right ventricular hypertrophy

RVHD rheumatic valvular heart disease

RVI relative value index; right ventricle infarction

RVIT right ventricular inflow tract

RVL right vastus lateralis

RVLG right ventrolateral gluteal

RVM right ventricular mean

RVO Regional Veterinary Officer; relaxed vaginal outlet; right ventricular outflow

RVOT right ventricular outflow tract

RVP red veterinary petrolatum; resting venous pressure; right ventricular pressure

RVPEP right ventricular pre-ejection period

RVPFR right ventricular peak filling rate

RVPRA renal vein plasma renin activity

RVR reduced vascular response; renal vascular resistance; repetitive ventricular response; resistance to venous return

RVRA renal vein rein activity; renal venous renin assay

RVRC renal vein renin concentration

RVS rectovaginal space; relative value scale/study; reported visual sensation; retrovaginal space

RVSO right ventricular stroke output
RVSW right ventricular stroke work
RVSWI right ventricular stroke work index
RVT renal vein thrombosis
RVTE recurring venous thromboembolism
RV/TLC residual volume/total lung capacity
RVU relative valve unit
RVV rubella vaccine-like virus; Russell viper venom
RW radiological warfare; ragweed; respiratory work; Romano-Ward [syndrome]; round window

R-W Rideal-Walker [coefficient]
RWAGE ragweed antigen E
RWIS restraint and water immersion stress
RWM regional wall motion
RWP ragweed pollen; R-wave progression
RWS ragweed sensitivity
Rx drug; medication; pharmacy; prescribe, prescription, prescription drug; take [Lat. *recipe*]; therapy; treatment
r(X) right X chromosome
RXLI recessive X-linked ichthyosis
RXN reaction
RXT right exotropia
R-Y Roux-en-Y [anastomosis]

S

S apparent power; in electrocardiography, a negative deflection that follows an R wave [wave]; entropy; exposure time; half [Lat. *semis*]; left [Lat. *sinister*]; mean dose per unit cumulated activity; the midpoint of the sella turcica [point]; sacral; saline; *Salmonella*; saturated; *Schistosoma*; schizophrenia; second; section; sedimentation coefficient; sella [turcica]; semilente [insulin]; senile, senility; sensation; sensitivity; septum; serine; serum; *Shigella*; siderocyte; siemens; signature [prescription]; silicate; single; small; smooth [colony]; soft [diet]; solid; soluble; solute; sone [unit]; space; spatial; specificity; spherical; *Spirillum*; spleen; standard normal deviation; *Staphylococcus*; stem [cell]; stimulus; *Streptococcus*; streptomycin; subject; subjective findings; substrate; sulfur; sum of an arithmetic series; supravergence; surface; surgery; suture; Svedberg [unit]; swine; Swiss [mouse]; synthesis; systole; without [Lat. *sine*]; write, let it be written [Lat. *signa*]

S1-S5 first to fifth sacral nerves

S₁-S₄ first to fourth heart sounds

s atomic orbital with angular momentum quantum number 0; distance; left [Lat. *sinister*]; length of path; sample standard deviation; satellite [chromosome]; scruple; second; section; sedimentation coefficient; sensation; series; signed; suckling

s without

s⁻¹ cycles per second

s² sample variance

Σ see *sigma*

σ see *sigma*

SA according to art [Lat. *secundum artem*]; salicylic acid; saline [solution]; salt added; sarcoidosis; sarcoma; scalenus anticus; secondary amenorrhea; secondary anemia; secondary arrest; self-analysis; semen analysis; sensitizing antibody; serum albumin; serum aldolase; sexual addict; simian adenovirus; sinoatrial; sinus arrest; sinus arrhythmia; skin-adipose [unit]; sleep apnea; slightly active; slowly adapting [receptors]; soluble in alkaline medium; specific activity; spectrum analysis; spiking activity; standard accuracy; stimulus artifact; Stokes-Adams [syndrome]; subarachnoid; succinylacetone; suicide attempt; surface antigen; surface area; sustained action; sympathetic activity; systemic aspergillosis

S-A sinoatrial; sinoauricular

S&A sickness and accident [insurance]; sugar and acetone

Sa the most anterior point of the anterior contour of the sella turcica [point]; saline; *Staphylococcus aureus*

sA statampere

sa according to art [Lat. *Secundum artem*]

SAA serum amyloid A; severe aplastic anemia

SAARD slow-acting antirheumatic drug

SAAST self-administered alcohol screening test

SAB serum albumin; significant asymptomatic bacteriuria; sinoatrial block; Society of American Bacteriologists; spontaneous abortion; subarachnoid block

SABP spontaneous acute bacterial peritonitis

SAC saccharin; sacrum; screening and acute care; Self-Assessment of Communication [scale]; short-arm cast; subarea advisory council

sacch saccharin

SACD subacute combined degeneration

SACE serum angiotensin–converting enzyme

SACH small animal care hospital; solid ankle cushioned heel

SACS secondary anticoagulation system

SACSF subarachnoid cerebrospinal fluid

SACT sinoatrial conduction time

SAD Scale of Anxiety and Depression; seasonal affective disorder; Self-Assessment Depression [scale]; small airway disease; source-to-axis distance; sugar, acetone, and diacetic acid; suppressor-activating determinant

SADD Short-Alcohol Dependence Data [questionnaire]; standardized assessment of depressive disorders

SADL simulated activities of daily living

SADR suspected adverse drug reaction

SADS Schedule for Affective Disorders and Schizophrenia

SADS-C Schedule for Affective Disorders and Schizophrenia–Change

SADS-L Schedule for Affective Disorders and Schizophrenia–Lifetime

SADT Stetson Auditory Discrimination Test

SAE short above-elbow [cast]; specific action exercise; subcortical arteriosclerotic encephalopathy; supported arm exercise

SAEB sinoatrial entrance block

SAEM Society for Academic Emergency Medicine

SAEP *Salmonella abortus equi* pyrogen

SAF scrapie-associated fibrils; self-articulating femoral; serum accelerator factor; simultaneous auditory feedback

SAFA soluble antigen fluorescent antibody

SAG salicyl acyl glucuronide; Swiss agammaglobulinemia

SAGM sodium chloride, adenine, glucose, mannitol

SAH S-adenosyl-L-homocysteine; subarachnoid hemorrhage

SAHA seborrhea–hypertrichosis/ hirsutism–alopecia [syndrome]

SAHH S-adenosylhomocysteine hydrolase

SAHIGES *Staphylococcus aureus* hyperimmunoglobulinemia E syndrome

SAHS sleep apnea–hypersomnolence [syndrome]

SAI Self-Analysis Inventory; Sexual Arousability Inventory; Social Adequacy Index; systemic active immunotherapy; without other qualification [Lat. *sine altera indicatione*]

SAID specific adaptation to imposed demand [principle]

SAIDS sexually acquired immunodeficiency syndrome; simian acquired immune deficiency syndrome

SAL sensorineural activity level; suction-assisted lipectomy

Sal salicylate, salicylic; *Salmonella*

sAl serum aluminum [level*]*

sal according to the rules of art [Lat. *secundum artis leges*]; salicylate, salicylic; saline; saliva

Salm *Salmonella*

SAM S-adenosyl-L-methionine; scanning acoustic microscope; sex arousal mechanism; staphylococcal absorption method; sulfated acid mucopolysaccharide; surface active material; systolic anterior motion

SAMA Student American Medical Association

SAMD S-adenosyl-L-methionine decarboxylase

SAM-DC S-adenosyl-L-methionine decarboxylase

SAMe S-adenosyl-L-methionine

SAMO Senior Administrative Medical Officer

S-AMY serum amylase

SAN sinoatrial node; sinoauricular node; slept all night; solitary autonomous nodule

Sanat sanatorium

SANDR sinoatrial nodal reentry

sang sanguinous

sanit sanitary, sanitation

SANS scale for the assessment of negative symptoms

SANWS sinoatrial node weakness syndrome

SAO small airway obstruction; splanchnic artery occlusion

S$_{AO2}$ oxygen saturation in alveolar gas

S_{aO2} oxygen saturation in arterial blood

SAP sensory action potential; serum acid phosphatase; serum alkaline phosphatase; serum amyloid P; situs ambiguus with polysplenia; *Staphylococcus aureus* protease; surfactant-associated protein; systemic arterial pressure

saph saphenous

SAPHO synovitis-acne-pustulosis hyperostosis-osteomyelitis [syndrome]

SAPX salivary peroxidase

SAQ short arc quadriceps [muscle]

SAQC statistical analysis of quality control

SAR seasonal allergic rhinitis; sexual attitude reassessment; structure-activity relationship

Sar sulfarsphenamine

SARA sexually acquired reactive arthritis; Superfund Amendments and Reauthorization

SAS self-rating anxiety scale; short arm splint; Sklar Aphasia Scale; sleep apnea syndrome; small animal surgery; small aorta syndrome; sodium amylosulfate; space-adaptation syndrome; statistical analysis system; sterile aqueous solution; sterile aqueous suspension; subaortic stenosis; sulfasalazine; supravalvular aortic stenosis; surface-active substance; synchronous atrial stimulation

SASE self-addressed stamped envelope

SASMAS skin-adipose superficial musculoaponeurotic system

SASP salicylazosulfapyridine

SASPP syndrome of absence of septum pellucidum with preencephaly

SAST Self-administered Alcoholism Screening Test; selective arterial secretin injection test; serum aspartate aminotransferase

SAT satellite; serum antitrypsin; single-agent chemotherapy; slide agglutination test; sodium ammonium thiosulfate; spermatogenic activity test; spontaneous activity test; subacute thyroiditis; symptomless autoimmune thyroiditis; systematic assertive therapy

Sat, sat saturation, saturated

SATA spatial average, temporal average

SATB special aptitude test battery

satd saturated

SATL surgical Achilles tendon lengthening

SATP spatial average temporal peak

SAU statistical analysis unit

SAV sequential atrioventricular [pacing]

SAVD spontaneous assisted vaginal delivery

SB Bachelor of Science; Schwartz-Bartter [syndrome]; serum bilirubin; shortness of breath; sick bay; sideroblast; single blind [study]; single breath; sinus bradycardia; small bowel; sodium balance; soybean; spina bifida; spontaneous blastogenesis; spontaneous breathing; Stanford-Binet [Intelligence Scale]; stereotyped behavior; sternal border; stillbirth; surface binding

Sb antimony [Lat. *stibium*]; strabismus

sb stilb

SBA serum bile acid; soybean agglutinin; spina bifida aperta

SBB stimulation-bound behavior

SBC serum bactericidal concentration; strict bed confinement

SBD senile brain disease

S-BD seizure-brain damage

SbDH sorbitol dehydrogenase

SBE breast self-examination; short below-elbow [cast]; shortness of breath on exertion; subacute bacterial endocarditis

S/ß sickle cell beta-thalassemia

SBF serologic-blocking factor; specific blocking factor; splanchnic blood flow

SBFT small bowel follow-through

SBG selenite brilliant green

SBH sea-blue histiocyte

SBI soybean trypsin inhibitor

SBIS Stanford-Binet Intelligence Scale

SBL soybean lecithin

sBL sporadic Burkitt's lymphoma

SBLA sarcoma, breast and brain tumors, leukemia, laryngeal and lung cancer, and adrenal cortical carcinoma

SB-LM Stanford-Binet Intelligence Test-Form LM

SBN₂ single-breath nitrogen test]

SBNS Society of British Neurological Surgeons

SBNT single-breath nitrogen test

SBNW single-breath nitrogen washout

SBO small bowel obstruction; spina bifida occulta

SBOM soybean oil meal

SBP schizobipolar; serotonin-binding protein; spontaneous bacterial peritonitis; steroid-binding plasma [protein]; sulfobromophthalein; systemic blood pressure; systolic blood pressure

SBQ Smoking Behavior Questionnaire

SBR small bowel resection; spleen-to-body [weight] ratio; strict bed rest; styrene-butadiene rubber

SBRN sensory branch of radial nerve

SBS shaken baby syndrome; short bowel syndrome; sick building syndrome; sinobronchial syndrome; small bowel series; social breakdown syndrome; straight back syndrome

SBSS Seligmann's buffered salt solution

SBT serum bactericidal titer; single-breath test; sulbactam

SBTI soybean trypsin inhibitor

SBTPE State Boards Test Pool Examination

SBTT small bowel transit time

SBV singular binocular vision

SC conditioned stimulus; sacrococcygeal; Sanitary Corps; scalenus [muscle]; scapula; Schwann cell; sciatica; science; secondary cleavage; secretory component; self care; semicircular; semilunar valve closure; serum complement; serum creatinine; service-connected; sex chromatin; Sézary cell; short circuit; sick call; sickle cell; silicone-coated; single chemical; skin conduction; slow component; Snellen's chart; sodium citrate; soluble complex; special care; spinal canal; spinal cord; squamous carcinoma; statistical control; sternoclavicular; stratum corneum; subcellular; subclavian; subcor-

neal; subcortical; subcutaneous; succinylcholine; sugar-coated; superior colliculus; supportive care; surface colony; systemic candidiasis; systolic click

S-C sickle cell

S&C sclerae and conjunctivae

Sc scandium; scapula; science, scientific; screening

sC statcoulomb

SCA self-care agency; severe congenital anomaly; sickle-cell anemia; single-channel analyzer; sperm-coating antigen; steroidal-cell antibody; subclavian artery; superior cerebellar artery; suppressor cell activity

SCAA Skin Care Association of America; sporadic cerebral amyloid angiopathy

SCABG single coronary artery bypass

SCAG Sandoz Clinical Assessment-Geriatric [Rating]

SCAMC Symposium on Computer Applications in Medical Care

SCAMIN Self-Concept and Motivation Inventory

SCAN suspected child abuse and neglect; systolic coronary artery narrowing

SCAP scapula

SCARF skeletal abnormalities, cutis laxa, craniostenosis, psychomotor retardation, facial abnormalities [syndrome]

SCAT sheep cell agglutination test; sickle cell anemia test; Sports Competition Anxiety Test

Scat orig original package, manufacturer's package [Lat. *scatula originalis*]

SCB strictly confined to bed

SCBA self-contained breathing apparatus

SCBF spinal cord blood flow

SCBG symmetric calcification of the basal cerebral ganglia

SCBH systemic cutaneous basophil hypersensitivity

SCBP stratum corneum basic protein

SCC sequential combination chemotherapy; services for crippled children; short-course chemotherapy; small-cell carcinoma; small cleaved cell; spinal cord compression; squamous cell carcinoma

SCCA single-cell cytotoxicity assay

SCCB small-cell carcinoma of the bronchus

SCCC squamous cell cervical carcinoma

SCCH sternocostoclavicular hyperostosis

SCCHN squamous cell carcinoma of the head and neck

SCCHO sternocostoclavicular hyperostosis

SCCL small cell carcinoma of the lung

SCCM Sertoli cell culture medium

SCCT severe cerebrocranial trauma

SCD service-connected disability; sickle-cell disease; spinocerebellar degeneration; subacute combined degeneration; subacute coronary disease; sudden cardiac death; systemic carnitine deficiency

ScD Doctor of Science

ScDA right scapuloanterior [fetal position] [Lat. *scapulodextra anterior*]

ScDP right scapuloposterior [fetal position] [Lat. *scapulodextra posterior*]

SCE secretory carcinoma of the endometrium; sister chromatid exchange; split hand–cleft lip/palate ectodermal [dysplasia]; subcutaneous emphysema

SCe somatic cell

SCEP sandwich counterelectrophoresis

SCER sister chromatid exchange rate

SCF Skin Cancer Foundation

SCFA short-chain fatty acid

SCFE slipped capital femoral epiphysis

SCG serum chemistry graft; serum chemogram; sodium cromoglycate; superior cervical ganglion

SCh succinylchloride; succinylcholine

SChE serum cholinesterase

schiz schizophrenia

SCHL subcapsular hematoma of the liver

SCI Science Citation Index; spinal cord injury; structured clinical interview

Sci science, scientific

SCID, SCIDS severe combined immunodeficiency [syndrome]

SCII Strong-Campbell Interest Inventory

SCIS spinal cord injury service

scint scintigram

SCIU spinal cord injury unit

SCIV subcutaneous intravenous

SCIWORA spinal cord injury without radiographic abnormality

SCJ squamocolumnar junction; sternoclavicular joint; sternocostal joint

SCK serum creatine kinase

SCL scleroderma; serum copper level; sinus cycle length; soft contact lens; symptom checklist; syndrome checklist

scl sclerosis, sclerotic, sclerosed

ScLA left scapuloanterior [fetal position] [Lat. *scapulolaeva anterior*]

SCLC small cell lung carcinoma

SCLD sickle-cell chronic lung disease

SCLE subacute cutaneous lupus erythematosus

scler sclerosis, scleroderma

ScLP left scapuloposterior [fetal position] [Lat. *scapulolaeva posterior*]

SCLS systemic capillary leak syndrome

SCM Schwann cell membrane; sensation, circulation, and motion; Society of Computer Medicine; soluble cytotoxic medium; spleen cell-conditioned medium; spondylitic caudal myelopathy; State Certified Midwife; streptococcal cell membrane; sternocleidomastoid; surface-connecting membrane

SCMC spontaneous cell-mediated cytotoxicity

SCMO Senior Clerical Medical Officer

SCN special care nursing; suprachiasmatic nucleus

SCNS subcutaneous nerve stimulation

SCO sclerocystic ovary; somatic crossing-over; subcommissural organ

SCOP scopolamine

SCP single-celled protein; standard care plan; sodium cellulose phosphate; soluble cytoplasmic protein; submucous cleft palate; superior cerebral peduncle

scp spherical candle power

SCPK serum creatine phosphokinase

SCPNT Southern California Postrotary Nystagmus Test

SCR Schick conversion rate; silicon-controlled rectifier; skin conductance response; slow-cycling rhodopsin; spondylitic caudal radiculopathy

SCr serum creatinine

scr scruple

SCRAM speech-controlled respirometer for ambulation measurement

scRNA small cytoplasmic ribonucleic acid

SCS Saethre-Chotzen syndrome; shared computer system; silicon-controlled switch; Society of Clinical Surgery; spinal cord stimulation; systolic click syndrome

SCSB static charge sensitive bed

SCSIT Southern California Sensory Integration Test

SCT sex chromatin test; sexual compatibility test; sickle-cell trait; sperm cytotoxicity; spinal computed tomography; spinocervicothalamic; staphylococcal clumping test; sugar-coated tablet

SCTAT sex cord tumor with annular tubules

SCTx spinal cervical traction

SCU self-care unit; special care unit

SCUBA self-contained underwater breathing apparatus

SCUD septicemic cutaneous ulcerative disease

SCUF slow continuous ultrafiltration therapy

SCU-PA single-chain urokinase plasminogen activator

SCV sensory nerve conduction velocity; smooth, capsulated, virulent; subclavian vein; squamous-cell carcinoma of the vulva

SCV-CPR simultaneous compression ventilation–cardiopulmonary resuscitation

SD Sandhoff disease; senile dementia; septal defect; serologically defined; serologically detectable; serologically determined; serum defect; Shine-Dalg-

arno [sequence]; short dialysis; shoulder disarticulation; Shy-Draper [syndrome]; skin destruction; skin dose; somatization disorder; sphincter dilatation; spontaneous delivery; sporadic depression; Sprague-Dawley [rat]; spreading depression; stable disease; standard deviation; statistical documentation; Stensen duct; Still's disease; stone disintegration; strength duration; streptodornase; sudden death; superoxide dismutase; systolic discharge

S-D sickle-cell hemoglobin D; suicide-depression

S/D sharp/dull; systolic/diastolic

Sd stimulus drive

S^d discriminative stimulus

SDA right sacroanterior [fetal position] [Lat. *sacrodextra anterior*]; sialodacryoadenitis; specific dynamic action; succinic dehydrogenase activity

SDAT senile dementia of Alzheimer type

SDB sleep-disordered breathing

SDBP seated (or standing, or supine) diastolic blood pressure

SDC serum digoxin concentration; sodium deoxycholate; subacute combined degeneration; subclavian hemodialysis catheter; succinyldicholine

SDCL symptom distress check list

SDD sporadic depressive disease; sterile dry dressing

SDDS 2-sulfamoyl-4,4′-diaminodiphenylsulfone

SDE specific dynamic effect

SDEEG sterotactic depth electroencephalography

SDES symptomatic diffuse esophageal spasm

SDF slow death factor; stress distribution factor

SDG sucrose density gradient

SDH serine dehydrase; sorbitol dehydrogenase; spinal dorsal horn; subdural hematoma; succinate dehydrogenase

SDHD sudden death heart disease

SDI standard deviation interval; survey diagnostic instrument

SDIHD sudden death ischemic heart disease

SDILINE Selective Dissemination of Information On-Line [data bank]

SDL serum digoxin level; speech discrimination level

sdl sideline; subline

SDM sensory detection method; standard deviation of the mean

SDN sexually dimorphic nucleus

SDO sudden dosage onset

SDP right sacroposterior [fetal position] [Lat. *sacrodextra posterior*]

SDR spontaneously diabetic rat; surgical dressing room

SDS same day surgery; school dental services; self-rating depression scale; sensory deprivation syndrome; sexual differentiation scale; Shy-Drager syndrome; single-dose suppression; sodium dodecylsulfate; specific diagnosis service; standard deviation score; sudden death syndrome; sulfadiazine silver; sustained depolarizing shift

SD-SK streptodornase-streptokinase

SDS/PAGE, SDS-PGE sodium dodecylsulfate–polyacrylamide gel electrophoresis

SDT right sacrotransverse [fetal position] [Lat. *sacrodextra transversa*]; single-donor transfusion; speech detection threshold

SD$_t$ standard deviation of total scores

SDU standard deviation unit; step-down unit

SDUB short double upright brace

SE saline enema; sanitary engineering; side effect; smoke exposure; solid extract; sphenoethmoidal; spin-echo; spongiform encephalopathy; Spurway-Eddowes [syndrome]; standard error; staphylococcal endotoxin; staphylococcal enterotoxin; starch equivalent; Starr-Edwards [prosthesis]; status epilepticus; subendothelial

S&E safety and efficiency

Se secretion; selenium

SEA sheep erythrocyte agglutination;

shock-elicited aggression; soluble egg antigen; spontaneous electrical activity; staphylococcal enterotoxin A

SEAT sheep erythrocyte agglutination test

SEB seborrhea; staphylococcal enterotoxin B

SEBA staphylococcal enterotoxin B antiserum

SEBL self-emptying blind loop

SEBM Society of Experimental Biology and Medicine

SEC secretin; Singapore epidemic conjunctivitis; soft elastic capsule

Sec Seconal

sec second; secondary; section

sec-Bu sec-butyl

SECG stress electrocardiography

SECSY spin-echo correlated spectroscopy

sect section

SED sedimentation rate; skin erythema dose; spondyloepiphyseal dysplasia; standard error of deviation; staphylococcal enterotoxin D

sed sedimentation; stool [Lat. *sedes*]

sed rt sedimentation rate

SEE standard error of estimate

SEEG stereotactic electroencephalography

SEER Surveillance Epidemiology and End Results [Program]

SEF somatically-evoked field; staphylococcal enterotoxin F

SEG segment; soft elastic gelatin; sonoencephalogram

segm segment, segmented

SEGNE secretory granules of neural and endocrine [cells]

SEH subependymal hemorrhage

SEI Self-Esteem Inventory

SELF Self-Evaluation of Life Function [scale]

SEM sample evaluation method; scanning electron microscopy; secondary enrichment medium; standard error of the mean; systolic ejection murmur

sem one-half [Lat. *semis*]; semen, seminal

SEMI subendocardial myocardial infarction

SEMDJL spondyloepimetaphyseal dysplasia with joint laxity

semid half a dram

semih half an hour [Lat. *semihora*]

SEN scalp-ear-nipple [syndrome*]*; State Enrolled Nurse

sen sensitive, sensitivity

SENSOR Sentinel Event Notification System for Occupational Risks

sens sensation, sensorium, sensory

SEP sensory-evoked potential; septum; somatosensory evoked potential; sperm entry point; spinal evoked potential; surface epithelium; systolic ejection period

separ separation, separation

sept seven [Lat. *septem*]

SEQ side effects questionnaire

seq sequence; sequel, sequela, sequelae; sequestrum

seq luce the following day [Lat. *sequenti luce*]

SER sebum excretion rate; sensory evoked response; service; smooth endoplasmic reticulum; smooth-surface endoplasmic reticulum; somatosensory evoked response; supination, external rotation [fracture]; systolic ejection rate

Ser serine; serology; serous; service

sER smooth endoplasmic reticulum

ser series, serial

SER-IV supination external rotation, type 4 fracture

SerCl serum chloride

SERHOLD National Biomedical Serials Holding Database

SERLINE Serials on Line

sero, serol serological, serology

SERS Stimulus Evaluation/Response Selection [test]

SERT sustained ethanol release tube

serv keep, preserve [Lat. *serva*]; service

SERVHEL Service and Health Records

SES Society of Eye Surgeons; socio-economic status; spatial emotional stimulus; subendothelial space

SESAP Surgical Educational and Self-Assessment Program

sesquih an hour and a half [Lat. *sesquihora*]

sesunc an ounce and a half [Lat. *sesuncia*]

SET systolic ejection time

sev severe; severed

SEWHO shoulder-elbow-wrist-hand orthosis

s expr without expressing [Lat. *sine expressio*]

SF Sabin-Feldman [test]; safety factor; salt-free; scarlet fever; seminal fluid; serosal fluid; serum factor; serum ferritin; serum fibrinogen; sham feeding; shell fragment; shunt flow; sickle cell-hemoglobin F [disease]; simian foam-virus; skin fibroblast; soft feces; spinal fluid; spontaneous fibrillation; stable factor; sterile female; stress formula; sugar-free; superior facet; suppressor factor; suprasternal fossa; Svedberg flotation [unit]; swine fever; symptom-free; synovial fluid

Sf *Streptococcus faecalis*

S$_f$ Svedberg flotation unit

SFA saturated fatty acid; seminal fluid assay; serum folic acid; stimulated fibrinolytic activity; superior femoral artery

SFB Sanfilippo syndrome type B; saphenofemoral bypass; surgical foreign body

SFBL self-filling blind loop

SFC soluble fibrin complex; soluble fibrin–fibrinogen complex; spinal fluid count

SFD silo filler's disease; skin-film distance; spectral frequency distribution

SFEMG single fiber electromyography

SFFA serum free fatty acid

SFFF sedimentation field flow fractionation

SFFV spleen focus-forming virus

SFG subglottic foreign body

SFH schizophrenia family history; serum-free hemoglobin; stroma-free hemoglobin

SFI Sexual Function Index; Social Function Index

SFL synovial fluid lymphocyte

SFM serum-free medium

SFMC soluble fibrin monomer complex

SFP screen filtration pressure; simultaneous foveal perception; spinal fluid pressure; stopped flow pressure

SFR screen filtration resistance; stroke with full recovery

SFS serial foveal seizures; skin and fascia stapler; split function study

SFT Sabin-Feldman test; sensory feedback therapy; skinfold thickness

SFU surgical follow-up

SFV Semliki Forest virus; shipping fever virus; Shope fibroma virus; squirrel fibroma virus

SFW sexual function of women; shell fragment wound; slow-filling wave

SG Sachs-Georgi [test]; salivary gland; serum globulin; serum glucose; signs; skin graft; soluble gelatin; specific gravity; subgluteal; substantia gelatinosa; Surgeon General

SGA small for gestational age

SG$_{AW}$ specific airway conductance

SGB sparsely granulated basophil

SGC spermicide-germicide compound

SGD specific granule deficiency

SGE secondary generalized epilepsy

SGF sarcoma growth factor; skeletal growth factor

SGH subgluteal hematoma

SGL salivary gland lymphocyte

SGM Society for General Microbiology

SGO Surgeon General's Office; surgery, gynecology, and obstetrics

SGOT serum glutamate oxaloacetate transaminase (aspartate aminotransferase)

SGP serine glycerophosphatide; sialoglycoprotein; Society of General Physiologists; soluble glycoprotein

SGPT serum glutamate pyruvate transaminase (alanine aminotransferase)

SGR Sachs-Georgi reaction; Shwartzman generalized reaction; skin galvanic reflex; submandibular gland renin; substantia gelatinosa Rolandi

S-Gt Sachs-Georgi test

SGTT standard glucose tolerance test

SGV salivary gland virus; selective gastric vagotomy

SGVHD syngeneic graft-versus-host disease

SH Salter-Harris [fracture]; Schönlein-Henoch [purpura]; self-help; serum hepatitis; sexual harassment; sex hormone; Sherman [rat]; sick in hospital; sinus histiocytosis; social history; somatotropic hormone; spontaneously hypertensive [rat]; state hospital; sulfhydryl; surgical history; symptomatic hypoglycemia; syndrome of hyporeninemic hypoaldosteronism; systemic hyperthermia

S/H sample and hold

S&H speech and hearing

Sh sheep; Sherwood number; *Shigella*; shoulder

sh shoulder

SHA staphylococcal hemagglutinating antibody

sHa suckling hamster

SHAA serum hepatitis associated antigen; Society of Hearing Aid Audiologists

SHAA-Ab serum hepatitis associated antigen antibody

SHAFT sad, hostile, anxious, frustrating, tenacious [patient] syndrome

SHARP school health additional referral program

SHB sequential hemibody [irradiation]

S-Hb sulfhemoglobin

SHBD serum hydroxybutyric dehydrogenase

SHBG sex hormone binding globulin

SHCC State Health Coordinating Council

SHCO sulfated hydrogenated castor oil

SHE Syrian hamster embryo

SHEENT skin, head, eyes, ears, nose, and throat

SHF simian hemorrhagic fever

shf super-high frequency

SHG synthetic human gastrin

SHH syndrome of hyporeninemic hypoaldosternonism

SHHD Scottish Home and Health Department

SHHV Society for Health and Human Values

Shig *Shigella*

SHL sensorineural hearing loss

SHLA soluble human lymphocyte antigen

SHLD shoulder

SHML sinus histiocytosis with massive lymphadenopathy

SHMP Senior Hospital Medical Officer

SHMT serine-hydroxymethyl transferase

SHN spontaneous hemorrhagic necrosis; subacute hepatic necrosis

SHO secondary hypertrophic osteoarthropathy; Senior House Officer

SHORT, S-H-O-R-T short stature, hyperextensibility of joints or hernia or both, ocular depression, Rieger anomaly, teething delayed

SHP Schönlein-Henoch purpura; secondary hyperparathyroidism; state health plan

SHPDA State Health Planning and Development Agency

SHR spontaneously hypertensive rat

SHS Sayre head sling; sheep hemolysate supernatant

SHSP spontaneously hypertensive stroke-prone [rat]

SHSS Stanford Hypnotic Susceptibility Scale

SHT simple hypocalcemic tetany; subcutaneous histamine test

SHUR System for Hospital Uniform Reporting

SHV simian herpes virus

SI International System of Units [Fr. *le Système International d'Unités*]; sacro-iliac; saline infusion; saline injection; saturation index; self-inflicted; sensory integration; septic inflammation; serious illness; serum iron; severity index; sex inventory; Singh Index; single injection; small intestine; soluble insulin; spirochetosis icterohaemorrhagica; stimulation index; stress incontinence; stroke index; suppression index

Si the most anterior point on the lower contour of the sella turcica [point]; silicon

S&I suction and irrigation

SIA serum inhibitory activity; stress-induced analgesia; stress-induced anesthesia; subacute infectious arthritis

SIADH syndrome of inappropriate secretion of antidiuretic hormone

SIB self-injurious behavior

sib, sibs sibling, siblings

SIC serum insulin concentration; Standard Industrial Classification

sic dry [Lat. *siccus*]

SICD serum isocitrate dehydrogenase

SICU spinal intensive care unit; surgical intensive care unit

SID single intradermal [test]; Society for Investigative Dermatology; sucrase-isomaltase deficiency; sudden inexplicable death; sudden infant death; suggested indication of diagnosis; systemic inflammatory disease

SIDS sudden infant death syndrome

SIE stroke in evolution

SIECUS Sex Information and Education Council of the United States

SIF serum-inhibition factor

SIFT selector ion flow tube

SIg, sIg surface immunoglobulin

sig let it be labeled [Lat. *signa, signetur*]; sigmoidoscopy; significant

S-IgA secretory immunoglobulin A

Σ Greek capital letter *sigma*; syphilis; summation of series

σ Greek lower case letter *sigma*; conductivity; cross section; millisecond; molecular type or bond; population standard deviation; stress; surface tension; wave number

sig n pro label with the proper name [Lat. *signa nomine proprio*]

SIH stimulation-induced hypalgesia; stress-induced hyperthermia

SIHE spontaneous intramural hematoma of the esophagus

SIJ sacroiliac joint

SIL soluble interleukin; speech interference level

SILD Sequenced Inventory of Language Development

SIM selected ion monitoring; Society of Industrial Microbiology

SIMA single internal mammary artery

SIMS secondary ion mass spectroscopy

simul simultaneously

SIMV synchronized intermittent mandatory ventilation

sin six times a night [Lat. *sex in nocte*]

sing of each [Lat. *singulorum*]

si non val if it is not enough [Lat. *si non valeat*]

SIO sacroiliac orthosis

si op sit if it is necessary [Lat. *si opus sit*]

SIP Sickness Impact Profile; slow inhibitory potential; surface inductive plethysmography

sIPTH serum immunoreactive parathyroid hormone

SIQ Symptom Interpretation Questionnaire

SIR single isomorphous replacement; specific immune release; standardized incidence ratio; syndrome of immediate reactivities

SIRA Scientific Instrument Research Association

SIREF specific immune response enhancing factor

SIRF severely impaired renal function

SIRS soluble immune response suppressor; Structured Interview of Reported Symptoms

SIS serotinin irritation syndrome; simian sarcoma; simulator-induced syndrome; social information system; spontaneous interictal spike; sterile injectable solution; sterile injectable suspension

SISI short increment sensitivity index

SISS small inducible secreted substances

SISV, SiSV simian sarcoma virus

SIT serum inhibiting titer; Slosson Intelligence Test; sperm immobilization test; suggested immobilization test

SIV simian immunodeficiency virus; Sprague-Dawley-Ivanovas [rat]

SIVagm simian immunodeficiency virus from African green monkeys

si vir perm if the strength will permit [Lat. *si vires permitant*]

SIVMAC simian immunodeficiency virus of macaques

SIW self-inflicted wound

SIWIP self-induced water intoxication and psychosis

SIWIS self-induced water intoxication and schizophrenic disorders

SJR Shinowara-Jones-Reinhart [unit]

S$_J$ Jaccard coefficient

SJS Stevens-Johnson syndrome; stiff joint syndrome; Swyer-James syndrome

SjS Sjögren syndrome

SK seborrheic keratosis; senile keratosis; Sloan-Kettering [Institute for Cancer Research]; spontaneous killer [cell]; streptokinase; swine kidney

Sk skin

SKA supracondylar knee-ankle [orthosis]

SKAT Sex Knowledge and Attitude Test

skel skeleton, skeletal

SKI Sloan-Kettering Institute

SKL serum killing level

SKSD, SK-SD streptokinase-streptodornase

sk trx skeletal traction

SL according to the rules [Lat. *secundum legem*]; sarcolemma; sclerosing leukoencephalopathy; secondary leukemia; sensation level; sensory latency; short-leg [brace]; Sibley-Lehninger [unit]; signal level; Sinding Larsen [syndrome]; Sjögren-Larsson [syndrome]; slit lamp; small lymphocyte; sodium lactate; solidified liquid; sound level; Stein-Leventhal [syndrome]; streptolysin; sublingual

Sl Steel [mouse]

sl in a broad sense [Lat. *sensu lato*]; stemline; sublingual

SLA left sacroanterior [fetal position] [Lat. *sacrolaeva anterior*]; single-cell liquid cytotoxic assay; slide latex agglutination; soluble liver antigen; surfactant-like activity

SLAC scapholunate advanced collapse [wrist]

SLAM scanning laser acoustic microscope

s lat in a broad sense [Lat. *sensu lato*]

SLAP serum leucine aminopeptidase

SLB short-leg brace

SLC short-leg cast

SLCC short-leg cylinder cast

SLD, SLDH serum lactate dehydrogenase

SLE slit lamp examination; St. Louis encephalitis; systemic lupus erythematosus

SLEA sheep erythrocyte antibody

SLEP short latent evoked potential

SLEV St. Louis encephalitis virus

SLHR sex-linked hypophosphatemic rickets

SLI selective lymphoid irradiation; somatostatin-like immunoreactivity; splenic localization index

SLIR somatostatin-like immunoreactivity

SLK superior limbic keratoconjunctivitis

SLKC superior limbic keratoconjunctivitis

SLM sound level meter

SLMC spontaneous lymphocyte-mediated cytotoxicity

SLN sublentiform nucleus; superior laryngeal nerve

SLNWBC short-leg nonweightbearing cast

SLNWC short-leg nonwalking cast

SLO Smith-Lemli-Opitz syndrome; streptolysin O

SLOS Smith-Lemli-Opitz syndrome

SLP left sacroposterior [fetal position] [Lat. *sacrolaeva posterior*]; segmental limb systolic pressure; sex-limited protein; short luteal phase; subluxation of the patella

SLPP serum lipophosphoprotein

SLR Shwartzman local reaction; single lens reflex; straight leg raising

SLRT straight leg raising test

SLS segment long-spacing; short-leg splint; single limb support; Sjögren-Larsson syndrome; stagnant loop syndrome; Stein-Leventhal syndrome

SLT left sacrotransverse [fetal position] [Lat. *sacrolaeva transversa*]; solid logic technology

SLUD salivation, lacrimation, urination, defecation

SLWC short-leg walking cast

SM Master of Science; sadomasochism; self-monitoring; simple mastectomy; skim milk; smooth muscle; somatomedin; space medicine; sphingomyelin; splenic macrophage; sports medicine; streptomycin; Strümpell-Marie [syndrome]; submandibular; submaxillary; submucous; suckling mouse; sucrose medium; suction method; superior mesenteric; sustained medication; symptoms; synaptic membrane; synovial membrane; systolic motion; systolic murmur

S/M sudomasochism

Sm samarium; *Serratia marcescens*

sm smear

sM suckling mouse

SMA sequential multiple analysis; sequential multichannel autoanalyzer; simultaneous multichannel autoanalyzer; smooth muscle antibody; Society for Medical Anthropology; somatomedin A; spinal muscular atrophy; spontaneous motor activity; standard method agar; superior mesenteric artery; supplementary motor area

SM-A somatomedin A

SMA-6 Sequential Multiple Analysis—six different serum tests

SMA-6/60 Sequential Multiple Analysis—six tests in 60 minutes

SMABF superior mesenteric artery blood flow

SMAC Sequential Multiple Analyzer Computer

SMAE superior mesenteric artery embolism

SMAF smooth muscle activating factor; specific macrophage arming factor

SMAG Special Medical Advisory Group

SMAL serum methyl alcohol level

sm an small animal

SMAO superior mesenteric artery occlusion

SMART simultaneous multiple angle reconstruction technique

SMAS submuscular aponeurotic system; superior mesenteric artery syndrome

SMAST Short Michigan Alcoholism Screening Test

SMB selected mucosal biopsy; standard mineral base

sMb suckling mouse brain

SMBFT small bowel follow-through

SMC Scientific Manpower Commission; smooth muscle cell; somatomedin C; succinylmonocholine

SM-C, Sm-C somatomedin C

SMCA smooth muscle contracting agent; suckling mouse cataract agent

SMCD senile macular choroidal degeneration; systemic mast cell disease; systemic meningococcal disease

SM-C/IGF somatomedin C/insulin-like growth factor

SMD senile macular degeneration; submanubrial dullness

SMDA Safe Medical Devices Act [of 1990]; starch methylenedianiline

SMDC sodium-N-methyl dithiocarbamate

SMDS secondary myelodysplastic syndrome

SME severe myoclonic epilepsy

SMEDI stillbirth-mummification, embryonic death, infertility [syndrome]

SMEI severe myoclonic epilepsy of infancy

SMEM supplemented Eagle's minimum essential medium

SMF streptozocin, mitomycin C, and 5-fluorouracil

smf sodium motive force

SMFP state medical facilities plan

SMG submandibular gland

SMH state mental hospital; strongyloidiasis with massive hyperinfection

SMI Self-Motivation Inventory; senior medical investigator; severe mental impairment; small volume infusion; stress myocardial image; Style of Mind Inventory; supplementary medical insurance; sustained maximum inspiration

SmIg surface membrane immunoglobulin

SML smouldering leukemia

SMMD specimen mass measurement device

SMN second malignant neoplasm

SMNB submaximal neuromuscular block

SMO Senior Medical Officer

SMOH Senior Medical Officer of Health; Society of Medical Officers of Health

SMON subacute myeloopticoneuropathy

SMP slow moving protease; standard medical practice; submitochondrial particle; sulfamethoxypyrazine

SMR senior medical resident; sensorimotor rhythm; severe mental retardation; skeletal muscle relaxant; somnolent metabolic rate; standardized mortality ratio; stroke with minimum residuum; submucosal resection

SMRR submucosal resection and rhinoplasty

SMRV squirrel monkey retrovirus

SMS senior medical student; serial motor seizures; Shared Medical Systems; somatostatin; stiff-man syndrome; supplemental minimum sodium

SMSA standard metropolitan statistical area

SMSV San Miguel sea lion virus

SMT spontaneous mammary tumor; stereotactic mesencephalic tractomy

SMuLV Scripps murine leukemia virus

SMV superior mesenteric vein

SMX, SMZ sulfamethoxazole

SN sclerema neonatorum; scrub nurse; sensorineural; sensory neuron; serum neutralization; sinus node; spontaneous nystagmus; staff nurse; student nurse; subnormal; substantia nigra; supernatant; suprasternal notch

S/N signal/noise [ratio]

Sn subnasale; tin [Lat. *stannum*]

sn according to nature [Lat. *secundum naturam*]

SNA specimen not available; Student Nurses Association

SNa serum sodium concentration

SNagg serum normal agglutinator

SNAP sensory nerve action potential

SNB scalene node biopsy

SNC spontaneous neonatal chylothorax

SNCL sinus node cycle length

SNCS sensory nerve conduction studies

SNCV sensory nerve conduction velocity

SND sinus node dysfunction; striatonigral degeneration

SNDA Student National Dental Association

SNDO Standard Nomenclature of Diseases and Operations

SNE sinus node electrogram; subacute necrotizing encephalomyelography

SNES suprascapular nerve entrapment syndrome

SNF sinus node formation; skilled nursing facility

SNGBF single nephron glomerular blood flow

SNGFR single nephron glomerular filtration rate

SNHL sensorineural hearing loss

SNM Society of Nuclear Medicine; sulfanilamide

SNMA Student National Medical Association

SNMT Society of Nuclear Medical Technologists

SNOBOL String-Oriented Symbolic Language

SNODO Standard Nomenclature of Diseases and Operations

SNOMED Symmetrical Nomenclature of Medicine

SNOP Systematized Nomenclature of Pathology

SNP school nurse practitioner; sinus node potential; sodium nitroprusside

SNR signal-to-noise ratio; substantia nigra zona reticulata; supernumerary rib

SNRB selective nerve root block

snRNA small nuclear ribonucleic acid

snRNP small nuclear ribonucleoprotein

SNRT sinus node recovery time

SNRTd sinus node recovery time, direct measuring

SNRTi sinus node recovery time, indirect measuring

SNS Senior Nursing Sister; Society of Neurological Surgeons; sympathetic nervous system

SNSA seronegative spondyloarthropathy

SNST sciatic nerve stretch test

SNT sinuses, nose, and throat

SNV spleen necrosis virus

SNW slow negative wave

SO salpingo-oophorectomy; Schlatter-Osgood [test]; second opinion; sex offender; spheno-occipital [synchondrosis]; sphincter of Oddi; standing orders; superior oblique [muscle]; supraoptic; supraorbital

S&O salpingo-oophorectomy

SO₂ oxygen saturation

SOA swelling of ankles

SoA symptoms of asthma

SOAA signed out against advice

SOAMA signed out against medical advice

SOA-MCA superficial occipital artery to middle cerebral artery

SOAP subjective, objective, assessment, and plan [problem-oriented record]

SOAPIE subjective, objective, assessment, plan, implementation, and evaluation [problem-oriented record]

SOB see order blank; shortness of breath

SOC sequential oral contraceptive; Standard Occupational Classification; standards of care; syphilitic osteochondritis

SoC state of consciousness

SocSec Social Security

SocServ social services

S-OCT serum ornithine carbamyl transferase

SOD septo-optic dysplasia; superoxide dismutase

sod sodium

sod bicarb sodium bicarbonate

SODAS spheroidal oral drug absorption system

SODH sorbitol dehydrogenase

SOF superior orbital fissure

SOH sympathetic orthostatic hypotension

SOHN supraoptic hypothalamic nucleus

SOL solution; space-occupying lesion

sol soluble, solution

SOLEC stand on one leg eyes closed

Soln solution

solv dissolve [Lat. *solve*]

SOM secretory otitis media; sensitivity of method; serous otitis media; somatotropin; superior oblique muscle; suppurative otitis media

SOMA Student Osteopathic Medical Association

somat somatic

SOMI sternal occipital mandibular immobilization

SON superior olivary nucleus; supraoptic nucleus

SOP standard operating procedure

SoP standard of performance

SOPA syndrome of primary aldosteronism

SOPCA sporadic olivopontocerebellar ataxia

s op s if it is necessary [Lat. *si opus sit*]

SOQ Suicide Opinion Questionnaire

SOR stimulus-organism response; superoxide release

SOr supraorbitale

Sorb, sorb sorbitol

SORD sorbitol dehydrogenase

SOS self-obtained smear; supplemental oxygen system

sos if it is necessary [Lat. *si opus sit*]

SOSF single organ system failure

SOT sensory organization test; systemic oxygen transport

SOWS subjective opiate withdrawal scale

SP sacroposterior; sacrum to pubis; salivary progesterone; schizotypal personality; semi-private [room]; senile plaque; septum pellucidum; seropositive; serum protein; shunt pressure; shunt procedure; silent period; skin potential; sleep deprivation; soft palate; solid phase; speech pathology; spleen; spontaneous proliferation; standard practice; standard procedure; staphylococcal protease; status post; stool preservative; subliminal perception; substance P; suprapatellar; suprapubic; surfactant protein; symphisis pubis; systolic pressure

Sp the most posterior point on the posterior contour of the sella turcica; species; sphenoid; spine; *Spirillum*; summation potential

sP senile parkinsonism

sp space; species; specific; spine, spinal; spirit, alcohol [Lat. *spiritus*]

s/p status post

SPA human albumin [salt-poor albumin]; sheep pulmonary adenomatosis; sperm penetration assay; spinal progressive amyotrophy; spondyloarthropathy; spontaneous platelet aggregation; staphylococcal protein A; suprapubic aspiration

SP-A surfactant protein A

sp act specific activity

SPAD stenosing peripheral arterial disease

SPAG small particle aerosol generator

SPAI steroid protein activity index

SPAM scanning photoacoustic microscopy

sp an spinal anesthesia

SPAR sensitivity prediction by acoustic reflex

SPAT slow paroxysmal atrial tachycardia

SP-B surfactant protein B

SPBI serum protein-bound iodine

SPC salicylamide, phenacetin, and caffeine; seropositive carrier; single palmar crease; single photoelectron count; spleen cell; statistical process control; synthetizing protein complex

SPCA serum prothrombin conversion accelerator; Society for Prevention of Cruelty to Animals

SPCC Spill Prevention, Control, and Countermeasure plan

SPCD syndrome of primary ciliary dyskinesia

sp cd spinal cord

SPD schizotypal personality disorder; sociopathic personality disorder; specific paroxysmal discharge; standard peak dilution; storage pool deficiency

SPDC strio-pallido-dentate calcinosis

SPE septic pulmonary edema; serum protein electrolytes; serum protein electrophoresis; streptococcal pyrogenic exotoxin; sucrose polyester; sustained physical exercise

SPEAR selective parenteral and enteral anti-sepsis regimen

SPE-C streptococcal pyrogenic exotoxin type C

Spec specialist, specialty

spec special; specific; specimen

spec gr specific gravity

SPECT single photon emission computed tomography

SPEG serum protein electrophoretogram

SPEM smooth pursuit eye movement

SPEP serum protein electrophoresis

SPF skin protection factor; specific-pathogen free; spectrophotofluorometer; S-phase fraction; split products of fibrin; standard perfusion fluid; Stuart-Prower factor; sun protection factor; systemic pulmonary fistula

sp fl spinal fluid

SPG serine phosphoglyceride; sucrose, phosphate, and glutamate; symmetrical peripheral gangrene

SpG specific gravity

spg sponge

SPGA Bovarnik's solution; sucrose

sp gr specific gravity

SPH secondary pulmonary hemosiderosis; severely and profoundly handicapped; spherocyte; spherocytosis; sphingomyelin

Sph sphenoidale; sphingomyelin

sph spherical; spherical lens; spheroid

sp ht specific heat

SPI Self-Perception Inventory; serum precipitable iodine; serum protein index; Shipley Personal Inventory

SPIA solid-phase immunoabsorption; solid-phase immunoassay

SPICU surgical pulmonary intensive care unit

SPID summed pain intensity difference

SPIF solid-phase immunoassay fluorescence

spin spine, spinal

sp indet indeterminate species [Lat. *species indeterminata*]

spir spiral; spirit, alcohol [Lat. *spiritus*]

spiss dried [Lat. *spissus*]; inspissated, thickened by evaporation [Lat. *spissatus*]

SPK serum pyruvate kinase; superficial punctate keratitis

SPL skin potential level; sound pressure level; splanchnic; spontaneous lesion; staphylococcal phage lysate; superior parietal lobule

SPLATT split anterior tibial tendon

sPLM sleep-related periodic leg movements

SPLV serum parvovirus-like virus

SPM shocks per minute; subhuman primate model; suspended particulate matter; synaptic plasma membrane

SpM spiriformis medialis [nucleus]

SPMA spinal progressive muscular atrophy

SPMR standard proportionate mortality ratio (or rate)

SPMSQ Short Portable Mental Status Questionnaire

SPN solitary pulmonary nodule; supplemental parental nutrition; sympathetic preganglionic neuron

sp n, sp nov new species [Lat. *species novum*]

SpO₂ pulse oximetry

SPOD spouse's perception of disease

spon, spont spontaneous

SPOOL simultaneous peripheral operation on-line

SPP plural of *species*; Sexuality Preference Profile; skin perfusion pressure; suprapubic prostatectomy

spp plural of *species*

SPPP, sppp plural of *subspecies*

SPPS solid phase peptide synthesis; stable plasma protein solution

SPPT superprecipitation response

SPR serial probe recognition; Society for Pediatric Radiology; Society for Pediatric Research; solid phase radioimmunoassay

Spr scan projection radiography

spr sprain

SPRIA solid phase radioimmunoassay

SPROM spontaneous premature rupture of membrane

SPS scapuloperoneal syndrome; shoulder pain and stiffness; simple partial seizures; slow-progressive schizophrenia; Society of Pelvic Surgeons; sodium polyanethol sulfonate; sound production sample; stimulated protein synthesis; Suicide Probability Scale; systemic progressive sclerosis

SpS sphenoid sinus

spSHR stroke-prone spontaneously hypertensive rat

SPST Symonds Picture-Story Test

SPT secretin-pancreazymin [test]; single

patch technique; sleep period time; station pull-through [technique]

SpT spinal tap

Spt spirit, alcohol [Lat. *spiritus*]

Sp tap spinal tap

SPTI systolic pressure time index

SPTS subjective posttraumatic syndrome

SPTx static pelvic traction

SPU short procedure unit; Society of Pediatric Urology

SPV selective proximal vagotomy; Shope papilloma virus; sulfophosphovanillin

SPZ sulfinpyrazone

SQ social quotient; status quo; subcutaneous; survey question; symptom questionnaire

Sq subcutaneous

sq square; squamous

SQC statistical quality control

sq cell ca squamous cell carcinoma

SQUID superconducting quantum interference device

SR sarcoplasmic reticulum; scanning radiometer; screen; secretion rate; sedimentation rate; seizure resistant; sensitivity response; sensitization response; service record; sex ratio; shorthair [guinea pig]; short range; side rails; sigma reaction; sinus rhythm; skin resistance; slow release; smooth-rough [colony]; specific release; specific response; spontaneous respiration; steroid resistance; stimulus response; stomach rumble; stress related; stretch reflex; sulfonamide-resistant; superior rectus; sustained release; systemic resistance; systems research; systems review

S-R smooth-rough [bacteria]

Sr strontium

sr steradian

SRA segmental renal artery; serum renin activity; spleen repopulating activity

SRAM static random access memory

SR_AW, SR_aw specific airway resistance

SRBC sheep red blood cells

SRBD sleep-related breathing disorder

SRC sedimented red cells; sheep red cells

src Rous sarcoma oncogene

SRCA specific red cell adherence

SRCBC serum reserve cholesterol binding capacity

SR/CP schizophrenic reaction, chronic paranoid

SRD service-related disability; Society for the Relief of Distress; Society for the Right to Die; sodium-restricted diet; specific reading disability

SRDS severe respiratory distress syndrome

SRDT single radial diffusion test

SRE Schedule of Recent Experiences

sREM stage rapid eye movement

SRF severe renal failure; skin reactive factor; somatotropin-releasing factor; split renal function; subretinal fluid

SRF–A slow-reacting factor–anaphylaxis

SRFS split renal function study

SRH single radial hemolysis; somatotropin-releasing hormone; spontaneously responding hyperthyroidism; stigmata of recent hemorrhage

SRI severe renal insufficiency; Stanford Research Institute

SRID single radial immunodiffusion

SRIF somatotropin-release inhibiting factor

SRM spontaneous rupture of membranes; Standard Reference Material; superior rectus muscle

SMRD stress-related mucosal damage

SRN State Registered Nurse

sRNA soluble ribonucleic acid

SRNG sustained release nitroglycerin

SRNS steroid-responsive nephrotic syndrome

SRO sex-ratio organism; smallest region of overlap; Steele-Richardson-Olszewski [syndrome]

SROM spontaneous rupture of membrane

SRP short rib–polydactyly [syndrome]; signal recognition particle; Society for Radiological Protection; State Registered Physiotherapist; synchronized retroperfusion

SRPS short rib–polydactyly syndrome

SRQ Self-Reporting Questionnaire

SRR standardized rate ratio; surgery recovery room

SRRS Social Readjustment Rating Scale

SR-RSV Schmidt-Ruppin strain Rous sarcoma virus

SRS schizophrenic residual state; sex reassignment surgery; Silver-Russell syndrome; slow-reacting substance; Social and Rehabilitation Service; Symptom Rating Scale

SRSA, SRS-A slow-reacting substance of anaphylaxis

SRT sedimentation rate test; simple reaction time; sinus node recovery time; speech reception test; speech reception threshold; spontaneously resolving thyrotoxicosis; surfactant replacement therapy; sustained-release theophylline; symptom rating test

SRU sample ratio units; side rails up; solitary rectal ulcer; structural repeating unit

SRUS solitary rectal ulcer syndrome

SRV Schmidt-Ruppin virus; simian retrovirus; superior radicular vein

SRVT sustained re-entrant ventricular tachyarrhythmia

SRW short ragweed [test]

SS disulfide; sacrosciatic; saline soak; saline solution; saliva sample; saliva substitute; Salmonella-Shigella [agar]; salt substitute; saturated solution; Schizophrenia Subscale; seizure-sensitive; selective shunt; serum sickness; Sézary syndrome; short sleep; siblings; sickle cell; side-to-side; signs and symptoms; single-stranded; Sjögren syndrome; skull series [radiographs]; soap suds; Social Security; social services; somatostatin; sparingly soluble; stainless steel; standard score; statistically significant; steady state; sterile solution; steroid sensitivity; Stickler syndrome; subaortic stenosis; subscapular; substernal; suction socket; sum of squares; supersaturated; support and stimulation; Sweet syndrome; systemic sclerosis

S/S salt substitute

S&S signs and symptoms

Ss *Shigella sonnei*; subjects

ss in the strict sense [Lat. *sensu stricto*]; one half [Lat. *semis*]; single-stranded; soap suds; subspinale

SSA salicylsalicylic acid; skin-sensitizing antibody; skin sympathetic activity; Sjögren syndrome A; Smith surface antigen; Social Security Administration; sperm-specific antiserum; sulfosalicylic acid

SSA1 Smallest Space Analysis

SSAV simian sarcoma-associated virus

SSB short spike burst; single-stranded binding [protein]; stereospecific binding

SS-B Sjögren syndrome B

SSBG sex steroid-binding globulin

SSC sister strand crossover; somatosensory cortex; standard saline citrate; standard sodium citrate; syngeneic spleen cell

SSc systemic scleroderma; systemic sclerosis

SSCA spontaneous suppressor cell activity

SSCCS slow spinal cord compression syndrome

ss(c)DNA single-stranded circular deoxyribonucleic acid

SSCF sleep stage change frequency

SSCr stainless steel crown

SSD single saturating dose; source-skin distance; source-surface distance; speech-sound discrimination; succinate semialdehyde dehydrogenase; sum of square deviations; syndrome of sudden death

SSDBS symptom schedule for the diagnosis of borderline schizophrenia

ssDNA single-stranded DNA

SSE saline solution enema; skin self-examination; soapsuds enema; steady state exercise; subacute spongiform encephalopathy

SSEA stage-specific embryonic antigen

SSEP somatosensory evoked potential

S seq without sequel [Lat. *sme sequela*]

SSER somatosensory evoked response

SSES Sexual Self-Efficacy Scale

SSF soluble suppressor factor; supplemental sensory feedback

SSG sublabial salivary gland

SSHL severe sensorineural hearing

SSI segmental sequential irradiation; shoulder subluxation inhibition; small-scale integration; Somatic Symptom Inventory; subshock insulin; Supplemental Security Income; System Sign Inventory

SSIDS sibling of sudden infant death syndrome [victim]

SSIE Smithsonian Science Information Exchange

SSKI saturated solution of potassium iodide

SSL skin surface lipid; sufficient sleep

SSLI serum sickness–like illness

SSM subsynaptic membrane; superficial spreading melanoma

SSMS saturated solution of magnesium iodide

SSN severely subnormal; subacute sensory neuropathy; suprasternal notch

SSNS steroid-sensitive nephrotic syndrome

SSO Society of Surgical Oncology; special sense organ

SSOP Second Surgical Opinion Program

SSP Sanarelli-Shwartzman phenomenon; subacute sclerosing panencephalitis; subspecies; supersensitivity perception

ssp subspecies

SSPE subacute sclerosing panencephalitis

SSPG steady state plasma glucose

SSPI steady state plasma insulin

SSPL saturation sound pressure level

SSPP subsynaptic plate perforation

SSPS side-to-side portacaval shunt

SS-PSE Schizophrenic Subscale of the Present State Examination

SSQ Social Support Questionnaire

SSR site-specific recombination; somatosensory response; surgical supply room

ssRNA single-stranded ribonucleic acid
SSS scalded skin syndrome; secondary Sjögren syndrome; sick sinus syndrome; specific soluble substance; Stanford Sleepiness Scale; sterile saline soak; systemic sicca syndrome
sss layer upon layer [Lat. *stratum super stratum*]
SSSS staphylococcal scalded skin syndrome
SSST superior sagittal sinus thrombosis
SSSV superior sagittal sinus velocity
SST sodium sulfite titration; somatostatin
s str in the strict sense [Lat. *sensu stricto*]
SSU self-service unit; sterile supply unit
SSV Schoolman-Schwartz virus; simian sarcoma virus; under a poison label [Lat. *sub signo veneni*]
SSX sulfisoxazole
ST esotropia; scala tympani; sclerotherapy; sedimentation time; semitendinosus; shock therapy; sickle [cell] thalassemia; sinus tachycardia; sinus tympani; skin test; skin thickness; slight trace; slow twitch; spastic torticollis; speech therapist; sphincter tone; stable toxin; standard test; starting time; sternothyroid; stimulus; store; stress test; stria terminalis; striation; subtalar; subtotal; surface tension; surgical treatment; survival time; syndrome of the trephined; systolic time
S-T [*segment*] in electrocardiography, the portion of the segment between the end of the S wave and the beginning of the T wave; sickle-cell thalassemia
St, st let it stand [Lat. *stet*]; let them stand [Lat. *stent*]; stage [of disease]; status; stere; sterile; stimulation; stokes; stone [unit]; straight; stroke; stomach; stomion; subtype
STA second trimester abortion; serum thrombotic accelerator; superficial temporal artery
Sta staphylion
stab stabilization; stabnuclear neutrophil
STAG slow-target attaching globulin; split-thickness autogenous graft

STA-MCA superficial temporal artery to middle cerebral artery
STAI State Trait Anxiety Inventory
StanPsych standard psychiatric [nomenclature]
Staph, staph *Staphylococcus*, staphylococcal
stat immediately [Lat. *statim*]; radiation emanation unit [German]
Stb stillborn
STC serum theophylline concentration; soft tissue calcification; stroke treatment center; subtotal colectomy
STD sexually transmitted disease; skin-to-tumor distance; skin test dose; sodium tetradecyl sulfate; standard test dose
std saturated; standardized
STDH skin test for delayed hypersensitivity
STEL short-term exposure limit
STEM scanning transmission electron microscope
sten stenosis, stenosed
stereo stereogram
STESS subject's treatment emergent symptom scale
STET submaximal treadmill exercise test
STF serum thymus factor; slow-twitch fiber; special tube feeding; specialized treatment center; sudden transient freezing
STFM Society of Teachers of Family Medicine
STEV short-term exposure value
STG split-thickness graft
STH somatotropic hormone; subtotal hysterectomy
STh sickle cell thalassemia
STHRF somatotropic hormone releasing factor
STI Scientific and Technical Information; serum trypsin inhibitor; soybean trypsin inhibitor; systolic time interval
STIC serum trypsin inhibition capacity; solid-state transducer intracompartment
stillat drop by drop [Lat. *stillatim*]
stillb stillborn
stim stimulated, stimulation; stimulus

STK streptokinase

STL serum theophylline level; status thymicolymphaticus; swelling, tenderness and limited motion

STLOM swelling, tenderness, and limitation of motion

STLS subacute thyroiditis-like syndrome

STLV simian T-lymphotropic virus

STM scanning tunneling microscope; short-term memory; streptomycin

STN subthalamic nucleus; supratrochlear nucleus

sTNM TNM (see p. 305) staging of tumors as determined by surgical procedures

STNR symmetric tonic neck reflex

STNV satellite tobacco necrosis virus

STO store

stom stomach

STORCH syphilis, toxoplasmosis, rubella, cytomegalovirus, and herpesvirus

STP scientifically treated petroleum; sodium thiopental; standard temperature and pressure; standard temperature and pulse

STPD a volume of gas at standard temperature and pressure that contains no water vapor

STPS specific thalamic projection system

STQ superior temporal quadrant

STR soft tissue relaxation; stirred tank reactor

Str, str *Streptococcus*, streptococcal

strab strabismus

Strep *Streptococcus*; streptomycin

STRT skin temperature recovery time

struct structure, structural

STS serologic test for syphilis; sodium tetradecyl sulfate; sodium thiosulfate; standard test for syphilis; steroid sulfatase

STSA Southern Thoracic Surgical Association

STSE split-thickness skin excision

STSG split-thickness skin graft

STSS staphylococcal toxic shock syndrome

STT scaphotrapeziotrapezoid [joint]; serial thrombin time; skin temperature test

STU skin test unit

STV superior temporal vein

STVA subtotal villose atrophy

STVS short-term visual storage

STX saxitoxin

STZ streptozocin; streptozyme

SU salicyluric acid; secretory unit; sensation unit; solar urticaria; sorbent unit; spectrophotometric unit; status uncertain; subunit; sulfonamide; sulfonylurea; supine

Su sulfonamide

su let him take [Lat. *sumat*]

SUA serum uric acid; single umbilical artery; single unit activity

subac subacute

subclav subclavian; subclavicular

subcut subcutaneous

sub fin coct toward the end of boiling [Lat. *sub finem coctionis*]

subling sublingual

SubN subthalamic nucleus

subq subcutaneous

subsp subspecies

substd substandard

suc juice [Lat. *succus*]

Succ succinate, succinic

SUD skin unit dose; sudden unexpected death

SUDH succinyldehydrogenase

SUI stress urinary incontinence

SUID sudden unexplained infant death

sulf sulfate

sulfa sulfonamide

SULF-PRIM sulfamethoxazole and trimethoprim

sum let him take [Lat. *sumat*]; to be taken [Lat. *sumendum*]

SUMA sporadic ulcerating and mutilating acropathy

SUMIT streptokinase-urokinase myocardial infarct test

SUN standard unit of nomenclature; serum urea nitrogen
SUO syncope of unknown origin
SUP schizo-unipolar; supination
sup above [Lat. *supra*]; superficial; superior; supinator; supine
supin supination, supine
suppl supplement, supplementary
suppos suppository
surg surgery, surgeon, surgical
SURS solitary ulcer of rectum syndrome
SUS Saybolt Universal Seconds; solitary ulcer syndrome; stained urinary sediment; suppressor sensitive
susp suspension, suspended
SUTI symptomatic urinary tract infection
SUUD sudden unexpected unexplained death
SUV small unilamellar vessel
SUX succinylcholine
SV saphenous vein; sarcoma virus; satellite virus; selective vagotomy; semilunar valve; seminal vesicle; severe; sigmoid volvulus; simian virus; single ventricle; sinus venosus; snake venom; splenic vein; spontaneous ventilation; stroke volume; subclavian vein; subventricular; supravital
S/V surface/volume ratio
SV40 simian vacuolating virus 40
Sv sievert
sv sievert; single vibration; spirit of wine [Lat. *spiritus vini*]
SVA selective vagotomy and antrectomy; selective visceral angiography; sequential ventriculoatrial [pacing]; subtotal villous atrophy
SVAS supravalvular aortic stenosis; supraventricular aortic stenosis
SVB saphenous vein bypass
SVBG saphenous vein bypass grafting
SVC segmental venous capacitance; selective venous catheterization; slow vital capacity; subclavian vein catheterization; superior vena cava
SVCCS superior vena cava compression syndrome

SVCG spatial vectorcardiogram
SVCO superior vena-caval obstruction
SVCP Special Virus Cancer Program
SVCR segmental venous capacitance ratio
SVCS superior vena cava syndrome
SVD single vessel disease; singular value decomposition; small vessel disease; spontaneous vaginal delivery; spontaneous vertex delivery; swine vesicular disease
SVE slow volume encephalography; soluble viral extract; sterile vaginal examination
SVG saphenous vein graft
SVI stroke volume index
SVL superficial vastus lateralis
SVM seminal vesicle microsome; syncytiovascular membrane
SVN sinuvertebral nerve; small volume nebulizer
SvO_2 venous oxygen saturation
SVOM sequential volitional oral movement
SVP selective vagotomy and pyloroplasty; small volume parenteral [infusion]; standing venous pressure; superior vascular plexus
SVPB supraventricular premature beat
SVR sequential vascular response; systemic vascular resistance
svr alcohol; rectified spirit of wine [Lat. *spiritus vini rectificatus*]
SVRI systemic vascular resistance index
SVS slit ventricle syndrome
SVT sinoventricular tachycardia; subclavian vein thrombosis; supraventricular tachyarrhythmia; supraventricular tachycardia
svt proof spirit [Lat. *spiritus vini tenuis*]
SW seriously wounded; short waves; sinewave; slow wave; soap and water; social worker; spike wave; spiral wound; stab wound; sterile water; stroke work; Sturge-Weber [syndrome]; Swiss Webster [mouse]
Sw swine
SWA seriously wounded in action
SWC submaximal working capacity

SWD short wave diathermy
SWE slow wave encephalography
SWG silkworm gut; standard wire gauge
SWI sterile water for injection; stroke work index; surgical wound infection
SWIM sperm-washing insemination method
SWIORA spinal cord injury without radiologic abnormality
SWM segmental wall motion
SWO superficial white onychomycosis
SWR serum Wassermann reaction
SWS slow-wave sleep; spike-wave stupor; steroid-wasting syndrome; Sturge-Weber syndrome
SWT sine-wave threshold
SWU septic work-up
Sx, S$_x$ signs; symptoms
Sxs serological sex-specific [antigen/
SXT sulfamethoxazole-trimethoprim [mixture]

SY syphilis, syphilitic
SYA subacute yellow atrophy
SYDS stomach yin deficiency syndrome
sym symmetrical; symptom
sympath sympathetic
symph symphysis
sympt symptom
SYN synovitis
syn synergistic; synonym; synovial
synd syndrome
syph syphilis, syphilitic
SYR Syrian [hamster]
syr syrup [Lat. *syrupus*]; syringe
SYS stretching-yawning syndrome
sys system, systemic
SYS-BP systolic blood pressure
syst system, systemic; systole, systolic
SZ streptozocin
Sz seizure; schizophrenia
SZN streptozocin

T

T absolute temperature; an electrocardiographic wave corresponding to the repolarization of the ventricles [wave]; life [time]; period [time]; ribosylthymine; tablespoonful; *Taenia*; tamoxifen; telomere or terminal banding; temperature; temporal electrode placement in electroencephalography; temporary; tenderness; tension [intraocular]; tera; tesla; testosterone; tetra; tetracycline; theophylline; therapy; thoracic; thorax; threatened [animal]; threonine; thrombosis; thrombus; thymidine; thymine; thymus [cell]; thymus-derived; thyroid; tidal gas; tidal volume; time; tincture; tocopherol; topical; torque; total; toxicity; training [group]; transition; transmittance; transverse; treatment; *Treponema*; *Trichophyton*; tritium; tryptamine; *Trypanosoma*; tuberculin; tuberculosis; tumor; turnkey system; type

$T_{1/2}$, $t_{1/2}$ half-life

T1-T12 first to twelfth thoracic vertebrae

T_1 spin-lattice or longitudinal relaxation time; tricuspid first sound

T + 1, T + 2, T + 3 first, second, and third stages of increased intraocular tension

T-1, T-2, T-3 first, second, and third stages of decreased intraocular tension

T_2 diiodothyronine; spin-spin or transverse relaxation time

2,4,5-T 2,4,5-trichlorophenoxyacetic acid

T_3 triiodothyronine

T_4 thyroxine

T-7 free thyroxine factor

t duration; Student t test; teaspoonful; temperature; temporal; terminal; tertiary; test of significance; three times [Lat. *ter*]; time; tissue; tonne; translocation

T_{90} time required for 90% mortality in a population of microorganisms exposed to a toxic agent

TA alkaline tuberculin; arterial tension; axillary temperature; tactile afferent; Takayasu arteritis; teichoic acid; temporal arteritis; terminal antrum; therapeutic abortion; thermophilic *Actinomyces*; thymocytotoxic autoantibody; thyroglobulin autoprecipitation; thyroid antibody; thyroid autoimmunity; tibialis anterior; titratable acid; total alkaloids; total antibody; toxic adenoma; toxinantitoxin; traffic accident; transactional analysis; transaldolase; transantral; transplantation antigen; transposition of aorta; trapped air; triamcinolone acetonide; tricuspid atresia; trophoblast antigen; true anomaly; truncus arteriosus; tryptamine; tryptose agar; tube agglutination; tumor-associated

T/A time and amount

T-A toxin-antitoxin

T&A tonsillectomy and adenoidectomy; tonsils and adenoids

Ta tantalum; tarsal

TAA thioacetamide; total ankle arthroplasty; tumor-associated antigen

TAAF thromboplastic activity of the amniotic fluid

TA-AIDS transfusion-associated acquired immunodeficiency syndrome

TAB total autonomic blockage; typhoid, paratyphoid A, and paratyphoid B [vaccine]

TAb therapeutic abortion

tab tablet

TABC total aerobic bacteria count; typhoid, paratyphoid A, paratyphoid B, and paratyphoid C [vaccine]

TABP type A behavior pattern

Tabs tablets

TABT typhoid, paratyphoid A, paratyphoid B, and tetanus toxoid [vaccine]

TABTD typhoid, paratyphoid A, paratyphoid B, tetanus toxoid, and diphtheria toxoid [vaccine]

TAC terminal antrum contraction; time-activity curve; total abdominal colectomy; total aganglionosis coli; triamcinolone cream

TACE chlorotrianicene; teichoic acid crude extract

tachy tachycardia

TAD test of auditory discrimination; thoracic asphyxiant dystrophy; transient acantholytic dermatosis

TADAC therapeutic abortion, dilatation, aspiration, curettage

TAF albumose-free tuberculin [Ger. *Tuberculin Albumose frei*]; tissue angiogenesis factor; toxin-antitoxin floccules; toxoid-antitoxin floccules; transabdominal hysterectomy; trypsinaldehyde-fuchsin; tumor angiogenesis factor

TAG target attaching globulin; technical advisory group; thymine, adenine, and guanine

TAGH triiodothyronine, amino acids, glucagon, and heparin

TAH total abdominal hysterectomy; total artificial heart

TAH BSO total abdominal hysterectomy and bilateral salpingo-oophorectomy

TAI Test Anxiety Inventory

TAL tendon of Achilles lengthening; thymic alymphoplasia

tal such a one [Lat. *talis*]

talc talcum

TALH thick ascending limb of Henle's loop

TALL, T-ALL T-cell acute lymphoblastic leukemia

TALLA T-cell acute lymphoblastic leukemia antigen

TAM tamoxifen; teen-age mother; thermoacidurans agar modified; total active motion; toxin-antitoxoid mixture; transient abnormal myelopoiesis

TAME toluenesulfonylarginine methyl ester

TAMIS Telemetric Automated Microbial Identification System

TAN total adenine nucleotide; total ammonia nitrogen

tan tandem translocation; tangent

TANI total axial [lymph] node irradiation

TAO thromboangiitis obliterans; triacetyloleandomycin

TAP transesophageal atrial pacing

TAPS trial assessment procedure scale

TAPVC total anomalous pulmonary venous connection

TAPVD total anomalous pulmonary venous drainage

TAPVR total anomalous pulmonary venous return

TAQW transient abnormal Q wave

TAR thoracic aortic rupture; thrombocytopenia with absent radii [syndrome]; tissue-air ratio; total abortion rate; transaxillary resection

TARA total articular replacement arthroplasty; tumor-associated rejection antigen

TARS threonyl-tRNA synthetase

TAS tetanus antitoxin serum; therapeutic activities specialist; thoracoabdominal syndrome; traumatic apallic syndrome

TASA tumor-associated surface antigen

Tase tryptophan synthetase

TASS thyrotoxicosis–Addison disease-Sjögren syndrome–sarcoidosis [syndrome]

TAT tetanus antitoxin; thematic apperception test; thematic aptitude test; thrombin-antithrombin complex; thromboplastin activation test; total antitryptic activity; toxin-antitoxin; transactivator; transaxial tomography; tray agglutination test; tumor activity test; turnaround time; tyrosine aminotransferase

TATA Pribnow [box]; tumor-associated transplantation antigen

TATR tyrosine aminotransferase regulator

τ Greek lower case letter *tau*; life [of radioisotope]; relaxation time; shear stress; spectral transmittance; transmission coefficient

TATST tetanus antitoxin skin test

TAV trapped air volume

TB Taussig-Bind [syndrome]; term birth; terminal bronchiole; terminal bronchus; thromboxane B; thymol blue; toluidine blue; total base; total bilirubin; total body; tracheal bronchiolar [region]; tracheobronchitis; trapezoid body; tub bath; tubercle bacillus; tuberculin; tuberculosis; tumor-bearing

Tb Tbilisi [phage]; terbium; tubercle bacillus; tuberculosis

T_b biological half-life; body temperature

tb tuberculosis

TBA tertiary butylacetate; testosterone-binding affinity; thiobarbituric acid; to be absorbed; to be added; total bile acids; trypsin-binding activity; tubercle bacillus; tumor-bearing animal

TBAB tryptose blood agar base

TBAN transbronchial aspiration needle

TBB transbronchial biopsy

TBBM total body bone minerals

TBC thyroxine-binding coagulin; total body calcium; total body clearance; tuberculosis

Tbc tubercle bacillus; tuberculosis

TBD total body density; Toxicology Data Base

TBE tick-borne encephalitis; tuberculin bacillin emulsion

TBF total body fat

TBFB tracheobronchial foreign body

TBFVL tidal breathing flow-volume loops

TBG testosterone-binding globulin; thyroglobulin; thyroxine-binding globulin; tracheobronchography; tris-buffered Gey's solution

TBGI thyroxine-binding globulin index

TBGP total blood granulocyte pool

TBH total body hematocrit

tBHP terbutyl hydroperoxide

TBHT total-body hyperthermia

TBI thyroid-binding index; thyroxine-binding index; tooth-brushing instruction; total-body irradiation; traumatic brain injury

TBII thyroid-stimulating hormone-binding inhibitory immunoglobulin

T bili total bilirubin

TBK total body potassium

tbl tablet

TBLB transbronchial lung biopsy

TBLC term birth, living child

TBLI term birth, living infant

TBM total body mass; tracheobronchiomegaly; trophoblastic basement membrane; tuberculous meningitis; tubular basement membrane

TBMN thin basement membrane nephropathy

TBN bacillus emulsion; total body nitrogen

TBNA total body neutron activation; treated but not admitted

TBNAA total body neutron activation analysis

TBP bithionol; testosterone-binding protein; thyroxine-binding protein; total bypass; tributyl phosphate; tuberculous peritonitis

TBPA thyroxine-binding prealbumin

TBPT total body protein turnover

TBR tumor-bearing rabbit

TB-RD tuberculosis and respiratory disease

TBS total body solids; total body solute; total body surface; total burn size; tracheobronchial submucosa; tracheobronchoscopy; tribromosalicylanilide; triethanolamine-buffered saline

tbs, tbsp tablespoon

TBSA total body surface area

TBSV tomato bushy stunt virus

TBT tolbutamide test; tracheobronchial toilet; tracheobronchial tree

TBTT tuberculin time test

TBV total blood volume

TBW total body water; total body weight

TBX thromboxane; total body irradiation

TBZ tetrabenazine; thiabendazole

TC target cell; taurocholate; temperature compensation; teratocarcinoma; tertiary cleavage; tetracycline; thermal conductivity; thoracic cage; throat culture; thyrocalcitonin; tissue culture; to contain; total calcium; total capacity; total cholesterol; total colonoscopy; total correction; transcobalamin; transcutaneous; transplant center; transverse colon; Treacher Collins [syndrome]; true conjugate; tuberculin contagiosum; tubocurarine; tumor cell; tumor of cerebrum; type and crossmatch

T&C turn and cough; type and crossmatch

T$_4$(C) serum thyroxine measured by column chromatography

TC$_{50}$ medium toxic concentration

Tc technetium; tetracycline; transcobalamin

T$_c$ cytotoxic T-cell; the generation time of a cell cycle

t(°C) temperature on the Celsius scale

tc transcutaneous; translational control

TCA T-cell A locus; terminal cancer; tetracyclic antidepressant; total cholic acid; total circulating albumin; total circulatory arrest; tricalcium aluminate; tricarboxylic acid; trichloroacetic acid; tricyclic antidepressant; thyrocalcitonin

TCAB 3,3',4,4'-tetrachloroazobenzene

TCABG triple coronary artery bypass graft

TCAD tricyclic antidepressant

TCAG triple coronary artery graft

TCAOB 3,3',4,4'-tetrachloroazoxybenzene

TCAP trimethyl-cetyl-ammonium pentachlorophenate

TCB tetrachlorobiphenyl; total cardiopulmonary bypass transcatheter biopsy; tumor cell burden

TCAR t-cell antigen receptor

TCBS thiosulfate–citrate–bile salts–sucrose [agar]

TCC terminal complement complex; thromboplastic cell component; transitional-cell carcinoma; trichlorocarbanilide

Tcc triclocarban

TCCA, TCCAV transitional cell cancer-associated [virus]

TCCL T-cell chronic lymphoblastic leukemia

TCD thermal conductivity detector; tissue culture dose; transverse cardiac diameter

TCD$_{50}$ median tissue culture dose

TCDB turn, cough, deep breathe

TCDC taurochenodeoxycholate

TCDD 2,3,7,8-tetrachlorodibenzo-p-dioxin

TCE T-cell enriched; tetrachlorodiphenyl ethane; trichloroethylene

TCES transcutaneous cranial electrical stimulation

TCESOM trichloroethylene-extracted soybean oil meal

TCET transcerebral electrotherapy

TCF tissue coding factor; total coronary flow

T-CFC T-colony forming cell

TCFU tumor colony-forming unit

TCGF T-cell growth factor

TCH thiophen-2-carboxylic acid hydrazide; total circulating hemoglobin; turn, cough, hyperventilate

TChE total cholinesterase

TCI total cerebral ischemia; transient cerebral ischemia

TCi teracurie

TCID tissue culture infective dose; tissue culture inoculated dose

TCID$_{50}$ median tissue culture infective dose

TCIE transient cerebral ischemic episode

TCL thermochemiluminescence; total capacity of the lung; transverse carpal ligament

T-CLL T-cell chronic lymphatic leukemia

TC$_{Lo}$ toxic concentration low

TCM tissue culture medium; transcutaneous monitor

Tc 99m technetium-99m

TCMA transcortical motor aphasia

TCMP thematic content modification program

TCMZ trichloromethiazide

TCN tetracycline

TĉNM tumor with lymph node metastases

TCNS transcutaneous nerve stimulation/stimulator

TCNV terminal contingent negative variation

T_{CO_2} total carbon dioxide

TCP therapeutic continuous penicillin; total circulating protein; tranylcypromine; tricalcium phosphate; trichlorophenol; tricresyl phosphate

tcPCO₂, tcPCO₂ transcutaneous carbon dioxide pressure

tcP₀₂, tcPO₂ transcutaneous oxygen pressure

2,4,5-TCPPA 2-(2,4,5-trichlorophenoxy)-propionic acid

TCPA tetrachlorophthalic anhydride

TCPS total cavopulmonary shunt

TCR T-cell reactivity; T-cell receptor; T-cell rosette; thalamocortical relay; total cytoplasmic ribosome

tcRNA translational control ribonucleic acid

TCRP total cellular receptor pool

TCRV total red cell volume

TCS T-cell supernatant; tethered cord syndrome; total coronary score

TCSA tetrachlorosalicylanilide

TCSF T-colony-stimulating factor

TCT thrombin clotting time; thyrocalcitonin; trachial cytotoxin; transmission computed tomography

Tct tincture

TCV thoracic cage volume; three concept view

TD tardive dyskinesia; T-cell dependent; temporary disability; terminal device; tetanus and diphtheria [toxoid]; tetrodotoxin; therapy discontinued; thermal dilution; thoracic duct; three times per day; threshold of detectability; threshold of discomfort; threshold dose; thymus-dependent; timed disintegration; toco-

pherol deficiency; to deliver; tone decay; torsion dystonia; total disability, total discrimination; totally disabled; total dose; toxic dose; tracheal diameter; transdermal; transverse diameter; traveler's diarrhea; treatment discontinued; tumor dose; typhoid dysentery

T/D treatment discontinued

T_D the time required to double the number of cells in a given population; thermal death time

Td tetanus-diphtheria toxoid

$T_4(D)$ serum thyroxine measured by displacement analysis

TD_{50} median toxic dose

td three times daily [Lat. *ter die*]

TDA thyroid-stimulating hormone-displacing antibody

TDB Toxicology Data Bank

TDC taurodeoxycholic acid; total dietary calories

TDD telecommunication device for the deaf; tetradecadiene; thoracic duct drainage; total digitalizing dose; toxic doses of drugs

TDE tetrachlorodiphenylethane; total digestible energy; triethylene glycol diglycidyl

TDF thoracic duct fistula; thoracic duct flow; time-dose fractionation; tissue-damaging factor; tumor dose fractionation

TDH threonine dehydrogenase

TDI temperature difference integration; three-dimensional interlocking [hip]; toluene 2,4-diisocyanate; total dose infusion; total dose insulin

TDL thoracic duct lymph; thymus-dependent lymphocyte; toxic dose level

TDM therapeutic drug monitoring

TDN total digestible nutrients

tDNA transfer deoxyribonucleic acid

TDO tricho-dento-osseous [syndrome]

TDP thermal death point; thoracic duct pressure; thymidine diphosphate; total degradation products

TdR thymidine

TDS temperature, depth, salinity; thiamine disulfide; transduodenal sphincteroplasty

tds to be taken three times a day [Lat. *ter die sumendum*]

TDSD transient digestive system disorder

TDT terminal deoxynucleotidyl transferase; thermal death time; tone decay test; tumor doubling time

TdT terminal deoxynucleotidyl transferase

TDZ thymus-dependent zone

TE echo-time; expiratory time; tennis elbow; test ear; tetanus; tetracycline; threshold energy; thromboembolism; thymus epithelium; thyrotoxic exophthalmos; tick-borne encephalitis; time estimation; tissue-equivalent; tonsillectomy; tooth extracted; total estrogen; toxic epidermolysis; *Toxoplasma* encephalitis; trace element; tracheoesophageal; transepithelial; treadmill exercise; trial error

T&E testing and evaluation; trial and error

Te effective half-life; tellurium; tetanic contraction; tetanus

T_E expiratory phase time

TEA temporal external artery; tetraethylammonium; thermal energy analyzer; thromboendarterectomy; total elbow arthroplasty; triethanolamine

TEAB tetraethylammonium bromide

TEAC tetraethylammonium chloride

TEAE triethylammonioethyl

TEAM Training in Expanded Auxiliary Management

teasp teaspoon

TEBG, TeBG testosterone-estradiol-binding globulin

TEC total electron count; total eosinophil count; total exchange capacity; transient erythroblastopenia of childhood; transluminal extraction catheter

T&EC trauma and emergency center

TECV traumatic epiphyseal coxa vara

TED Tasks of Emotional Development; threshold erythema dose; thromboembolic disease

TEDS anti-embolism stockings

TEE thermic effect of exercise; transesophageal echocardiography; tyrosine ethyl ester

TEEP tetraethyl pyrophosphate

TEF thermic effect of food; tracheoesophageal fistula; trunk extension-flexion [unit]

T_{eff} effective half-life

TEFRA Tax Equity and Fiscal Responsibility Act

TEFS transmural electrical field stimulation

TEG thromboelastogram; triethyleneglycol

TEIB triethyleneiminobenzoquinone

TEL tetraethyl lead

TEM transmission electron microscope/microscopy; triethylenemelamine

temp temperature; temple, temporal

temp dext to the right temple [Lat. *tempori dextro*]

temp sinist to the left temple [Lat. *tempori sinistro*]

TEN total enteral nutrition; total excretory nitrogen; toxic epidermal necrolysis; transepidermal neurostimulation

TENS transcutaneous electrical nerve stimulation

TEP tetraethylpyrophosphate; tracheoesophageal puncture; transesophageal pacing

TEPA triethylenephosphamide

TEPP tetraethyl pyrophosphate; triethylene pyrophosphate

TER teratogen; total endoplasmic reticulum; transcapillary escape rate

ter rub [Lat. *tere*]; terminal or end; ternary; tertiary; three times; threefold

ter in die three times a day

term terminal

tert tertiary

TES thymic epithelial supernatant; toxic epidemic syndrome; transcutaneous electrical stimulation; transmural electrical stimulation

TESPA thiotepa

TET tetracycline; total ejection time; total

exchange thyroxine; treadmill exercise test

Tet tetralogy of Fallot

tet tetanus

TETD tetraethylthiuram disulfide

TETA triethylenetetramine

tet tox tetanus toxoid

TEV tadpole edema virus; talipes equinovarus

TEWL transepidermal water loss

TEZ transthoracic electric impedance respirogram

TF free thyroxine; tactile fremitus; tail flick [reflex]; temperature factor; testicular feminization; tetralogy of Fallot; thymol flocculation; thymus factor; tissue-damaging factor; to follow; total flow; transfer factor; transferrin; transformation frequency; transfrontal; tube feeding; tuberculin filtrate; tubular fluid; tuning fork

t(°F) temperature on the Fahrenheit scale

Tf transferrin

T_f freezing temperature

TFA total fatty acids; transverse fascicular area; trifluoroacetic acid

TFC common form of transferrin

TFCC triangular fibrocartilage complex

TFd dialyzable transfer factor

TFE polytetrafluoroethylene

TFF tube-fed food

TFM testicular feminization male; testicular feminization mutation; total fluid movement; transmission electron microscopy

TFMPP 1-(trifluoromethylphenyl)-piperazine

TFN total fecal nitrogen; transferrin

TFP tubular fluid plasma

TFPZ trifluoroperazine

TFR total fertility rate; total flow resistance; transferrin receptor

TFS testicular feminization syndrome; thyroid function study; tube-fed saline

TFT thrombus formation time; thyroid function test; tight filum terminale; trifluorothymidine

TFX toxic effects

TG tendon graft; testosterone glucuronide; tetraglycine; thioglucose; thioglycolate; thioguanine; thromboglobulin; thyroglobulin; total gastrectomy; toxic goiter; transmissible gastroenteritis; treated group; triacylglycerol; trigeminal ganglion; triglyceride; tumor growth

Tg generation time; thyroglobulin; *Toxoplasma gondii*

T_g glass transition temperature

6-TG thioguanine

tG_1 the time required to complete the G_1 phase of the cell cycle

tG_2 the time required to complete the G_2 phase of the cell cycle

TGA taurocholate gelatin agar; thyroglobulin activity; total glycoalkaloids; total gonadotropin activity; transient global amnesia; transposition of great arteries; tumor glycoprotein assay

TgAb thyroglobulin antibody

TGAR total graft area rejected

TBG thyroid-binding globulin

TGBG dimethylglyoxal bis-guanylhydrazone

TGC time pain compensation

TGD thermal-green dye

TGE theoretical growth evaluation; transmissible gastroenteritis [virus]; tryptone glucose extract

TGF T-cell growth factor; transforming growth factor; tuboglomerular feedback; tumor growth factor

TGFA triglyceride fatty acid

TGG turkey gamma globulin

TGL triglyceride; triglyceride lipase

TGP tobacco glycoprotein

6-TGR 6-thioguanine riboside

TGS tincture of green soap

TGT thromboplastin generation test/time; tolbutamide-glucagon test

TGV thoracic gas volume; transposition of great vessels

TGY tryptone glucose yeast [agar]

TGYA tryptone glucose yeast agar

TH tension headache; tetrahydrocortisol; T helper [cell]; theophylline; thorax; thrill; thyrohyoid; thyroid hormone; topical hypothermia; total hysterectomy; tyrosine hydroxylase

T$_H$, T$_h$, Th T-helper [lymphocyte]; thenar; therapy; thoracic, thorax; thorium; throat

th thenar; thermie; thoracic; thyroid; transhepatic

THA tetrahydroaminoacridine; total hip arthroplasty; total hydroxyapatite; *Treponema* hemagglutination

ThA thoracic aorta

THAL thalassemia

THAM tris(hydroxymethyl)aminomethane

THB Todd-Hewitt broth; total heart beats

THb total hemoglobin

THBI thyroid hormone binding inhibitor

THBP 7,8,9,10-tetrahydrobenzo[a]pyrene

THC terpin hydrate and codeine; tetrahydrocannabinol; tetrahydrocortisol; thiocarbanidin; transhepatic cholangiogram; transplantable hepatocellular carcinoma

THCA alpha-trihydroxy-5-beta-cholestannic acid

THD transverse heart diameter

Thd ribothymidine

THDOC tetrahydrodeoxycorticosterone

THE tetrahydrocortisone E; tonic hind limb extension; transhepatic embolization; tropical hypereosinophilia

theor theory, theoretical

ther therapy, therapeutic; thermometer

therap therapy, therapeutic

Θ Greek capital letter *theta*; thermodynamic temperature

θ Greek lower case letter *theta*; an angular coordinate variable; customary temperature; temperature interval

ther ex therapeutic exercise

therm thermal; thermometer

THF tetrahydrocortisone F; tetrahydrofolate; tetrahydrofuran; thymic humoral factor

THFA tetrahydrofolic acid; tetrahydrofurfuryl alcohol

Thg thyroglobulin

THH telangiectasia hereditaria haemorrhagica

Thi thiamine

THIP tetrahydroisoxazolopyridinol

Thio-TEPA thiotriethylenephosphamide

THM total heme mass

thor thorax, thoracic

THO titrated water

thou thousandth

THP Tamm-Horstall protein; tetrahydropapaveroline; tissue hydrostatic pressure; total hip replacement; total hydroxyproline; trihexphenidyl

THPA tetrahydropteric acid

THPP thiamine pyrophosphate; trihydroxy propriophenone

ThPP thiamine pyrophosphate

THPV transhepatic portal vein

THQ tetraquinone

THR targeted heart rate; threonine; total hip replacement; transhepatic resistance

Thr thrill; threonine

thr thyroid, thyroidectomy

THRF thyrotropic hormone-releasing factor

throm, thromb thrombosis, thrombus

THS tetrahydro-compound S; thrombohemorrhagic syndrome

THSC totipotent hematopoietic stem cell

THTH thyrotropic hromone

THU tetrahydrouridine

THUG thyroid uptake gradient

THVO terminal hepatic vein obliteration

Thx thromboxane

Thy thymine

thy thymus, thymectomy

THz terahertz

TI inversion time; temporal integration; terminal ileum; thalassemia intermedia; therapeutic index; thoracic index; thymus-independent; time interval; tonic immobility; transischial; translational inhibition; transverse inlet; tricuspid incompetence; tricuspid insufficiency; tumor induction

T$_I$ inspiration time

Ti titanium

TIA transient ischemic attack; tumor-induced angiogenesis; turbidimetric immunoassay

TIAH total implantation of artificial heart

TIB tibia; time in bed; tumor immunology bank

TIBC total iron-binding capacity

TIC Toxicology Information Center; trypsin inhibitory capability; tubulo-interstitial cell; tumor-inducing complex

TID time interval difference [imaging]; titrated initial dose

tid three times a day [Lat. *ter in die*]

TIDA tuberoinfundibular dopaminergic system

TIE transient ischemic episode

TIF tumor-inducing factor; tumor-inhibiting factor

TIg tetanus immunoglobulin

TIH time interval histogram

TIL tumor-infiltrating leukocyte; tumor-infiltrating lymphocyte

TIM transthoracic intracardiac monitoring

TIMC tumor-induced marrow cytotoxicity

TIMP tissue inhibitor of metalloproteinases

TIN tubulointerstitial nephropathy

tin three times a night [Lat. *ter in nocte*]

tinc, tinct tincture

TINU tubulo-interstitial nephritis–uveitis [syndrome]

TIP thermal inactivation point; Toxicology Information Program; translation-inhibiting protein; tumor-inhibiting principle

TIPI time-insensitive predictive instrument

TIPPS tetraiodophenylphthalein sodium

TIR terminal innervation ratio

TIS tetracycline-induced steatosis; transdermal infusion system; trypsin-insoluble segment; tumor in situ

TISP total immunoreactive serum pepsinogen

TISS Therapeutic Intervention Scoring System

TIT *Treponema* immobilization test

TIT, TITh triiodothyronine

TIU trypsin-inhibiting unit

TIUV total intrauterine volume

TIVC thoracic inferior vena cava

TJ tetrajoule; thigh junction; triceps jerk

TJR total joint replacement

TK thymidine kinase; transketolase; triose-kinase

T(°K) absolute temperature on the Kelvin scale

TKA total knee arthroplasty; transketolase activity; trochanter, knee, ankle

TKD thymidine kinase deficiency; tokodynamometer

TKG tokodynagraph

TKLI tachykinin-like immunoreactivity

TKR total knee replacement

TL temporal lobe; terminal limen; thermolabile; thermoluminescence; threat to life; thymus-leukemia [antigen]; thymus lymphocyte; thymus lymphoma; time lapse; time-limited; total lipids; total lung [capacity]; tubal ligation

T-L thymus-dependent lymphocyte

Tl thallium

TLA tissue lactase activity; tongue-to-lip adhesion; translaryngeal aspiration; translumbar aortogram; transluminal angioplasty

TLAA T-lymphocyte-associated antigen

TLam thoracic laminectomy

TLC tender loving care; thin-layer chromatography; total L-chain concentration; total lung capacity; total lung compliance; total lymphocyte count

TLD thermoluminescent dosimeter; thoracic lymphatic duct; tumor lethal dose

T/LD$_{100}$ minimum dose causing 100% deaths or malformations

TLE temporal lobe epilepsy; thin-layer electrophoresis; total lipid extract

TLI thymidine labeling index; total lymphoid irradiation; trypsin-like immune activity

TLm median tolerance limit

TLQ total living quotient

TLR tonic labyrinthine reflex

TLS thoracolumbosacral; Tourette-like syndrome

TLSO thoracolumboscral orthosis

TLSSO thoracolumbosacral spinal orthosis

TLT tryptophan load test

TLV threshold limit value; total lung volume

TLW total lung water

TLX trophoblast-lymphocyte cross-reactivity

TM tectorial membrane; temperature by mouth; temporalis muscle; temporomandibular; tender midline; tendomyopathy; teres major; thalassemia major; Thayer-Martin [medium]; time-motion; tobramycin; trademark; traditional medicine; transitional mucosa; transatrial membranotomy; transmediastinal; transmetatarsal; transport mechanism; transport medium; transverse myelitis; tropical medicine; tuberculous meningitis; twitch movement; tympanic membrane

T-M Thayer-Martin [medium]

T&M type and crossmatch

Tm thulium; tubular maximum excretory capacity of kidneys

T_m melting temperature; temperature midpoint; tubular maximum excretory capacity of kidneys

tM the time required to complete the M phase of the cell cycle

tm transport medium; true mean

TMA tetramethylammonium; thrombotic microangiopathy; thyroid microsomal antibody; transcortical mixed aphasia; transmetatarsal amputation; trimellitic anhydride; trimethoxyamphetamine; trimethoxyphenyl aminopropane; trimethylamine

TMAH trimethylphenylammonium (anilinium) hydroxide

TMAI trimethylphenylammonium (anilinium) iodide

TMAS Taylor Manifest Anxiety Scale

T_{max} maximum threshold; time of maximum concentration

TMBA trimethoxybenzaldehyde

TMC triamcinolone and terramycin capsules

TMD trimethadione

t-MDS therapy-related myelodysplastic syndrome

TME total metabolizable energy; transmissible mink encephalopathy; transmural enteritis

TMET treadmill exercise test

TMF transformed mink fibroblast; transmitral flow

TM_g maximum tubular reabsorption rate for glucose

TMH tetramethylammonium hydroxide

TM-HSA trimellityl-human serum albumin

TMI testing motor impairment; transmural myocardial infarction

TMIC Toxic Materials Information Center

TMIF tumor-cell migratory inhibition factor

TMIS Technicon Medical Information System

TMJ temporomandibular joint; trapeziometacarpal joint

TMJS temporomandibular joint syndrome

TML terminal midline; terminal motor latency; tetramethyl lead

TMNST tethered median nerve stress test

TMP thiamine monophosphate; thymidine monophosphate; thymolphthalein monophosphate; transmembrane potential; transmembrane pressure; trimethoprim; trimethylpsoralen

TM_{PAH} maximum tubular excretory capacity for para-aminohippuric acid

TMPD tetramethyl-p-phenylinediamine

TMPDS temporomandibular pain and dysfunction syndrome; thiamine monophosphate disulfide

TMP-SMX trimethoprim-sulfamethoxazole

TMR tissue maximum ratio; topical magnetic resonance; trainable mentally retarded

TMS thalium myocardial scintigraphy;

thread mate system; trapezoidoce-phaly–multiple synostosis [syndrome]; trimethylsilane

TMST treadmill stem test

TMT tarsometatarsal; Trail-Making Test; trimethyllin

TMTD tetramethylthiuram disulfide

TMU tetramethyl urea

TMV tobacco mosaic virus

TMX tamoxifen

TMZ transformation zone

TN talonavicular; tarsonavicular; team nursing; temperature normal; trigeminal nucleus; total negatives; trochlear nucleus; true negative

T/N tar and nicotine

Tn normal intraocular tension; transposon

TND term normal delivery

t-NE total norepinephrine

TNEE titrated norepinephrine excretion

T$_4$N normal serum thyroxine

TNF true negative fraction; tumor necrosing factor

tng tongue

TNH transient neonatal hyperammonemia

TNI total nodal irradiation

TNM primary tumor, regional nodes, metastasis [tumor staging]; thyroid node metastases; tumor node metastasis

TNMR tritium nuclear magnetic resonance

TNP total net positive

TNR tonic neck reflex; true negative rate

TNS total nuclear score; transcutaneous nerve stimulation; tumor necrosis serum

TNT tetranitroblue tetrazolium; 2,4,6-trinitrotoluene

TNTC too numerous to count

TNV tobacco necrosis virus

TO old tuberculin; oral temperature; original tuberculin; target organ; telephone order; thoracic orthosis; tincture of opium; total obstruction; tracheoesophageal; tubo-ovarian; turnover

T(O) oral temperature

TO$_2$ oxygen transport

to tincture of opium

TOA tubo-ovarian abscess

TOAP thioguanine, oncovin, cytosine arabinoside, and prednisone

TOB tobramycin

TobRV tobacco ringspot virus

TOC total organic carbon

TOCP tri-o-cresyl phosphate

TOD right eye tension [Lat. *oculus dexter*]; Time-Oriented Data [Bank]; titanium optimized design [plate]

TODS toxic organic dust syndrome

TOE tracheoesophageal

TOES toxic oil epidemic syndrome

TOF tetralogy of Fallot; train of four [monitor]; tracheo[o]esophageal fistula

T of F tetralogy of Fallot

TOH transient osteoporosis of hip

TOL trial of labor

tol tolerance, tolerated

TOLB, tolb tolbutamine

TOM toxic oxygen metabolite

tonoc tonight

top topical

TOPV trivalent oral poliovaccine

TORCH toxoplasmosis, other [congenital syphilis and viruses], rubella, cytomegalovirus, and herpes simplex virus

TORP total ossicular replacement prosthesis

torr mm Hg pressure

TOS left eye tension [Lat. *oculus sinister*]; thoracic outlet syndrome; toxic oil syndrome

TOT total operating time

TOV trial of voiding

tox toxicity, toxic

TOXICON Toxicology Information Conversational On-Line Network

TOXLINE Toxicology Information On-Line [data bank]

TOXLIT Toxicology Liturature [data bank]

TOXNET Toxicology Network (NLM) [data bank]

TP temperature and pressure; temperature probe; temporal peak; temporoparietal; terminal phalanx; testosterone propionate; thick padding; threshold potential; thrombocytopenic purpura; thrombophlebitis; thymopentin; thymus polypeptide; thymus protein; torsades de pointes; total positives; total protein; transforming principle; transition point; transverse polarization; transverse process; *Treponema pallidum*; trigger point; triphosphate; true positive; tryptophan; tryptophan pyrrolase; tube precipitin; tuberculin precipitate

6-TP 6-thiopurine

T + P temperature and pulse

Tp *Treponema pallidum*; tryptophan

T$_p$ physical half-life

TPA tannic acid, polyphosphomolybdic acid, and amino acid; 12-0-tetradecanoyl-phorbol-13-acetate; third-party administrator; tissue plasminogen activator; total parenteral alimentation; *Treponema pallidum* agglutination; tumor polypeptide antigen

t-PA tissue-type plasminogen activator

TPB tetraphenyl borate; tryptone phosphate broth

TBPF total pulmonary blood flow

TPBS three-phase radionuclide bone scanning

TPC thromboplastic plasma component; total patient care; total plasma catecholamines; total plasma cholesterol; *Treponema pallidum* complement

TPCF *Treponema pallidum* complement fixation

TPCV total packed cell volume

TPD temporary partial disability; thiamine propyl disulfide; tripotassium phenolphthalein disulfate; tumor-producing dose

TPDS tropical pancreatic diabetes syndrome

TPE therapeutic plasma exchange; totally protected environment; typhoid-parathyroid enteritis

T^{Pe} expiratory pause time

TPEY tellurite polymyxin egg yolk [agar]

TPF thymus permeability factor; thymus to peak flow; true positive fraction

TPG transmembrane potential gradient; transplacental gradient; tryptophan peptone glucose [broth]

TPGYT trypticase-peptone-glucose-yeast extract-trypsin [medium]

TPH transplacental hemorrhage

TPHA *Treponema pallidum* hemagglutination

TPI time period integrator; treponemal immobilization test; *Treponema pallidum* immobilization; triosephosphate isomerase

T^{Pi} inspiratory pause time

TPIA *Treponema pallidum* immune adherence

TPIIA time of postexpiratory inspiratory activity

TPL titanium proximal loading; tyrosine phenol-lyase

TPLV transient pulmonary vascular lability

TPM temporary pacemaker; thrombophlebitis migrans; total particulate matter; total passive motion; triphenylmethane

TPMT thiopurine methyltransferase

TPN thalamic projection neuron; total parenteral nutrition; triphosphopyridine nucleotide

TPNH reduced triphosphopyridine nucleotide

TPO thyroid peroxidase; tryptophan peroxidase

TPP thiamine pyrophosphate; transpulmonary pressure; treadmill performance test; triphenyl phosphite

TPPase thiamine pyrophosphatase

TPPD thoracic-pelvic-phalangeal dystrophy

TPPN total peripheral parenteral nutrition

TPQ Threshold Planning Quantity

TPR temperature; temperature, pulse, and respiration; testosterone production rate; total peripheral resistance; total pulmonary resistance; true positive rate

TPRI total peripheral resistance index

TPS trypsin; tumor polysaccharide substance

TPSE 2-(p-triphenyl)sulfonylethanol

TPST true positive stress test

TPT tetraphenyl tetrazolium; total protein tuberculin; typhoid-paratyphoid [vaccine]

TPTE 2-(p-triphenyl)thioethanol

TPTX thyro-parathyroidectomized

TPTZ tripyridyltriazine

TPV tetanus-pertussis vaccine

TPVR total peripheral vascular resistance; total pulmonary vascular resistance

TPZ thioproperazine

TQ tocopherolquinone; tourniquet

TQM total quality management

TR recovery time; rectal temperature; repetition time; residual tuberculin; terminal repeat; tetrazolium reduction; therapeutic radiology; time release; total resistance; total response; trachea; transfusion reaction; tricuspid regurgitation; tuberculin R [new tuberculin]; tuberculin residue; turbidity-reducing; turnover ratio

T(°R) absolute temperature on the Rankine scale

Tr trace; tragion; transferrin; trypsin

T$_r$ radiologic half-life; retention time

tr tincture; trace; traction; transaldolase; trauma, traumatic; tremor; triradial

TRA total renin activity; tumor-resistant antigen

tra transfer

TRAb thyrotoxin receptor antibody

trach trachea, tracheal, tracheostomy

TRAJ time repetitive ankle jerk

TRALT transfusion-related acute lung injury

TRAM Treatment Rating Assessment Matrix; Treatment Response Assessment Method

TRAMPE tricho-rhino-auriculophalangeal multiple exostoses

trans transference; transverse

trans D transverse diameter

transm transmitted, transmission

transpl transplantation, transplanted

TRAP tartrate-resistant acid phosphatase; transport and rapid accessioning for additional procedures

trap trapezius

TRAS transplanted renal artery stenosis

traum trauma, traumatic

TRB terbutalone

TRBF total renal blood flow

TRC tanned red cell; therapeutic residential center; total renin concentration; total respiratory conductance; total ridge count

TRCA tanned red cell agglutination

TRCH tanned red cell hemagglutination

TRCHI tanned red cell hemagglutination inhibition

TRCV total red cell volume

TRD tongue-retaining device

TRDN transient respiratory distress of the newborn

TRE thymic reticuloendothelial; true radiation emission

TREA triethanolamine

treat treatment

Trend Trendelenburg [position]

Trep Treponema

TRF T-cell replacing factor; thyrotropin-releasing factor; tubular rejection fraction

TRFC total rosette-forming cell

TRH tension-reducing hypothesis; thyrotropin-releasing hormone

TRH-ST thyrotropin-releasing hormone stimulation test

TRI tetrazolium reduction inhibition; Thyroid Research Institute; total response index; Toxic Chemical Release Inventory; tubuloreticular inclusion

tri tricentric

T$_3$RIA, T$_3$(RIA) triiodothyronine radioimmunoassay

T$_4$RIA, T$_4$(RIA) thyroxine radioimmunoassay

TRIC trachoma inclusion conjunctivitis [organism]

TRICB trichlorobiphenyl

Trich Trichomonas

Trid three days [Lat. *triduum*]

trig trigger; triglycerides; trigonum

TRIMIS Tri-Service Medical Information System

TRIS tris-hydroxymethyl-amino methane

TRIT triiodothyronine

trit triturate

TRITC tetrarhodamine isothiocyanate

TRK transketolase

TRLP triglyceride-rich lipoprotein

TRMC trimethylrhodamino-isothiocyanate

TRML, Trml terminal

TRM-SMX trimethoprim-sulfamethoxazole

TRN tegmental reticular nucleus

tRNA transfer ribonucleic acid

TRO tissue reflectance oximetry

Trop tropical

TRP total refractory period; trichorhinophalangeal [syndrome]; tubular reabsorption of phosphate

Trp tryptophan

TRPA tryptophan-rich prealbumin

TrPl treatment plan

TRPS trichorhinophalangeal syndrome

TRPT theoretical renal phosphorus threshold

TRR total respiratory resistance

TRS total reducing sugars; tubuloreticular structure

TrS trauma surgery

TRSV tobacco ringspot virus

TRU turbidity-reducing unit

T₃RU triiodothyronine resin uptake

TRUS transrectal ultrasonography

TRV tobacco rattle virus

Tryp tryptophan

trx traction

TS Tay-Sachs; temperature sensitivity; temperature, skin; temporal stem; tensile strength; test solution; thermal stability; thoracic surgery; tissue space; total solids [in urine]; Tourette syndrome; toxic substance; toxic syndrome; tracheal sound; transitional sleep; transsexual; transverse section; transverse sinus; trauma score; treadmill score; tricuspid stenosis; triple strength; tropical sprue;

trypticase soy [plate]; T suppressor [cell]; tuberous sclerosis; tumor-specific; Turner syndrome; type-specific

T + S type and screen

Ts skin temperature; tosylate

T_s T-cell suppressor

tS time required to complete the S phase of the cell cycle

ts, tsp teaspoon

TSA technical surgical assistance; toluene sulfonic acid; total shoulder arthroplasty; total solute absorption; toxic shock antigen; transcortical sensory aphasia; trypticase-soy agar; tumor-specific antigen; tumor surface antigen; type-specific antibody

T₄SA thyroxine-specific activity

TSAb thyroid-stimulating antibody

TSAP toxic-shock-associated protein

TSAS total severity assessment score

TSAT tube slide agglutination test

TSB total serum bilirubin; trypticase soy broth; tryptone soy broth

TSBA total serum bile acids

TSBB transtracheal selective bronchial brushing

TSC technetium sulfur colloid; thiosemicarbazide; transverse spinal sclerosis

TSCA Toxic Substances Control Act

TSD target-skin distance; Tay-Sachs disease; theory of signal detectability

TSE testicular self-examination; total skin examination; trisodium edetate

TSEB total skin electron beam

T sect transverse section

TSEM transmission scanning electron microscopy

TSES Target Symptom Evaluation Scale

T-set tracheotomy set

TSF testicular feminization syndrome; thrombopoiesis-stimulating factor; total systemic flow; triceps skinfold

TSG, TSGP tumor-specific glycoprotein

TSH thyroid-stimulating hormone; transient synovitis of the hip

TSH-RF thyroid-stimulating hormone-releasing factor

TSH-RH thyroid-stimulating hormone-releasing hormone
TSI thyroid stimulating immunoglobulin; triple sugar iron [agar]
TSIA total small intestine allotransplantation; triple sugar iron agar
tSIDS totally unexplained sudden infant death syndrome
TSL terminal sensory latency
TSM type-specific M protein
TSP thrombin-sensitive protein; total serum protein; total suspended particulate; trisodium phosphate; tropical spastic paraparesis
tsp teaspoon
TSPA thiotepa
TSPAP total serum prostatic acid phosphatase
TSPP tetrasodium pyrophosphate
TSR theophylline sustained release; thyroid to serum ratio; total systemic resistance
TSS toxic shock syndrome; tropical splenomegaly syndrome
TSSA tumor-specific cell surface antigen
TSSE toxic shock syndrome exotoxin
TSST toxic shock syndrome toxin
TST thromboplastin screening test; total sleep time; treadmill stress test; tumor skin test
TSTA toxoplasmin skin test antigen; tumor-specific tissue antigen; tumor-specific transplantation antigen
TSU triple sugar urea [agar]
TSV total stomach volume
TSY trypticase soy yeast
TT tablet triturate; tactile tension; tendon transfer; test tube; tetanus toxin; tetanus toxoid; tetrathionate; tetrazol; thrombin time; thymol turbidity; tibial tubercle; tilt table; tolerance test; total thyroxine; total time; transient tachypnea; transferred to; transit time; transthoracic; transtracheal; tuberculin test; tube thoracostomy; tumor thrombus; turnover time
T&T time and temperature; touch and tone

TT₂ total diiodothyronine
TT_2 total diiodothyronine
TT₃ total triiodothyronine
TT₄ total thyroxine
TTA tetanus toxoid antibody; timed therapeutic absence; total toe arthroplasty; transtracheal aspiration
TTAP threaded titanium acetabular prosthesis
TTC triphenyltetrazolium chloride; T-tube cholangiogram
TTD temporary total disability; tissue tolerance dose; transient tic disorder; transverse thoracic diameter; trichothiodystrophy
TTFD tetrahydrofurfuryldisulfide
TTG tellurite, taurocholate, and gelatin
TTGA tellurite, taurocholate, and gelatin agar
TTH thyrotropic hormone; tritiated thymidine
TTI tension-time index; time-tension index; transtracheal insufflation
TTL total thymus lymphocytes; transistor-transistor logic
TTLC true total lung capacity
TTLD terminal transverse limb defect
TTN transient tachypnea of the newborn
TTNA transthoracic needle aspiration
TTNB transthoracic needle biopsy
TTP thrombotic thrombocytopenic purpura; thymidine triphosphate; time to peak
TTPA triethylene thiophosphoramide
TTR transthoracic resistance; transthyretin; triceps tendon reflex
TTS tarsal tunnel syndrome; temporary threshold shift; through the skin; tilt table standing; transdermal therapeutic system; twin transfusion syndrome
TTT thymol turbidity test; tolbutamide tolerance test; total twitch time; tuberculin tine test
TTTT test tube turbidity test
TTV tracheal transport velocity; transfusion-transmitted virus
TTX tetrodotoxin
TU thiouracil; thyroid uptake; Todd unit; toxin unit; transmission unit; transurethral; tuberculin unit; turbidity unit

T₃U triiodothyronine uptake
tuberc tuberculosis
TUD total urethral discharge
TUG total urinary gonadotropin
TUI transurethral incision
TUR transurethral resection
TURB, TURBT transurethral resection of bladder [tumor]
turb turbidity, turbid
TURP transurethral prostatectomy
TURS transurethral resection syndrome
TURV transurethral resection of valves
tus cough [Lat. *tussis*]
TV talipes varus; television; tetrazolium violet; thoracic vertebra; tickborne virus; tidal volume; total volume; toxic vertigo; transvenous; transverse; trial visit; *Trichomonas vaginalis*; tricuspid valve; trivalent; true vertebra; truncal vagotomy; tuberculin volutin; tubovesicular typhoid vaccine
Tv Trichomonas vaginalis
TVA truncal vagotomy and antrectomy
TVC timed vital capacity; total viable cells; total volume capacity; transvaginal cone; triple voiding cystogram; true vocal cords
TVD transmissible virus dementia; triple vessel disease
TVF tactile vocal fremitus
TVG time-varied gain
TVH total vaginal hysterectomy; turkey virus hepatitis
TVL tenth value layer; tunica vasculosa lentis
TVP tensor veli palatini [muscle]; textured vegetable protein; transvenous pacemaker; tricuspid valve prolapse; truncal vagotomy and pyloroplasty
TVR tonic vibratory reflex; total vascular resistance; tricuspid valve replacement
TVSS transient voltage surge suppressor
TVT transmissible venereal tumor; tunica vaginalis testis
TVU total volume of the urine
TW tap water; terminal web; test weight; total body water
Tw twist
TWA time weighted average
TWBC total white blood cells; total white blood count
TWD total white and differential [cell count]
TWE tap water enema; tepid water enema
TWL transepidermal water loss
TWS tranquilizer withdrawal syndrome
TWs triphasic waves
TWWD tap water wet dressing
TX a derivative of contagious tuberculin; thromboxane; thyroidectomized; transplantation; treatment
T&X type and crossmatch
Tx, Tₓ treatment; therapy, traction
tx traction
TXA, TxA thromboxane A
TXA2, TXA₂ thromboxane A2 (A₂)
TXB2, TXB₂ thromboxane B2 (B₂)
TXDS qualifying toxic dose
Ty type, typhoid; tyrosine
Tymp tympanum, tympanic
TYMV turnip yellow mosaic virus
Tyr tyrosine
TyRIA thyroid radioisotope assay
TZ zymoplastic tuberculin [the dried residue which is soluble in alcohol] [Ger. *Tuberculin zymoplastische*]

U congenital limb absence; in electro-cardiography, an undulating deflection that follows the T wave; internal energy; International Unit of enzyme activity; Mann-Whitney rank sum statistic; potential difference (in volts); ulcer; ulna; ultralente [insulin]; umbilicus; uncertain; unerupted; unit; unknown; upper; uracil; uranium; urea; urethra; uridine; uridylic acid; urinary concentration; urine; urology; uterus; uvula; volume velocity

u to be used [Lat. *utendus*]; unified atomic mass unit; velocity

U/2 upper half

U/3 upper third

UA ultra-audible; ultrasonic arteriography; umbilical artery; unauthorized absence; unit of analysis; unstable angina; upper airways; upper arm; urinalysis; uric acid; uridylic acid; urinalysis; urinary aldosterone; uronic acid; uterine aspiration

U/A urinalysis; uric acid

UAC umbilical artery catheter

UA/C uric acid/creatinine [ratio]

U-AMY urinary amylase

UAE unilateral absence of excretion; urine albumin excretion

UAI uterine activity interval

UAN uric acid nitrogen

UAO upper airway obstruction

UAP unstable angina pectoris; urinary acid phosphatase; urinary alkaline phosphatase

UAR upper airway resistance; uric acid riboside

UAS upper abdomen surgery; upstream activation site

UAU uterine activity unit

UB ultimobranchial body; Unna boot; upper back; urinary bladder

UB 82 universal billing document [1982]

UBA undenaturated bacterial antigen

UBBC unsaturated vitamin B12 binding capacity

UBC University of British Columbia [brace]

UBF uterine blood flow

UBG, Ubg urobilinogen

UBI ultraviolet blood irradiation

UBL undifferentiated B-cell lymphoma

UBN urobilin

UBP ureteral back pressure

UC ulcerative colitis; ultracentrifugal; umbilical cord; unchanged; unclassifiable; unconscious; undifferentiated cells; unit clerk; unsatisfactory condition; untreated cells; urea clearance; urethral catheterization; urinary catheter; urine concentrate; urine culture; uterine contractions

U&C urethral and cervical; usual and customary

UCB unconjugated bilirubin

UCBC umbilical cord blood culture

UCD urine collection device; usual childhood diseases

UCE urea cycle enzymopathy

UCG ultrasonic cardiography; urinary chorionic gonadotropin

UCHD usual childhood diseases

UCI unusual childhood illness; urethral catheter in; urinary catheter in

UCL ulnar collateral ligament; upper collateral ligament; upper confidence limit; urea clearance

UCLP unilateral cleft of lip and palate

UCO urethral catheter out; urinary catheter out

UCOD underlying cause of death

UCP urinary coproporphyrin; urinary C-peptide

UCPT urinary coproporphyrin test

UCR unconditioned response; usual, customary, and reasonable [fees]

UCS unconditioned stimulus; unconscious; uterine compression syndrome

ucs unconscious

UCTD unclassifiable connective tissue disease

uCTD undifferentiated connective tissue disease

UCV uncontrolled variable

UD ulcerative dermatosis; ulnar deviation; undetermined; underdeveloped; unit dose; urethral discharge; uridine diphosphate; uroporphyrinogen decarboxylase; uterine delivery

ud as directed [Lat. *ud dictum*]

UDC usual diseases of childhood

UDCA ursodeoxycholic acid

UDN ulcerative dermal necrosis

UDO undetermined origin

UDP uridine diphosphate

UDPG urine diphosphoglucose

UDPGA uridine diphosphate glucuronic acid

UDPGT uridine diphosphate glucuronosyl transferase

UDR-BMD ultradistal radius bone mineral density

UDRP urine diribose phosphate

UDS ultra-Doppler sonography; unscheduled deoxynucleic acid synthesis

UE uncertain etiology; under elbow; uninvolved epidermis; upper esophagus; upper extremity

uE$_s$ unconjugated estriol

UEG ultrasonic encephalography; unifocal eosinophilic granuloma

UEL upper explosive limit

UEM universal electron microscope

UEMC unidentified endosteal marrow cell

UES upper esophageal sphincter

u/ext upper extremity

UF ultrafiltrate; ultrafiltration; ultrafine; ultrasonic frequency; universal feeder; unknown factor; urinary formaldehyde

UFA unesterified fatty acid

UFB urinary fat bodies

UFC urinary free cortisol

UFD ultrasonic flow detector; unilateral facet dislocation

UFFI urea formaldehyde foam insulation

UFL upper flammable limit

UFP ultrafiltration pressure

UFR ultrafiltration rate; urine filtration rate

uFSH urinary follicle-stimulating hormone

UG urogastrone; urogenital

UGD urogenital diaphragm

UGDP University Group Diabetes Project

UGF unidentified growth factor

UGH uveitis-glaucoma-hyphema [syndrome]

UGH + uveitis-glaucoma-hyphema plus vitreous hemorrhage [syndrome]

UGI upper gastrointestinal [tract]

UGIH upper gastrointestinal hemorrhage

UGIS upper gastrointestinal series

UGS urogenital sinus

UGT urogenital tuberculosis

UH umbilical hernia; unfavorable histology; upper half

UHD unstable hemoglobin disease

UHF ultrahigh frequency

UHL universal hypertrichosis languinosa

UHMW ultrahigh molecular weight

UHR underlying heart rhythm

UHSC university health services clinic

UHT ultrahigh temperature

UI uroporphyrin isomerase

U/I unidentified

UIBC unsaturated iron-binding capacity

UICAO unilateral internal carotid artery occlusion

UIF undegraded insulin factor

UIP usual interstitial pneumonia

UIQ upper inner quadrant

UIS Utilization Information Service

UJT unijunction transistor

UK unknown; urinary kallikrein; urokinase

UKa urinary kallikrein

UKAEA United Kingdom Atomic Energy Authority

UKCCSG United Kingdom Children's Cancer Study Group
UKM urea kinetic modeling
UL ultrasonic; Underwriters' Laboratories; undifferentiated lymphoma; upper limb; upper limit; upper lobe
U&L upper and lower
U/l units per liter
ULBW ultralow birth weight
ULDH urinary lactate dehydrogenase
ULLE upper lid of left eye
ULN upper limits of normal
uln ulna, ulnar
ULP ultra low profile
ULPE upper lobe pulmonary edema
ULQ upper left quadrant
ULRE upper lid of right eye
ULT ultrahigh temperature
ult ultimate
ult praes last prescribed [Lat. *ultimum praescriptus*]
ULV ultralow volume
UM upper motor [neuron]; uracil mustard
UMA ulcerative mutilating acropathy; urinary muramidase activity
Umax maximum urinary osmolality
umb umbilicus, umbilical
UMC unidimensional chromatography
UMCV-TO ulnar motor conduction velocity across thoracic outlet
UMDNS Universal Medical Device Nomenclature System
UMI urinary meconium index
UMLS Unified Medical Language System
UMN upper motor neuron
UMNL upper motor neuron lesion
UMP uridine monophosphate
UMPK uridine monophosphate kinase
UMS urethral manipulation syndrome
UMT units of medical time
UN ulnar nerve; undernourished; unilateral neglect; urea nitrogen; urinary nitrogen
UNa urinary sodium
uncomp uncompensated
uncond unconditioned

unct smeared [Lat. *unctus*]
UNCV ulnar nerve conduction velocity
undet undetermined
UNE urinary norepinephrine
ung ointment [Lat. *unguentum*]
unilat unilateral
univ universal
unk, unkn unknown
UNL upper normal limit
unsat unsatisfactory; unsaturated
UNT untreated
UNTS unilateral nevoid telangiectasia syndrome
UNX uninephrectomy
UO under observation; undetermined origin; urethral orifice; urinary output
u/o under observation
UOQ upper outer quadrant
UOsm urinary osmolality
UOV units of variance
UP ulcerative proctitis; ultrahigh purity; unipolar; upright posture; ureteropelvic; uridine phosphorylase; uroporphyrin
U/P urine to plasma [ratio]
u-PA urinary type plasminogen activator
UPD urinary production
UPF Universal proximal femur [prosthesis]
UPEP urinary protein electrophoresis
UPG uroporphyrinogen
UPGMA unweighted pair group method with averages
UPI uteroplacental insufficiency; uteroplacental ischemia
UPJ ureteropelvic junction
UPL unusual position of limbs
UPP urethral pressure profile
UPPP uvulopalatopharyngoplasty
UPPRA upright peripheral plasma renin activity
UPS ultraviolet photoelectron spectroscopy; uninterruptible power supply; uroporphyrinogen synthetase; uterine progesterone system
Υ Greek capital letter *upsilon*
υ Greek lower case letter *upsilon*
UPSIT University of Pennsylvania Smell Identification Test

UQ ubiquinone; upper quadrant

UQS upper quadrant syndrome

UR unconditioned reflex; upper respiratory; uridine; urinal; urology; utilization review

Ur urine, urinary

URA, Ura uracil

URC upper rib cage; utilization review committee

URD unspecified respiratory disease; upper respiratory disease

Urd uridine

ureth urethra

URF unidentified reading frame; uterine relaxing factor

URI upper respiratory illness; upper respiratory infection

U-RNA uridylic acid ribonucleic acid

URO urology; uroporphyrin; uroporphyrinogen

URO-GEN urogenital

Urol urology, urologist

URQ upper right quadrant

URS ultrasonic renal scanning

URT upper respiratory tract

URTI upper respiratory tract infection

URVD unilateral renovascular disease

US ultrasonic, ultrasound; ultrasonography; unconditioned stimulus; unique sequence; unit separator; upper segment; upper strength; urinary sugar; Usher syndrome

USAFH United States Air Force Hospital

USAFRHL United States Air Force Radiological Health Laboratory

USAH United States Army Hospital

USAHC United States Army Health Clinic

USAIDR United States Army Institute of Dental Research

USAMEDS United States Army Medical Service

USAN United States Adopted Names

USASI United States of America Standards Institute

USB upper sternal border

USBS United States Bureau of Standards

USD United States Dispensary

USDA United States Department of Agriculture

USDHEW United States Department of Health, Education, and Welfare

USDHHS United States Department of Health and Human Services

USE ultrasonic echography; ultrasonography

USFMG United States foreign medical graduate

USFMS United States foreign medical student

USG ultrasonography

USHL United States Hygienic Laboratory

USHMAC United States Health Manpower Advisory Council

USI urinary stress incontinence

US/LS upper strength/lower strength [ratio]

USMG United States medical graduate

USMH United States Marine Hospital

USMLE United States Medical Licensing Examination

USN ultrasonic nebulizer; unilateral spatial neglect

USNCHS United States National Center for Health Statistics

USNH United States Naval Hospital

USO unilateral salpingo-oophorectomy

USP United States Pharmacopeia

USPDI United States Pharmacopeia Drug Information

USPHS United States Public Health Service

USPSTF United States Preventive Services Task Force

USPTA United States Phyical Therapy Association

USR unheated serum reagin

USS ultrasound scanning

ust burnt, calcined [Lat. *ustus*]

USVH United States Veterans Hospital

USVMD urine specimen volume measuring device

USW ultrashort waves

UT Ullrich-Turner [syndrome]; Unna-

Thost [syndrome]; untested; untreated; urinary tract; urticaria

uT unbound testosterone

UTBG unbound thyroxine-binding globulin

UTC upper thoracic compression

UTD up to date

ut dict as directed [Lat. *ut dictum*]

utend to be used [Lat. *utendus*]

UTI urinary tract infection; urinary trypsin inhibitor

UTO upper tibial osteotomy

UTP unilateral tension pneumothorax; uridine triphosphate

UTS Ullrich-Turner syndrome; ulnar tunnel syndrome; ultimate tensile strength

UTZ ultrasound

UU urinary urea; urine urobilinogen

UUN urinary urea nitrogen

UUO unilateral urethral obstruction

UUP urinary uroporphyrin

UV ultraviolet; umbilical vein; ureterovesical; Uppsala virus; urinary volume

UVA ureterovesical angle

UVB ultraviolet B

UVC umbilical venous catheter

UVER ultraviolet-enhanced reactivation

UVI ultraviolet irradiation

UVJ ureterovesical junction

UVL ultraviolet light

UVP ultraviolet photometry

UVR ultraviolet radiation

UW unilateral weakness

UWB unit of whole blood

UWD Urbach-Wiethe disease

UWSC unstimulated whole saliva collection

UX uranium X, proactinium

UYP upper yield point

V

V in cardiography, unipolar chest lead; coefficient of variation; electrical potential (in volts); in electroencephalography, vertex sharp transient; five; a logical binary relation that is true if any argument is true, and false otherwise; luminous efficiency; potential energy (joules); vaccinated, vaccine; vagina; valine; valve; vanadium; variable, variation, varnish; vector; vegetarian; vein [Lat. *vena*]; velocity; ventilation; ventral; ventricular [fibrillation]; verbal comprehension [factor]; vertebra; vertex; vestibular; *Vibrio*; violet; viral [antigen]; virulence; virus; vision; visual acuity; voice; volt; voltage; volume; vomiting

v or [Lat. *vel*]; rate of reaction catalyzed by an enzyme; see [Lat. *vide*]; specific volume; valve; vein [Lat. *vena*]; velocity; venous; ventral; ventricular; versus; very; virus; vision; volt; volume

VA vacuum aspiration; valproic acid; vasodilator agent; ventricular aneurysm; ventricular arrhythmia; ventriculoatrial; ventroanterior; vertebral artery; Veterans Affairs; viral antigen; visual acuity; visual aid; visual axis; volt-ampere; volume-average

V$_A$ alveolar ventilation

V/A volt/ampere

V$_a$ alveolar ventilation

VAB vincristine, actinomycin D, and bleomycin; violent antisocial behavior

VABP venoarterial bypass pumping

VAC ventriculoatrial conduction; vincristine, doxorubicin, and cyclophosphamide; virus capsid antigen

vac vacuum

VAcc visual acuity with correction

vacc vaccination

VACTERL vertebral abnormalities, anal atresia, cardiac abnormalities, tracheoesophageal fistula and/or esophageal atresia, renal agenesis and dysplasia, and limb defects [association]

VAD venous access device; ventricular assist device; vitamin A deficiency; virus-adjusting diluent

vag vagina, vaginal, vaginitis

VAG HYST vaginal hysterectomy

VAH vertebral ankylosing hyperostosis; Veterans Administration Hospital; virilizing adrenal hyperplasia

VAHS virus-associated hemophagocytic syndrome

VAIN vaginal intraepithelial neoplasm

Val valine

val valve

VALE visual acuity, left eye

VAM ventricular arrhythmia monitor

VAMC Veterans Affairs Medical Center

VAMP vincristine, amethopterine, 6-mercaptopurine; and prednisone

VAOD visual acuity right eye [Lat. *oculus dexter*]

VAOL visual acuity [Lat. *oculus sinister*]

VAP vaginal acid phosphatase; variant angina pectoris

vap vapor

V$_A$/Q$_C$ ventilation-perfusion [ratio]

VAR visual-auditory range

Var, var variable; variant, variation, variety

var varicose

VARE visual acuity, right eye

VAS vascular; vesicle attachment site; viral arthritis syndrome; Visual Analogue Scale

VASC Verbal Auditory Screen for Children; visual-auditory screening

VAsc visual acuity without correction

vasc vascular

VAS RAD vascular radiology

VAT variable antigen type; ventricular accommodation test; ventricular activation time; visual action time; visual apperception test; vocational apperception test

VATER vertebral defects, imperforate anus, tracheoesophageal fistula, and radial and renal dysplasia

VATS Veterans Administration medical center transference syndrome

VATs surface variable antigen

VB vaginal bulb; valence bond; venous blood; ventrobasal; Veronal buffer; vertebrobasilar; viable birth; vinblastine; virus buffer; voided bladder

VBAC vaginal birth after cesarean section

VBAIN vertebrobasilar artery insufficiency nystagmus

VBC vincristine, bleomycin, and cisplatin

VBD vanishing bile duct; Veronal-buffered diluent

VBG vagotomy and Billroth gastroenterostomy; venous blood gases; venous bypass graft; vertical-banded gastroplasty

VBI vertebrobasilar insufficiency; vertebrobasilar ischemia

VBL vinblastine

VBOS Veronal-buffered oxalated saline

VBP vagal body paraganglia; venous blood pressure; ventricular premature beat

VBR ventricular brain ratio

VBS Veronal-buffered saline; vertebrobasilar system

VBS:FBS Veronal-buffered saline-fetal bovine serum

VC color vision; vascular changes; vasoconstriction; vena cava; venereal case; venous capacitance; ventilatory capacity; ventral column; ventricular contraction; vertebral caval; Veterinary Corps; videocasette; vincristine; vinyl chloride; visual capacity; visual cortex; vital capacity; vocal cord

V/C ventilation/circulation [ratio]

V_C pulmonary capillary blood volume

VCA vancomycin, colistin, and anisomycin; viral capsid antigen

VCAP vincristine, cyclophosphamide, Adriamycin, and prednisone

vCBF venous cerebral blood flow

VCC vasoconstrictor center; ventral cell column

VCD vibrational circular dichroism

VCE vagina, ectocervix, and endocervix

VCFS velo-cardio-facial syndrome

VCG vectorcardiogram, vectorcardiography; voiding cystography, voiding cystourethrography

VCM vinyl chloride monomer

VCMP vincristine, cyclophosphamide, melphalan, and prednisone

VCN vancomycin, colistomethane, and nystatin; *Vibrio chloreae* neuraminidase

VCO, V_{CO} endogenous production of carbon monoxide

VCO_2, V_{CO2} carbon dioxide output

VCP vincristine, cyclophosphamide, and prednisone

VCR vasoconstriction rate; vincristine; volume clearance rate

VCS vasoconstrictor substance; vesicocervical space

VCSA viral cell surface antigen

VCSF ventricular cerebrospinal fluid

VCT venous clotting time

VCU videocystourethrography; voiding cystourethrogram, voiding cystourethrography

VCUG vesicoureterogram; voiding cystourethrogram

VD vapor density; vascular disease; vasodilation, vasodilator; venereal disease; venous dilatation; ventricular dilator; ventrodorsal; vertical deviation; vertical divergence; video-disk; viral diarrhea; voided; volume of dead space; volume of distribution

V_D dead space

Vd voided, voiding; volume dead space

V_d apparent volume of distribution

VDA visual discriminatory acuity

VDAC voltage-dependent anion channel

VdB van der Bergh [test]

VDBR volume of distribution of bilirubin

VDC vasodilator center

VDD atrial synchronous ventricular inhibited [pacemaker]; vitamin D-dependent

VDDR vitamin D-dependent rickets

VDEL Venereal Disease Experimental Laboratory

VDEM vasodepressor material

VDF ventricular diastolic fragmentation

VDG, VD-G venereal disease–gonorrhea

vdg voiding

VDH valvular disease of the heart

VDL vasodepressor lipid; visual detection level

VDM vasodepressor material

VDP ventricular premature depolarization

VDR venous diameter ratio

VDRL Venereal Disease Research Laboratory [test for syphilis]

VDRR vitamin D-resistant rickets

VDRS Verdun Depression Rating Scale

VDRT venereal disease reference test

VDS vasodilator substance; vindesine

VDS, VD-S venereal disease-syphilis

VDT vibration disappearance threshold; visual display terminal; visual distortion test

VDU video display unit

VDV ventricular end-diastolic volume

VD/VT dead space vantilation/total ventilation [ratio]

VE vaginal examination; Venezuelan encephalitis; venous emptying; venous extension; ventilation; ventilatory equivalent; ventricular elasticity; ventricular extrasystole; vertex; vesicular exanthema; viral encephalitis; visual efficiency; vitamin E; volume ejection; voluntary effort

V$_E$ environmental variance; respiratory minute volume

Ve ventilation

V&E Vinethine and ether

VEA ventricular ectopic activity; ventricular ectopic arrhythmia; viral envelope antigen

VEB ventricular ectopic beat

VECG vector electrocardiogram

VECP visually evoked cortical potential

VED vacuum erection device; ventricular ectopic depolarization; vital exhaustion and depression

VEE vagina, ectocervix, endocervix; Venezuelan equine encephalomyelitis

VEF ventricular ejection fraction; visually evoked field

VEGAS ventricular enlargement with gait apraxia syndrome

vehic vehicle

vel, veloc velocity

VEM vasoexcitor material

vent ventilation; ventral; ventricle, ventricular

vent fib ventricular fibrillation

ventric ventricle

VEP visual evoked potential

VER visual evoked response

Verc vervet (African green monkey) kidney cells

vert vertebra, vertebral

ves bladder [Lat. *vesica*]; vesicular; vessel

vesic a blister [Lat. *vesicula*]

vesp evening [Lat. *vesper*]

vest vestibular

ves ur urinary bladder [Lat. *vesica urinaria*]

VET vestigial testis

Vet veteran; veterinarian, veterinary

VetMB Bachelor of Veterinary Medicine

Vet Med veterinary medicine

VETS Veterans Adjustment Scale

Vet Sci veterinary science

VF left leg [electrode]; ventricular fibrillation; ventricular fluid; ventricular flutter; visual field; vitreous fluorophotometry; vocal fremitus

Vf visual frequency

V$_f$ variant frequency

vf visual field

VFA volatile fatty acid

VFC ventricular function curve

VFD visual feedback display

VFI visual field intact
V fib ventricular fibrillation
VFL ventricular flutter
VFP ventricular filling pressure; ventricular fluid pressure
VFR voiding flow rate
VFS vascular fragility syndrome
VFT venous filling time; ventricular fibrillation threshold
VG van Gieson [stain]; ventricular gallop; volume of gas
V_G genetic variance
VGCC voltage-gated calcium channels
VGH very good health
VGM venous graft myringoplasty
VGP viral glycoprotein
VH vaginal hysterectomy; venous hematocrit; ventricular hypertrophy; veterans hospital; viral hepatitis
V_H variable domain of heavy chain
VHD valvular heart disease; viral hematodepressive disease
VHDL very high density lipoprotein
VHF very high frequency; viral hemorrhagic fever; visual half-field
VHL von Hippel-Lindau [syndrome]
VHN Vickers hardness number
VI Roman numeral six; vaginal irrigation; variable interval; vastus intermedius; virgo intacta; virulence, virulent; viscosity index; visual impairment; visual inspection; vitality index; volume index
Vi virulence, virulent
VIA virus inactivating agent; virus infection-associated antigen
vib vibration
VIC vasoinhibitory center; voice intensity control
VI-CTS vibration-induced carpal tunnel syndrome
VID visible iris diameter
VIF virus-induced interferon
VIG, VIg vaccinia immunoglobulin
VIIag factor VII antigen
VIIIc factor VIII clotting activity
VIII_{vwf} von Willebrand factor
VIM video-intensification microscopy; vimentin

VIN vulvar intraepithelial neoplasm
vin vinyl
VIP vasoactive intestinal peptide; vasoinhibitory peptide; venous impedance plethysmography; voluntary interruption of pregnancy
VIPoma vasoactive intestinal polypeptide-secreting tumor
VIQ Verbal Intelligence Quotient
VIR virology
Vir virus, viral
vir green [Lat. *viridis*]; virulent
VIS vaginal irrigation smear; venous insufficiency syndrome; vertebral irritation syndrome; visible; visual information storage
vis vision, visual
VISC vitreous infusion suction cutter
visc viscera, visceral; viscosity
VISI volar intercalated segment instability
Vit vitamin
vit vital
vit cap vital capacity
vit ov sol dissolved in egg yolk [Lat. *vitello ovis solutus*]
VJ ventriculojugular
VJC ventriculojugularcardiac
VK vervet (African green monkey) kidney cells
VKH, VKHS Vogt-Koyanagi-Harada [syndrome]
VL left arm [electrode]; ventralis lateratis [nucleus]; ventrolateral; visceral leishmaniasis; vision, left [eye]
V_L variable domain of the light chain
VLA virus-like agent
VLB vinblastine; vincaleukoblastine
VLBR very low birth rate
VLBW very low birth weight
VLCFA very long chain fatty acid
VLD very low density
VLDL, VLDLP very low density lipoprotein
VLF very low frequency
VLG ventral nucleus of the lateral geniculate body

VLH ventrolateral nucleus of the hypothalamus

VLM visceral larva migrans

VLO vastus lateralis obliquus

VLP vincristine, L-asparaginase, and prednisone; virus-like particle

VLR vinleurosine

VLS vascular leak syndrome

VLSI very large scale integration

VM vasomotor; ventralis medialus; ventromedial; ventricular mass; ventriculometry; vestibular membrane; viomycin; viral myocarditis; voltmeter

V/m volts per meter

VMA vanillylmandelic acid

Vmax maximum velocity

VMC vasomotor center

VMCG vector magnetocardiogram

VMD Doctor of Veterinary Medicine

vMDV virulent Marek disease virus

VMF vasomotor flushing

VMGT Visual Motor Gestalt Test

VMH ventromedial hypothalamic [syndrome]

VMI, VMIT visual-motor integration [test]

VMN ventromedial nucleus

VMO vastus medialis obliquus [muscle]

VMR vasomotor rhinitis

VMS visual memory span

VMST visual motor sequencing test

VMT vasomotor tonus; ventilatory muscle training; ventromedial tegmentum

VN vesical neck; vestibular nucleus; virus neutralization; visceral nucleus; visiting nurse; vocational nurse; vomeronasal

VNA Visiting Nurse Association

VNDPT visual numerical discrimination pre-test

VNO vomeronasal organ

VNS visiting nursing service

VNTR variable number of tandem repeats

VO verbal order; volume overload; voluntary opening

Vo standard volume

VO$_2$, V$_{o2}$ volume of oxygen utilization

VOC volatile organic chemical

VOCC voltage-operated calcium channel

VOD veno-occlusive disease; vision, right eye [Lat. *visio, oculus dexter*]

vol volar; volatile; volume; voluntary, volunteer

VOM volt-ohm-milliammeter

VON Victorian Order of Nurses

V-ONC viral oncogene

VOO ventricular asynchronous (competitive, fixed-rate) [pacemaker]

VOP venous occlusion plethysmography

VOR vestibulo-ocular reflex

VOS vision, left eye [Lat. *visio, oculus sinister*]

vos dissolved in egg yolk [Lat. *vitello ovi solutus*]

VOT voice onset time

VOU vision, each eye [Lat. *visio oculus uterque*]

VP physiological volume; vapor pressure; variegate porphyria; vascular permeability; vasopressin; velopharyngeal; venipuncture; venous pressure; ventricular pacing; ventricular premature [beat]; ventriculoperitoneal; ventroposterior; vertex potential; vincristine and prednisone; viral protein; Voges-Proskauer [medium or test]; volume-pressure; vulnerable period

V/P ventilation/perfusion [ratio]

V&P vagotomy and pyloroplasty

Vp peak voltage; phenotype variance; plasma volume; ventricular premature [beat]

vp vapor pressure

VPA valproic acid

VPB ventricular premature beat

VPC vapor-phase chromatography; ventricular premature complex; ventricular premature contraction; volume-packed cells; volume percent

VPCT ventricular premature contraction threshold

VPD ventricular premature depolarization

VPF vascular permeability factor

VPG velopharyngeal gap

VPGSS venous pressure gradient support stockings

VPI vapor phase inhibitor; velopharyngeal insufficiency

VPL ventroposterolateral

VPM ventilator pressure manometer; ventroposteromedial

vpm vibrations per minute

VPN ventral pontine nucleus

VPO velopharyngeal opening; vertical pendular oscillation

VPP viral porcine pneumonia

VPR Voges-Proskauer reaction; volume/pressure ratio

VPRBC volume of packed red blood cells

VPRC volume of packed red cells

VPS ventriculoperitoneal shunt; visual pleural space

vps vibrations per second

VPT vibratory perception threshold

V/Q ventilation-perfusion; voice quality

VR right arm [electrode]; valve replacement; variable ratio; vascular resistance; venous reflux; venous return; ventilation rate; ventilation ratio; ventral root; ventricular rhythm; vesicular rosette; vision, right [eye]; vital records; vocal resonance; vocational rehabilitation

Vr volume of relaxation

VRA visual reinforcement audiometry

VRBC red blood cell volume

VRC venous renin concentration

VRCP vitreoretinochoroidopathy

VRD ventricular radial dysplasia

VR&E vocational rehabilitation and education

VRI viral respiratory infection

VRL Virus Reference Laboratory

VRNA viral ribonucleic acid

VROM voluntary range of motion

VRR ventral root reflex

VRS verbal rating scale

VRT vehicle rescue technician

VRV ventricular residual volume; viper retrovirus

VS vaccination scar; vaccine serotype; vagal stimulation; vasospasm; venesection; ventricular septum; vesicular stomatitis; veterinary surgeon; vibration syndrome; visual storage; vital sign; Vogt-Spielmeyer [syndrome]; volatile solid; volumetric solution; voluntary sterilization

Vs venesection

V•s vibration second; volt-second

V x s volts by seconds

vs see above [Lat. *vide supra*]; single vibration; versus; vibration seconds; vital signs

VSA variant-specific surface antigen

VsB bleeding in the arm [Lat. *venaesectio brachii*]

VSBE very short below-elbow [cast]

VSC voluntary surgical contraception

VSD ventricular septal defect; virtually safe dose

VSFP venous stop flow pressure

VSG variant surface glycoprotein

VSHD ventricular septal heart defect

VSINC Virus Subcommittee of the International Nomenclature Committee

VSM vascular smooth muscle

VSMS Vineland Social Maturity Scale

vsn vision

VSOK vital signs normal

VSP variable spine plating

VSR venous stasis retinopathy

VSS vital signs stable

VST ventral spinothalamic tract

VSV vesicular stomatitis virus

VSW ventricular stroke work

VT tetrazolium violet; total ventilation; vacuum tube; vacuum tuberculin; vasotonin; venous thrombosis; ventricular tachyarrhythmia; ventricular tachycardia; verocytotoxin; verotoxin; vibration threshold

V_T tidal volume; total ventilation

V&T volume and tension

VTA ventral tegmental area

V tach ventricular tachycardia

VTE venous thromboembolism; ventricular tachycardia event

VTEC verotoxin-producing *Escherichia coli*

VTG volume thoracic gas
VTI volume thickness index
VTM mechanical tidal volume; virus transport medium
VTR variable tandem repeats; videotape recording; vesicular transport system
VTSRS Verdun Target Symptom Rating Scale
VTVM vacuum tube voltmeter
VTX, vtx vertex
VU varicose ulcer; volume unit
vu volume unit
VUR vesicoureteral reflex
VUV vacuum ultraviolet
VV varicose veins; viper venom; vulva and vagina
V-V veno-venous [bypass]
vv varicose veins; veins
v/v percent volume in volume
VVD vaginal vertex delivery

VVFR vesicovaginal fistula repair
VVI ventricular inhibited [pacemaker]; vocal velocity index
vvMDV very virulent Marek disease virus
VVS vesicovaginal space; vesicovaginal space; vestibulo-vegetative syndrome
VVT ventricular triggered [pacemaker]
VW vascular wall; vessel wall; von Willebrand's [disease]
v/w volume per weight
vWD von Willebrand's disease
VWF velocity waveform; vibration-induced white finger
vWF, vWf von Willebrand's factor
VWM ventricular wall motion
vWS von Willebrand syndrome
Vx vertex
VZ varicella-zoster
VZIG, VZIg varicella zoster immuno-globulin
VZV varicella-zoster virus

W dominant spotting [mouse]; energy; section modulus; a series of small triangular incisions in plastic surgery [plasty]; tryptophan; tungsten [Ger. *wolfram*]; ward; water; watt; Weber [test]; week; wehnelt; weight; white; widowed; width; wife; Wilcoxson rank sum statistic; Wistar [rat]; with; word fluency; work; wound

w water; watt; while; with; velocity (m/s)

Wt weakly positive

WA when awake; white adult; Wiskott-Aldrich [syndrome]

W/A watt/ampere

W&A weakness and atrophy

WAADA Women's Auxiliary of the American Dental Association

WAB Western Aphasia Battery

WAF weakness, atrophy and fasciculation; white adult female

WAGR Wilms' tumor, aniridia, genitourinary abnormalities, and mental retardation

WAIS Wechsler Adult Intelligence Scale

WAIS-R revised Wechsler Adult Intelligence Scale

WAK wearable artificial kidney

WAM white adult male

WAP wandering atrial pacemaker

WAR Wasserman antigen reaction; without additional reagents

WARDS Welfare of Animals Used for Research in Drugs and Therapy

WARF warfarin [Wisconsin Alumni Research Foundation]

WAS weekly activities summary; Wiskott-Aldrich syndrome

WASP Weber Advanced Spatial Perception [test]

Wass Wasserman [reaction]

WAT word association test

WB waist belt; washable base; washed bladder; water bottle; Wechsler-Bellevue [Scale]; weight-bearing; well baby; Western blot [assay]; wet bulb; whole blood; whole body; Willowbrook [virus]; Wilson-Blair [agar]

Wb weber; well-being

WBA wax bean agglutinin; whole body activity

Wb/A webers/ampere

WBAPTT whole blood activated partial thromboplastin time

WBC well baby care/clinic; white blood cell; white blood cell count; whole blood cell count

WBCT whole-blood clotting time

WBDC whole-body digital scanner

WBE whole-body extract

WBF whole-blood folate

WBGT wet bulb global temperature

WBH whole-blood hematocrit; whole-body hyperthermia

Wb/m^2 weber per square meter

WBN whole-blood nitrogen

WBPTT whole-blood partial thromboplastin time

WBR whole-body radiation

WBRT whole-blood recalcification time

WBS Wechsler-Bellevue Scale; whole-blood serum; whole-body scan; Wiedemann-Beckwith syndrome; withdrawal body shakes

WBT wet bulb temperature

WC ward clerk; water closet; Weber-Christian [syndrome]; wheel chair; white cell; white cell casts; white cell count; white child; whooping cough; wild caught [animal]; work capacity; writer's cramp

WC' whole complement

wc wheel chair

WCC Walker's carcinosarcoma cells; white cell count

WCD Weber-Christian disease

WCE work capacity evaluation

WCL Wenckebach cycle length; whole cell lysate

w/cm² watts per square centimeter
WCS white clot syndrome; Wisconsin Card Sort [test]
WCST Wisconsin Card Sorting Test
WD wallerian degeneration; well developed; well differentiated; wet dressing; Whitney Damon [dextrose]; Wilson's disease; with disease; without dyskinesia; Wolman's disease; wrist disarticulation
W/D warm and dry
Wd ward
wd well developed; wound, wounded
WDCC well-developed collateral circulation
WDHA watery diarrhea, hypokalemia, achlorhydria [syndrome]
WDI warfarin dose index
WDL well-differentiated lymphocytic
WDLL well-differentiated lymphatic lymphoma
WDMF wall-defective microbial forms
WDS watery diarrhea syndrome; wet dog shakes [syndrome]
WDWN well developed and well nourished
WE wax ester; Wernicke encephalopathy; western encephalitis; western encephalomyelitis; wound of entry
We weber
WEE western equine encephalitis/encephalomyelitis
WER wheal erythema reaction
WF Weil-Felix reaction; white female; Wistar-Furth [rat]
W/F, wf white female
WFE Williams flexion exercise
WFI water for injection
WFL within function limits
WFOT World Federation of Occupational Therapists
WFR Weil-Felix reaction; wheal-and-flare reaction
WG water gauge; Wegener's granulomatosis; Wright-Giemsa [stain]
WGA wheat germ agglutinin
WH well hydrated; Werdnig-Hoffmann [syndrome]; whole homogenate; wound healing
Wh white
w•h watt-hour
wh white
WHA warm and humid air
wh ch wheel chair; white child
WHCOA White House Conference on Aging
WHD Werdnig-Hoffmann disease
WHML Wellcome Historical Medical Library
WHO World Health Organization; wrist-hand orthosis
whp whirlpool
WHR waist:hips girth ratio
whr watt-hour
WHRC World Health Research Centre
WHS Werdnig-Hoffmann syndrome
WHV woodchuck hepatic virus
WHVP wedged hepatic venous pressure
WI human embryonic lung cell line; walk-in [patient]; water ingestion; Wistar [rat]
WIA wounded in action
WIC women, infants, and children
WIPI Word Intelligibility Picture Identification
WIS Wechsler Intelligence Scale
WISC Wechsler Intelligence Scale for Children
WISC-R Wechsler Intelligence Scale for Children–Revised
WIST Whitaker Index of Schizophrenic Thinking
WITT Wittenborn [Psychiatric Rating Scale]
W-J Woodcock-Johnson [Psychoeducational Battery]
WK week; Wernicke-Korsakoff [syndrome]; Wilson-Kimmelstiel [syndrome]
wk weak; week; work
WKD Wilson-Kimmelstiel disease
W/kg watts per kilogram
WKS Wernicke-Korsakoff syndrome
WKY Wistar-Kyoto [rat]
WL waiting list; waterload; wavelength; withdrawal; working level; workload

wl wavelength
WLE wide local excision
WLF whole lymphocytic fraction
WLI weight-length index
WLM white light microscopy; working level month [radon]
WLS wet lung syndrome
WLT whole lung tomography
WM Waldenström's macroglobulinemia; ward manager; warm and moist; Wernicke-Mann [hemiplegia]; wet mount; white male; whole milk; Wilson-Mikity [syndrome]
W/M white male
wm white male; whole milk; whole mount
w/m² watts per square meter
WMA World Medical Association
WMC weight-matched control
WME Williams' medium E
WMO ward medical officer
WMP weight management program
WMR work metabolic rate; World Medical Relief
WMS Wechsler Memory Scale
WMX whirlpool, massage, exercise
WN, wn well nourished
WNE West Nile encephalitis
WNF well-nourished female
WNL within normal limits
WNM well-nourished male
WNPW wide, notched P wave
WNV West Nile virus
WO wash out; will order; written order
W/O water in oil [emulsion]
w/o without
wo weeks old
WOB work of breathing
WOE wound of entry
WOP without pain
WOU women's outpatient unit
WOWS weak opiate withdrawal scale
WOX wound of exit
WP weakly positive; wedge pressure; wet pack; wettable powder; whirlpool; white pulp; word processor; working point
W/P water/powder ratio
wp wettable powder
WPB whirlpool bath

WPCU weighted patient care unit
WPFM Wright peak flow meter
WPk Ward's pack; wet pack
WPPSI Wechsler Preschool and Primary Scale of Intelligence
WPRS Wittenborn Psychiatric Rating Scale
WPS wasting pig syndrome
WPW Wolff-Parkinson-White [syndrome]
WR Wassermann reaction; water retention; weakly reactive; weak response; whole response; wiping reaction; work rate
Wr wrist; writhe
WRAMC Walter Reed Army Medical Center
WRAML Wide Range Assessment of Memory and Learning
WRAT Wide Range Achievement Test
WRE wahole ragweed extract
WRC washed red cells; water retention coefficient
WRK Woodward's reagent K
WRMT Woodcock Reading Mastery Test
WRS Wiedemann-Rautenstrauch syndrome
WRVP wedged renal vein pressure
WS Waardenburg syndrome; ward secretary; Warkany syndrome; Warthin-Starry [stain]; water soluble; water swallow; Werner syndrome; West syndrome; Wilder's silver [stain]; Williams syndrome; Wolfram syndrome
W·s watt-second
WSB wheat-soy blend
w-sec watt-second
WSI Waardenburg syndrome type I
WSA water-soluble antibiotic
WSL Wesselsbron [virus]
WSP withdrawal seizure prone
WSR Westergren sedimentation rate; withdrawal seizure resistant
W/sr watts per steradian
WT wall thickness; water temperature; wild type [strain]; Wilms' tumor; wisdom teeth; work therapy
wt weight; white

WTE whole time equivalent
WTF weight transferral frequency
W/U workup
WV walking ventilation
W/V, w/v percent weight in volume, weight/volume
W^v variable dominant spotting [mouse]
WW Weight Watchers; wet weight

W/W, w/w weight; percent weight
W/wo with or without
WWU weighted work units [of DRGs]
WX wound of exit
WxB wax bite
WxP wax pattern
WY women years
WZa wide zone alpha

X androgenic [zone]; cross; crossbite; exophoria distance; extra; female sex chromosome; ionization exposure; Kienböck's unit of x-ray exposure; magnification; multiplication times; reactance; removal of; respirations [anesthesia chart]; Roman numeral ten; start of anesthesia; "times"; translocation between two X chromosomes; transverse; unknown quantity; X unit; xylene

X̄ sample mean

Ẋ ionization exposure rate

x except; extremity; horizontal axis of a rectangular coordinate system; mole fraction; multiplication times; roentgen [rays]; sample mean; unknown factor; xanthine

X3 orientation as to time, place, and person

XA xanthurenic acid

X-A xylene and alcohol

Xa chiasma

Xaa unknown amino acid

Xam examination

Xan xanthine

Xanth xanthomatosis

Xao xanthosine

x-mat crossmatch [blood]

XC, Xc excretory cystogram

X-CGD X-linked chronic granulomatous disease

XDH xanthine dehydrogenase

XDP xanthine diphosphate; xeroderma pigmentosum

XDR transducer

Xe electric susceptibility; xenon

XECT xenon-enhanced computed tomography

XEF excess ejection fraction

XES x-ray energy spectrometry

Xfb cross-linked Gibrin

XGP xanthogranulomatous pyelonephritis

Ξ Greek capital letter *xi*

ξ Greek lower case letter *xi*

XIP x-ray–induced polypeptide

XL excess lactate; X-linked [inheritance]; xylose-lysine [agar base]

X-LA X-linked agammaglobulinemia

XLAS X-linked aqueductal stenosis

XLD xylose-lysine-deoxycholate [agar]

XLH X-linked hypophosphatemia

XLI X-linked ichthyosis

XLMR X-linked mental retardation

XLP X-linked lymphoproliferative [syndrome]

XLR X-linked recessive

XLS X-linked recessive lymphoproliferative syndrome

XM crossmatch

Xm maternal chromosome X

xma chiasma

X-mas Christmas [factor]

X-match crossmatch

XMP xanthine monophosphate

XMR X-linked mental retardation

XN night blindness

XO presence of only one sex chromosome; xanthine oxidase

XOM extraocular movements

XOR exclusive operating room

XP xanthogranulomatous pyelonephritis; xeroderma pigmentosum

Xp paternal chromosome X; short arm of chromosome X

Xp- deletion of short arm of chromosome X

XPA xeroderma pigmentosum group A

XPC xeroderma pigmentosum group C

XPS x-ray photoemission spectroscopy

Xq long arm of chromosome X

Xq- deletion of long arm of chromosome X

XR X-linked recessive [inheritance]; x-ray

x-rays roentgen rays

XRD x-ray diffraction

XRF x-ray fluorescence

XRMR X-linked recessive mental retardation

XRS x-ray sensitivity

XRT x-ray therapy

XS cross-section; excessive; xiphisternum

XSA cross-section area

X-sect cross-section

XSP xanthoma striatum palmare

XT exotropia

Xta chiasmata

Xtab cross-tabulating

XTE xeroderma, talipes, and enamel defect [syndrome]

X-TEP crossed immunoelectrophoresis

XTM xanthoma tuberosum multiplex

XTP xanthosine triphosphate

XU excretory urogram; X unit

Xu X-unit

XuMP xylulose monophosphate

XX double strength; female chromosome type

46, XX 46 chromosomes, 2 X chromosomes (normal female)

XXL xylocaine

XX/XY sex karyotypes

49, XXXXY 49 chromosomes, 4 X and 1 Y chromosomes (XXXXY syndrome)

47, XXY 47 chromosomes, 2 X and 1 Y chromosomes (Klinefelter syndrome)

XY male chromosome type

46, XY 46 chromosomes, 1 X and 1 Y chromosome (normal male)

47, XY, +21 47 chromosomes, male, additional No. 21 chromosome (Down syndrome)

Xyl xylose

47, XYY 47 chromosomes, 1 X and 2 Y chromosomes (XYY syndrome)

Y a coordinate axis in a plane; male sex chromosome; tyrosine; year; yellow; yield; yttrium; *Yersinia*

y the vertical axis of a rectangular coordinate system

Y see *upsilon*

υ see *upsilon*

YA *Yersinia* arthritis

Y/A years of age

YACP young adult chronic patient

YADH yeast alcohol dehydrogenase

YAG yttrium aluminum garnet [laser]

Yb ytterbium

YCB yeast carbon base

yd yard

YDV yeast-derived hepatitis B vaccine

YDYES yin deficiency yang excess syndrome

YE yeast extract; yellow enzyme

YEH₂ reduced yellow enzyme

YEI *Yersinia enterocolitica* infection

Yel yellow

YF yellow fever

YFI yellow fever immunization

YFMD yellow fever membrane disease

YLC youngest living child

YM yeast and mannitol

Y$_{max}$ maximum yield

YNB yeast nitrogen base

YNS yellow nail syndrome

y/o years old

YOB year of birth

YP yeast phase; yield pressure

YPA yeast, peptone, and adenine sulfate

yr year

YRD Yangtze River disease

YS yellow spot; yolk sac

ys yellow spot; yolk sac

YST yolk sac tumor

YT, yt yttrium

Z

Z acoustic impedance; atomic number; complex impedance; contraction [Ger. *Zuckung*] the disk that separates sarcomeres [Ger. *Zwischenscheibe*, intermediate disk]; glutamine; impedance; ionic charge number; no effect; point formed by a line perpendicular to the nasion-menton line through the anterior nasal spine; proton number; section modulus; standard score; standardized deviate; zero; zone; a Z-shaped incision in plastic surgery

Z',Z" increasing degrees of contraction

z algebraic unknown or space coordinate; axis of a three-dimensional rectangular coordinate system; catalytic amount; standard normal deviate; zero

ZAP zymosan-activated plasma [rabbit]

ZAPF zinc adequate pair-fed

ZAS zymosan-activated autologous serum

ZB zebra body

ZCD zinc chloride poisoning

ZD zero defects; zero discharge; zinc deficiency

ZDDP zinc dialkyldithiophosphate

Z-DNA zig-zag (left-handed helical) deoxyribonucleic acid

ZDO zero differential overlap

ZDS zinc depletion syndrome

ZE Zollinger-Ellison [syndrome]

ZEC Zinsser-Engman-Cole [syndrome]

ZEEP zero end-expiratory pressure

Z-ERS zeta erythrocyte sedimentation rate

ZES Zollinger-Ellison syndrome

Z Greek capital letter *zeta*

ζ Greek lower case letter *zeta*

ZF zero frequency; zona fasciculata

ZFF Zinc Fume Fever

ZG zona glomerulosa

ZGM zinc glycinate marker

ZIFT zygote intrafallopian tube transfer

ZIG, ZIg zoster immunoglobulin

ZIP zoster immune plasma

ZK Zuelzer-Kaplan [syndrome]

ZLS Zimmerman-Laband syndrome

Zm zygomaxillare

ZMA zinc meta-arsenite

Zn zinc

ZnOE zinc oxide and eugenol

ZO Zichen-Oppenheim [syndrome]; Zuelzer-Ogden [syndrome]

ZOE zinc oxide-eugenol

Zool zoology

ZPA zone of polarizing activity

ZPC zero point of change

ZPG zero population growth

ZPO zinc peroxide

ZPP zinc protoporphyrin

ZR zona reticularis

Zr zirconium

ZS Zellweger syndrome

ZSR zeta sedimentation ratio

ZTS zymosan-treated serum

Z-TSP zephiran-trisodium phosphate

ZTT zinc turbidity test

ZVT Zehlenverbindungstest

Zy zygion

ZyC zymosan complement

zyg zygotene

Zz ginger [Lat. *zingibar*]